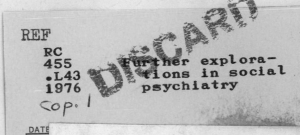

Further Explorations in Social Psychiatry

FURTHER EXPLORATIONS IN SOCIAL PSYCHIATRY

EDITED BY

Berton H. Kaplan, Robert N. Wilson,
& Alexander H. Leighton

BASIC BOOKS, INC., PUBLISHERS

NEW YORK

Library of Congress Cataloging in Publication Data
Main entry under title:

Further explorations in social psychiatry.

   Leighton's name appeared 1st on t. p. of earlier
ed., published in 1957 under title: Explorations
in social psychiatry.
   Includes bibliographies and index.
   1.   Social psychiatry.   I.   Kaplan, Berton H.,
1930–   II.   Wilson, Robert Neal, 1924–
III.   Leighton, Alexander Hamilton, 1908–
IV.   Leighton, Alexander Hamilton, 1908–   ed.
Explorations in social psychiatry.   [DNLM: 1.   Psy-
chiatry, Community.   WM440 F992]
RC455.L43   1976   362.2'04'2   74-25914
ISBN 0-465-02589-7

DEDICATION

WE DEDICATE this volume to Alexander H. Leighton, M.D. Although it is very unusual to dedicate a book to one of its co-editors, we do so because of the great significance of Alexander Leighton's contributions. This book is being published on the occasion of Dr. Leighton's official retirement from the Harvard School of Public Health. His creative work, notably in the Stirling County and other studies, has uniquely influenced the development of modern social science and social psychiatry. Indeed, he is one of the genuine pioneers in the study of human behavior in our times.

Since this is an extension of the original *Explorations in Social Psychiatry*, and since Dr. Leighton was the primary editor of that volume, we feel it is particularly appropriate to inscribe this book to him.

We do so, without Professor Leighton's knowledge, in recognition of an extraordinary scholar whose career has been marked by an inventive and concerned striving for the betterment of human health.

Berton H. Kaplan
Robert N. Wilson

CONTENTS

Contents

Part III

Part IV

Part V

CONTRIBUTORS

WILLIAM C. ACKERLY, M. D. Department of Psychiatry, Cambridge Hospital; Assistant Clinical Professor of Psychiatry, Harvard Medical School.

JOHN E. ADAMS, M.D. Professor and Chairman, Department of Psychiatry, University of Florida.

MORTON BEISER, M.D. Associate Professor of Social Psychiatry, Department of Behavioral Sciences, Harvard University School of Public Health.

ROBERT C. BENFARI, PH.D. Associate Professor of Psychology, Harvard University School of Public Health.

H. KEITH H. BRODIE, M.D. Chairman, Department of Psychiatry, Duke University School of Medicine.

VICTOR G. CARDOZA, Judge of the Court of Canadian Citizenship, Halifax, Nova Scotia; formerly Director, Community Program, Harvard Program in Social Psychiatry, Digby, Nova Scotia.

LEONARD S. COTTRELL, JR., PH.D. Formerly Secretary, Russell Sage Foundation; formerly Professor of Sociology and Psychology, University of North Carolina at Chapel Hill.

ALFRED DEAN, PH.D. Department of Psychiatry, Albany Medical School.

J. WILBERT EDGERTON, PH.D. Professor of Psychology, Department of Community Psychiatry, University of North Carolina at Chapel Hill.

DANA L. FARNSWORTH, M.D. Henry K. Oliver Professor of Hygiene, Emeritus, Harvard University.

JEROME D. FRANK, M.D. Professor Emeritus of Psychiatry, Johns Hopkins University School of Medicine.

MILTON GREENBLATT, M.D. Professor of Psychiatry, UCLA; Chief of Psychiatry, Veterans Administration Hospital, Sepulveda, California; formerly Commissioner, Massachusetts Department of Mental Health.

DAVID A. HAMBURG, M.D. Reed-Hodgson Professor of Human Biology and Psychiatry, Department of Psychiatry and Behavioral Sciences, Stanford University School of Medicine.

Contributors

WILLIAM G. HOLLISTER, M.D. Professor of Psychiatry and Director of the Community Psychiatry Division of the Department of Psychiatry, University of North Carolina School of Medicine.

BERTON H. KAPLAN, PH.D. Professor of Epidemiology, School of Public Health, University of North Carolina at Chapel Hill.

ARI KIEV, M.D. Clinical Associate Professor of Psychiatry, Cornell University Medical College.

ALEXANDER H. LEIGHTON, M.D. Professor of Social Psychiatry Emeritus, Department of Behavioral Science, Harvard University School of Public Health.

CHARLES J. MERTENS, M.D. Professor of Psychiatry, University of Louvain; Professor of Social Psychiatry, Harvard University.

JANE M. MURPHY, PH.D. Associate Professor of Anthropology, Department of Behavioral Science, Harvard University School of Public Health.

J. CHRISTOPHER PERRY, M.D., M.P.H. Resident in Psychiatry, Cambridge Hospital.

PATRICIA PERRI RIEKER, PH.D. Assistant Professor, Department of Sociology, University of North Carolina.

JOHN S. ROLLAND, M.D. Resident in Psychiatry, Yale University School of Medicine.

EDWARD A. SUCHMAN, PH.D. Formerly Graduate School of Public Health, Department of Public Health Practice, University of Pittsburgh.

MERVYN SUSSER, M.D. Professor and Head, Division of Epidemiology, Columbia University School of Public Health.

ROBERT N. WILSON, PH.D. Professor of Sociology, University of North Carolina at Chapel Hill.

PREFACE

PSYCHIATRIC DISORDER is certainly one of the major human problems of our time, perhaps of all time. (It has always intrigued me that Cain slew Abel very early in Genesis—Chapter 4, verse 8.) The classic epidemiological expression of the key problems in social psychiatry is more precise: Who has how much psychiatric disorder and why? In terms of magnitude, the tentative answer to that question is indeed that the population at risk to mental impairment is large. Three classic examples will suffice.

In Sweden, a clinical psychiatric survey of a "normal" population by Essen-Möller [1] found the following:

Psychiatric Ratings
(from Table IX)

PSYCHIATRIC ABNORMALITY IS:	MALE %	FEMALE %
Evident	9	8
Probable	13	24
Conceivable	28	26
Absent	50	42

The Midtown study initiated by Rennie, Srole, et al. [2] surveyed a sample of 1,660 adults (ages twenty to fifty–nine) and estimated the following overall results:

Midtown Findings

MENTAL HEALTH RATING	%
Well	19
Mild Symptoms	36
Moderate Symptoms	22
Impaired	23
Marked	13
Severe	7
Incapacitated	3

In a summary overview of Leighton's findings from the Stirling County Study,[3] the following table is an example of the magnitude of the epidemiology of psychiatric disorder.

Typology of Need for Psychiatric
Attention

TYPE	%
I / Most abnormal	3
II / Psychiatric disorder with significant impairment	17
III / Probable psychiatric disorder	37
IV / Doubtful	26
V / Probably well	17
	100%

Classified another way, in terms of acute distress, in Stirling 31 percent of the men were significantly impaired, and 33 percent of the women were likewise significantly impaired.

Although our present concepts and measures are imperfect, a reasonable inference is that the magnitude of psychiatric problems in "normal" populations is large. These three pioneering studies suggest approximately 20 percent with significant impairment. The level of serious distress is therefore probably large; the socio-psychosomatic issues loom large also in such major killers as heart disease, strokes, and accidents. A challenging issue emerges: can life styles be made more conducive to socio-emotional health?

Given the magnitude of the psychiatric problem, this book represents a continuity of concern around several issues: How do social processes relate to psychiatric disorder? (Part I) What is the evolution of the need for more effective care systems? (Part II) Can social environments be made more competence-promoting? (Part III) Can we do a better job of assessing social effectiveness and the treatment systems? (Part IV) Finally, what are the future conceptual and measurement problems for understanding the social risks to psychiatric distress? (Part V) These are the dominating questions for each part of this volume.

These five issues represent a synthesis of the dominant questions that have evolved as central problems in social psychiatry. These problems also represent the continuity issues since the first volume, *Explorations in Social Psychiatry*, edited by Alexander H. Leighton, John Clausen, and Robert N. Wilson.

Each contributor to this volume casts light on how Alexander H. Leighton's tree of hypotheses for studying social processes relates to psychiatric disorder. Leighton's frame of reference and the related issues of social psychiatry as fundamental problems to be solved are all set forth in Part I.

Part II revolves around the evolution of a more effective patient care system. Such topics as the diverse interferences in the sociocultural environment that lead to and require patient hospitalization, the problems of cultural diversity and treatment needs, the evolution of the healing-treatment role of the state hospital, and the problems of coordination and evaluation of community care are considered. These problems reflect the evolving contemporary conceptions of treatment, consumer needs, and program effectiveness. A focal point in this section is how people are labeled as patients and subsequently how that labeling process relates to entrance into the mental health treatment system. The key problems are: What is normality and what is abnormality? Who are the definers? How is this done? What indeed are the precise relationships between the sociocultural environment and psychiatric disorder? Can psychiatric disorder be prevented or at least treated early?

High risk groups and key parameters for mental health care system effectiveness may be identified by means of the patient register. Who is coming for treatment and why? The relationship of the environment to clinical definitions, the structure or need for restructuring of professional roles in the mental health area, the difficult problem of coordinating community care and more effective program evaluation are examined in light of this question. The evolution of the therapeutic process and its varying roles and techniques is discussed as it reflects changing scientific understanding and therapies in a changing environment. The adequacy of existing professional modes of treatment, the creation of more effective treatment, and means for better utilization of social restructuring in the treatment process are fundamental issues. In sum, therapeutic techniques should reflect the factors which go into the social-psychological breakdown process.

How does psychiatric disorder vary and how is it treated in different cultures? Is there indeed a set of essential strivings which, if interfered with in any social system, increases the probability of psychiatric disorder? We seek to enlarge our understanding of the relationship of the social environment to mental health and mental illness, and to understand the importance of cultural diversity, and, perhaps, the limits of psychological relativity.

Part III of the book is dominated by this problem: Can more effective individual and social competences be created? The kinds of preventions which can block the evolution of psychiatric disorder must be examined. How and where are coping techniques taught and provided? Indeed, how can more effective inner and outer coping methods be understood and realized?

For another perspective on competence, we ask which psychosocial assets are promotive of mental health. Perhaps the next decade's work will give increased emphasis to this question so that the process which leads to the evolution of psychiatric disorder can be impeded and more effective prevention created. Can we provide more effective conceptualization and measurement of the predictors for development and maintenance of mental health?

The questions of creating healthier social arrangements at the level of the community as a whole are also examined in this section. What are the issues which relate individual essential strivings and interpersonal life styles to community patterns? What in the community life styles are sources of need interference? Is it possible to create a healthier social system, taken as a whole, or in terms of its major components? Are there measures which may be taken to lower the risk of mental illness in the same way that the risk of heart disease may be lowered by decreasing levels of cholesterol and blood pressure? What are the parameters which define competence and normality? In a Durkheimian sense, we are posing the classic question of social integration: what is a healthy society?

Can the mental health of individuals be affected by community action, leadership, and sociocultural pattern changes? Questions are raised regarding the relationship of the social environment to mental health, problems of social manipulation and social engineering, changing professional roles for care and prevention, the imperatives of program evaluation, and the necessity of enlarging our knowledge of social change processes.

Attention is focused again on prevention and treatment of the system as a whole. Can consultation promote mental health in the educational process through early identification of problems and utilization of the contributions of the educational environment to emotional growth and development? What of the requirements and difficulties of social manipulation? Of changing professional roles? Where are the best places to provide care, particularly preventive care?

Means for revising work role relationships in the interest of healthier personal relationships and the betterment of mental health are presented. The reader is confronted with the ways in which social arrangements can be repaired. He is challenged to look at ways by which change can be brought about to enlarge the capacity to cope and therefore promote mental health in work settings. This second area is one of the most crucial for intervention in the interest of a healthier social environment. The noxious aspects of work are probably conducive to social change; for example, work overload, or role conflicts, can be demonstrated to be risk factors. In other words, how does the social environment affect mental health? How are preventive strategies best exerted?

Drug dependence is discussed as another setting for the enlargement of opportunities for timely intervention, in view of the preceding questions of competency skills, normality, prevention, and primary care within the socialization processes.

Part IV is devoted to the problems of evaluation of social systems and program effectiveness. The measurement of social system effectiveness is directly addressed in this section. A series of new concepts and instruments for measuring types of adaptation to the sociocultural environment and related mental health risks is presented. What are the parameters for measuring a healthy social structure of subsystems? In attempting to answer this question, new challenges are posed for defining normality in social system terms, for evaluating programs, and for enlarging the understanding of social contributions to coping styles and strategies.

The classic design questions for evaluating programs and program effectiveness are described. These tools provide ways of relating sociocultural patterns to psychiatric disorder, treatment programs, and treatment outcomes. The next decade may be dominated by the related questions of personal and socio-environmental competencies, and program effectiveness and evaluation.

Another model for evaluating the treatment process, the mental health center concept, is put under the microscope of evaluation. Has the community mental health center been oversold? The answer to that question lies in better evaluation of what it does. The problems of community care, social manipulation, and evaluation are examined in this light.

Epidemiological instruments to assess more specific entities for understanding and treating psychological problems are provided. We are moving beyond the global issues of high symptom level or the impaired, which have dominated so much of past psychiatric epidemiological measurement. Perhaps through the greater specificity of problems of psychiatric interest better treatment and preventive opportunities will emerge. Expanding our current notions of social and psychological normality, the relationship of social environment to mental health, and the distribution of very specific psychiatric entities in different cultures is one goal of this section. Another is evaluation of programs by focusing not only on the ill, but also on the distribution of other health indicators.

Part V concerns future issues. It is only through the more precise conceptualization and measurement of mental health and mental illness that better understanding of the predictors of mental illness will emerge. The crucial problem of the sociocultural environment and its relationship to mental health or mental illness is also examined. Again, it is through a more accurate approximation to the social predictors of psychological distress that we will understand mental disorders more clearly and develop better methods for reducing risk factors in the psychosocial environment.

The book relates to the basic issues of life styles and health, the paradoxes of the human condition. It asks what kind of society would be more socially and emotionally health promotive. The content of this volume is likewise relevant to current issues: racism and mental health; the changing roles of men and women; war and peace; exploitation and equity; opportunity and the protection of identity; social integration and the escape from social and emotional alienation. It may be summarized briefly around the hypothesis that social support, sexual identity, coping skills, and associated public and private self-esteem may relate to the level of mental health just as the combined predictive value of knowing the blood pressure, cholesterol level, and smoking behavior relate to the risk of developing coronary heart disease.

It is not necessary to document the importance that myth has played in the work of Sigmund Freud or to review the great importance that Carl Jung placed on myth as archetype. It is also clear from the works of a number of people, such as Henry A. Murray and Robert N. Wilson, that literature and myth are prototypes of fundamental social and psychological processes. As a matter of fact, Ernest Jones [4] points out that Freud was extremely indebted to writers such as Nietzsche, Dostoyevsky, Borne, and Schiller, whose work aided him in his understanding of the unconscious.

In keeping with an interest in the utilization of myth for the suggestion of basic ideas and especially for the refinement of concepts, it may be suggested that the prototype of issues in social psychiatry may be summed up in Moses' Difficulties. [5] The "Moses Complex" is one of the most universal complexes that confronts all human beings. The Moses Complex and related anxieties are deep and the resolutions usually difficult and probably never complete.

With such a pessimistic note, it is appropriate to ask, "What is the Moses Complex?" The Bible indicates that Moses had "four difficulties" (as revealed in Exodus, Chapters 3 and 4).

Moses' first difficulty, the first dimension of his complex, was the fear that he was unsuited for his mission. This is in Exodus 3:11–12. In modern parlance, Moses was plagued by the question "Who am I?" (Adequacy!)

Moses' second difficulty is what the Bible calls the name of God, which, when interpreted, apparently meant that Moses' insecurity was built on his lack of faith in his own power to convince others to heed his message. This is a version of a certain kind of personal anomie; a person does not really know how to say what he needs to say. Will people listen to him? Will he be rejected?

The third difficulty that confronted Moses was a deep fear that the Israelites might not believe his message of freedom. The essence of this is described in 4:1–9. Moses feared rejection.

The fourth difficulty was his sense of concern over his lack of eloquence. Hence, he hesitated to take the role of leader. Moses felt he was not eloquent; he was also not sure that he was fluent or convincing (Exodus 4:10–17).

The Moses Complex confronts all individuals throughout the life cycle. I became very aware of this in my work in Blue Ridge [6], a fundamentalist Christian culture. I had never before been exposed to individuals so concerned with the question "Am I worthy?" In this regard, the Moses Complex deals with the question of adequacy in the four fundamental ways: role fit, how to communicate, how others respond, and comfort with self-expression.

The Moses Complex could stimulate the reassessment of a definition of what role adequacy includes. This question is an often-overlooked concern in social psychiatry. What is role adequacy? Does Moses' Four Difficulties represent a prototype of role adequacy?

It is interesting to observe the four ways by which Moses coped with these Difficulties (Exodus 4–5). He learned to accept the pain, ambivalence, conflict, and inherent difficulty of his roles. He learned from experience. He accepted inevitable doubts through his ultimate dependency on God. And he gained support from his brother Aaron, who became his spokesman. Perhaps when confronted with a Moses complex, all individuals might profit from developing an "Aaron Complex," by learning how to depend on people who can help us through the labyrinth of the life experience (Exodus 4:11–31).

The questions of social psychiatry are ancient yet forever contemporary in that man will always seek health and well-being in his existence.

Berton H. Kaplan

REFERENCES

1. Essen-Möller, E. "Individual Traits and Morbidity in a Swedish Rural Population," *Acta Psychiatrica Scandinavia*, suppl. 100, 1956.

2. Srole, L., Langer, T. S., Michael, S. T., Opler, M. K., and Rennie, T. A. C. *Mental Health in the Metropolis*. New York: McGraw-Hill, 1962.

3. Leighton, D. C., Harding, J. S., Macklin, D. B., Macmillan, A. M., and Leighton, A. H. *The Character of Danger*. New York: Basic Books, 1963.

4. Jones, E. *The Life and Work of Sigmund Freud*. Edited and adapted by Lionel Trilling and Steven Marcus. New York: Basic Books, 1961.

5. Hertz, J. H. (Ed.) *The Pentateuch and Haftorahs*. London: Soncino Press, 1963. (Exodus 3–6)

6. Kaplan, B. H. *Blue Ridge*. Morgantown: University of West Virginia, 1971.

ACKNOWLEDGMENTS

WE WISH gratefully to acknowledge the following:

The Social Science Research Council, which made possible the original volume, *Explorations in Social Psychiatry*, edited by Alexander H. Leighton, John A. Clausen, and Robert N. Wilson.

It should be noted that several of the chapters in this volume draw upon the Stirling County Study, which was funded by the following organizations: The Andrew Carnegie Foundation, the Milbank Memorial Foundation, the National Institute of Mental Health, the Canadian Government, and the Ford Foundation.

Leonard J. Duhl, M.D., Harold M. Visotsky, M.D., Jack R. Ewalt, M.D., M. Brewster Smith, PH.D., Paul V. Lemkau, M.D., and John C. Cassel, M.D., for their support and help in the formulation and evaluation of our proposal.

Our wives, Ellen Kaplan, Joan Wilson, and Jane Murphy, who supported and encouraged this lengthy endeavor.

Arthur Rosenthal, the former publisher of Basic Books, who guided us through the early stages of development for this volume.

Herb Reich, Director of the Behavioral Science Program for Basic Books, for his perceptive comments, encouragement, patience, and commitment to excellence.

Kathy B. Murray and Mary Lee for editorial assistance.

Part I

Further Explorations in Social Psychiatry

THE FIRST PART of the book provides the reader with a preamble of the continuity of past and present key issues in social psychiatry, and a statement of the theoretical perspective that focuses on social processes and their contribution to psychiatric disorder.

What more challenging problem is there in social science than the nature of a health-promoting social system? More specifically, how can we better define the criteria of social arrangements that are most likely to be promotive of emotional well-being? What would a social system be like that maximizes one's potentiality for three score and ten? How do we escape the stress of malfunctioning social systems?

Indeed, the most fundamental problems of our time can be viewed in terms of a social psychiatric frame of reference: the search for healthier life styles; the social and psychological liberation of blacks and other minorities; the painful worldwide problems of poverty and development; the threat of nuclear war; the liberation of all individuals from ineffective social arrangements, such as the "pressure" syndrome of American life, or the need for positive role identification for the sexes; the indicators of social disintegration such as uncontrolled anger, widespread fear, delusional formations, and pathological leadership.

Another classic issue is the nature of shared sanity or shared, rewarded forms of psychopathology. For example, how do groups or subcultures form so as to encourage excessive competition, gross work overload, paranoid fears of strangers, or virtually no reassuring feedback? How do groups or subcultures form around shared psychopathology or shared healthy life styles?

1

Editorial Note

A field is known by the questions it asks. Progress in a field is demonstrated by the importance and relevance of those questions. In these regards, this volume builds on the key issues of social psychiatry that were covered extensively in Explorations in Social Psychiatry *by Alexander H. Leighton, John Clausen, and Robert N. Wilson. The four original key issues were the investigation and understanding of the concepts of normality and abnormality, the nature of the relationship of the social environment to personality development and to levels of mental well-being, the implications of cultural and cross-cultural diversity for understanding and preventing psychiatric disorder, and, finally, the effects of mental illness on the social environment.*

We build on those still-relevant topics, but deal with additional lively questions as well. The seven additional questions which represent our continuity with the above key issues are: a concern with the conflict between the model of clinical treatment and the model of social system intervention; the revision and innovation necessary for more effective treatment roles; the problem of coordination and continuity in community care; the necessity for better identification of effective modes of primary intervention, whether they be in school, family, work place, or neighborhood; the respective roles of expert and layman; the difficulty of program evaluation; and the model of effective coping and noncoping with life stress.

All these questions are examined in the context of Alexander Leighton's frame of reference for looking at the relationship between the social environment and psychiatric disorder. Leighton's frame of reference is built on a series of basic questions concerning the following: fundamental assumptions, evolution of psychiatric disorders, nonoccurrence of psychiatric disorder, interference with essential strivings, striving sentiments and the sociocultural environment, interpersonal patterns in the sociocultural environment, the nature of the society and culture, and sociocultural patterns and psychiatric disorder. These problems and propositions are still extremely timely and in need of refinement for the sake of a better understanding of the relationship between the social environment and mental disorder. Leighton's scheme, in sum, points us toward the clarification of what is meant by an effective social system for optimal psychological functioning.

B. H. K.

CHAPTER 1

Continuities in Social Psychiatry

ROBERT N. WILSON

IN 1957 the authors and editors of *Explorations in Social Psychiatry*,[2] the fore-runner of this book, viewed their task as that of articulating individual psycho-dynamics with group processes. Although the task remains unfinished today, the intervening years have been marked by growing acceptance of an essentially social psychiatric orientation to the problems of mental health and illness. Concepts of social etiology have been widely adopted, despite a paucity of well-substantiated causal links. The idea that our treatment of the disturbed individual is affected by, and affects in turn, the social institutions and cultural values in which we all—healthy and ill—are immersed, is today a truism.

The earlier volume identified four major spheres of investigation, termed "key issues," for social psychiatry:

1. Concepts of normality and abnormality;
2. The relation of social environment to personality development with reference to mental health;
3. Implications of cultural and cross-cultural diversity for effective understanding and prevention;
4. The effect of mental illness on social environment; modes of societal reaction to illness.

Since 1963 the community mental health movement, exemplified by legislation providing for the establishment of community centers throughout the nation, has made these issues manifest and meaningful to a degree scarcely foreseen seventeen years ago. Indeed, the centers themselves are a prominent "mode of societal reaction to illness." The first three issues continue to engage all who work in community mental health: dilemmas of defining health and illness have a tangible impact on the goals of preventive programs, and on the identification of target populations; the relation of social environment to personality development emerges especially in the effort to reach out to disadvantaged sectors of the community, an effort grounded in the hypothesis that general socio-economic deprivation heightens the risk of severe psychological disorder; implications of cultural, or perhaps better, subcultural diversity are made concrete in such matters as the relationship between middle-class professional treater and lower-class client.

The fourth original issue, the effect of mental illness on social environment, takes on added significance as the emphasis in mental health programing shifts to the community. Instead of being sequestered permanently in the "human warehouse" of the state mental hospital, increasing numbers of distressed individuals are being maintained at home or, if hospitalized, are returning more quickly and frequently to the local scene. One may well question the impact of disabled persons on familial, occupational, and other social institutions. How are these portions of the community's organized fabric, not explicitly designed for therapeutic functions, influenced by the challenge to cope with illness in their midst? In effect, the protagonists of community health say to the community: "Your wounded ones are your problems, not solely the province of specialized helping agents." But the consequences are less than clear; professionals are unable to counsel families or employers with precision about just what actions are called for vis-à-vis the ill. The propositions framing our discussion (see pp. 8–12) underline the effect of communal disintegration upon individual levels of health. Yet the other side of the coin may raise concerns of equal importance: Does the presence of numbers of disturbed individuals, only meagerly if at all capable of enacting their social roles, tend to promote disintegration of the community's organized networks of relationship? Even more pointedly, how often may the exemplary presence of a severely disturbed person play on the vulnerabilities of fragile kin or friends to induce a version of shared psychopathology?

Thus one might say that the community mental health movement has sharpened our earlier concerns, bringing them into focus not only for the psychiatrist or other helping agent but for the society at large.

We believe that although the key issues have a continuing vitality and validity, they must be supplemented in the 1970s by a series of corollary issues that have emerged as a result of the United States' determination to make social psychiatry operational in the local community. As in the earlier book,[2] these supplementary themes will be woven into the several topical contributions. They are pervasive, and we shall try to demonstrate their relevance to the diverse activities entailed in community mental health.

The additional issues, each the subject of lively debate and audacious experiment, may be sketched as follows:

5. Tension between alternative goals in community mental health, with its implications for professional roles. Most bluntly posed, the conflict is between a model of clinical treatment and a model of social system intervention, including the question of the professional's political involvement (the competent community and/or the competent individual).
6. Revision/innovation in helping roles, including extension of professional effectiveness through such techniques as consultation, and creation of new roles, such as the indigenous worker.
7. Coordination/continuity in community care, perhaps especially in aftercare of the individual returning from institutional treatment.
8. Identifying the modes of primary prevention: school, family, workplace, neighborhood, other?
9. What are the respective roles of expert and layman, professional and community representative, in policy formation/health planning? Provider dominance and consumer dominance?
10. The torment of program evaluation: Who is helped? How? By whom?
11. Models of coping/noncoping with life stress; polarities: creative competence, leadership vs. addictive withdrawal, "social breakdown."

The present discussion is organized about three primary divisions of current social psychiatric concern: patient care; habilitation and environmental enrichment; research and evaluation. These functions are readily endorsed by nearly all who work in the field, and by much of the informed lay public as well. Unfortunately, as is so often true in attempts at large-scale social amelioration in a democratic polity, our ideological and theoretical commitments are exceedingly difficult to translate into practical applications. Thus the initial enthusiasm for the community mental health center, an enthusiasm that was sometimes expressed with almost religious fervor, is already being tempered. As Leighton covers in some detail (pp. 14–23), a combination of shifts in administrative policy and public mood, financial stringencies, failure to evaluate centers' results, and interprofessional rivalries has dealt the high promise of community-focused care at least a temporary setback.

We hope that these assembled contributions will further the effective application of social psychiatric thought to the health problems of populations at risk.

A Conceptual Overview

There have been many attempts to define the nature of "community," to sketch its major parameters and then link these to the psychological health of its members. How do the requirements of a cohesive culture and a viable social system articulate with the personality needs of individuals? Analyses of these complex relationships range from the transcendental to the prosaic, from existential anxiety in the face of philosophic absurdity to explosive outbursts in the situation of crowded ghetto housing.

If we are to speak intelligently about a social psychiatry, we must be able to sort out the key components of group life and propose ways in which they are tied to the psychosocial interior of the person. At a minimum, one might identify the key components of community as consisting of, *material resources, human interaction*, and *symbolic expression*. That is, an ongoing group process must entail the physical bases to sustain life, the network of human relationships through which activities are patterned, and some symbol system to afford communication among the members and at least rudimentary coherence of goals and means. These three basic elements, or clusters of elements, that are necessary to perpetuate a *community* are also (not accidentally) critical to the fulfillment of the ten "essential striving sentiments" proposed by Leighton as integral to successful *individual* functioning. What have been termed the "functional prerequisites of a society" mesh compellingly with most conceptualizations of personality needs. The fit is clearly very far from perfect, in any place or time; the conflict Freud posed[1] remains—the delicate balancing of individual desire and collective regulation. But that there *is* a fit must be the first premise of a social psychiatry.

Leighton, primarily in the context of the Stirling County Study, has set forth a series of propositions concerning the manner in which psychological illness and health are engendered, and particularly the ways in which these processes of individual functioning are related to salient features of the social environment.[2] His propositions, which follow, provide an appropriate framework for thinking about the key issues, old and new, sketched above, and about the diverse contributions of this book.

Series A. The Fundamental Propositions

A1. All human beings exist in a state of psychological striving.
A2. Striving plays a part in the maintenance of an essential psychical condition.

A3. Interference with striving leads to a disturbance of the essential condition.

A4. Disturbance of the essential psychical condition gives rise to disagreeable feelings.

Series B.   Propositions Concerned with the Evolution of a Psychiatric Disorder

B1. Given a disturbance of the essential psychical condition, a personality may adopt patterns of sentiment and action which lead to some relief from the resultant disagreeable feelings (A4), but which fail to restore adequately the essential psychical condition.

B2. Because of the relief, each response facilitates its repetition, hence there is a tendency for a personality to persist in a maladaptive direction (B1) once this has been started, leading ultimately to the occurrence of psychiatric disorders.

B3. Given a disturbance of the essential psychical condition (A4), physiological symptoms may appear as part of a general disturbance of dynamic equilibrium in the organism.

B4. Given a disturbance of the essential psychical condition (A4), preexisting defect in personality may contribute toward the development of psychiatric disorder and/or the appearance of physiological symptoms.

B5. Given a disturbance of the essential psychical condition (A4), sociocultural conditions have a selective influence on the emergence and persistence of malfunctional patterns of personality leading to psychiatric disorder (B1, B2, and B3).

Series C.   Propositions Concerned with the Nonoccurrence of Psychiatric Disorder

C1. Given a disturbance of the essential psychical condition, a personality may adopt patterns of sentiment and action which lead to relief of the resultant disagreeable feelings (A4), by means of restoration of the essential psychical condition.

C2. Because of the relief, each response facilitates its repetition, hence there is a tendency for a personality system to persist in the constructive direction (C1) once this has been started, leading to adequate, or even superior, functions.

C3. Given a resolution of the disturbance to the essential psychical condition, and a consequent improvement in dynamic equilibrium of the organism, there will be nonoccurrence or disappearance of psychophysiological disorders.

C4. Given a disturbance of the essential psychical condition (A4), preexisting resources of the personality may contribute toward the development of adequate or superior functioning.

C5. Given a disturbance of the essential psychical condition (A4), sociocultural conditions have a selective influence on the emergence and persistence of personality patterns which do not lead to psychiatric disorder and which may lead to superior functioning (C1, C2, and C3).

Series BC. Combined Proposition

BC1. The trends indicated for the development of psychiatric disorder (B1, B2, B3, and B4) and for the maintenance of health or increasing capabilities (C1, C2, C3, and C4) can occur simultaneously in the same personality.

Series D. Propositions Concerning Interference with the Essential Striving Sentiments

D1. Given proposition A2, certain striving sentiments may be designated as essential because maximally concerned with the maintenance of the "essential" psychical condition.

D2. Essential striving sentiments may fail in this function due to interference imposed by the environment.

D3. Essential striving sentiments may fail in this function due to defects inherent in the objects of striving.

D4. Essential striving sentiments may fail in this function due to defect, inborn or acquired, in the personality.

Series E. Propositions Relating Essential Striving Sentiments and Sociocultural Environment

E1. Sociocultural situations which interfere with sentiments of physical security foster psychiatric disorder.

E2. Sociocultural situations which interfere with sentiments of securing sexual satisfaction foster psychiatric disorder.

E3. Sociocultural situations which interfere with sentiments bearing on the expression of hostility foster psychiatric disorder.

E4. Sociocultural situations which interfere with sentiments of giving love foster psychiatric disorder.

E5. Sociocultural situations which interfere with sentiments of securing love foster psychiatric disorder.

E6. Sociocultural situations which interfere with sentiments bearing on obtaining recognition foster psychiatric disorder.

E7. Sociocultural situations which interfere with sentiments bearing on the expression of spontaneity (positive force, creativity, volition) foster psychiatric disorder.

E8. Sociocultural situations which interfere with sentiments of orientation in the person regarding his place in society and the place of others foster psychiatric disorder.

E9. Sociocultural situations which interfere with the person's sentiments of membership in a definite human group foster psychiatric disorder.

E10. Sociocultural situations which interfere with sentiments of belonging to a moral order and of being right in what one does foster psychiatric disorder.

Series F. Proposition Relating Interpersonal Patterns and Sociocultural Environment

F1. Sociocultural situations which expose a growing personality to defective role relationships foster psychiatric disorder.

Series G. Propositions Regarding the Nature of Society and Culture

G1. Human society is composed of a network of interrelated sociocultural self-integrating units.

G2. Each self-integrating unit is an energy system and is in a constant state of performing functions upon which its existence depends.

G3. The functioning of the unit as a unit (G2) proceeds through patterns of interpersonal relationships based on the communication of shared symbols and coordinating sentiments.

Series H. Propositions Relating Sociocultural Patterns to Psychiatric Disorder

H1. Given that human society is composed of functioning self-integrating units based on patterns of interpersonal relationships which include communications, symbols, and sentiments (Series G), it follows that the different functional parts of a particular unit (such as associations, socioeconomic classes, and roles) may have differential effects on personalities exposed to them, and hence on mental health (B5, C5, D3, Series E and F1).

H2. Given that human society is composed of functioning self-integrating units based on patterns of interpersonal relationships which include communications, symbols, and sentiments (Series G), it follows that different units with different patterns of organization (culture) may have differential effects on personalities exposed to them, and hence on mental health (B5, C5, D2, Series E, and F1).

H3. Given that human society is composed of functioning self-integrating units based on patterns of interpersonal relationships which include communications, symbols, and sentiments (Series G), it follows that social disintegration will affect personalities in such a manner as to foster psychiatric disorder (B5, C5, D2, D3, Series E, and F1).

A close review of these propositions makes their articulation with the substance of this volume evident. For example, Series A, dealing with fundamental striving and its disruption, bears directly on the issue of environmental influences on personality development. It further aids in the interpretation of Chapter 6 (identifying vulnerable populations through the use of a psychiatric register) and Chapter 15 (the etiology of adolescent drug use), among others.

Series B and C provide a framework for understanding central aspects of psychiatric etiology; they trace the manner in which an individual copes or fails to cope with threats to the stability of the essential psychical condition. Hence they illuminate several key issues, notably those concerned with social etiology and with coping models. These series also pinpoint the questions posed in Chapter 5 (pathways to patienthood), Chapter 15 (adolescents' failure to cope with the stresses of emergent adulthood), and Chapter 9 (the analysis of successful coping responses).

Series E details the impact of the sociocultural environment on the fulfillment of individual needs. As such, it deals with virtually all of the identified key issues, perhaps especially with those clustered around the organization of a community network of helping processes. Series E is particularly helpful in the examination of problems of primary prevention (see Chapter 13 on consultation and education) and of traditional responses to illness (see Chapter 3 on the state mental hospital treatment model).

Finally, Series G and H address the broad sweep of community organization in its juncture with population states of health. Again, these propositions are relevant to each key issue; they appear especially germane to the dilemma of alternative goals in mental health policy, and to the search for feasible modes of primary prevention. Series G and H are valuable to the analysis of "community competence," as exemplified in Chapters 11, 12, and 13, each of which deals with aspects of concerted local action: How may we work with and on the social system to foster health-promoting behaviors?

The editors, then, believe that the present volume represents important continuities with the 1957 book.[3] At least some of the hopes of that early symposium seem to have been redeemed; most significant, perhaps, has been devoted and widespread thought and action addressed to the challenges sketched then. Today our tone of voice is probably somewhat less optimistic, somewhat more realistically attuned to the observed hazards entailed in moving from social psychiatric theory and ideology to community mental health operations. Yet an unrelieved pessimism would be equally inappropriate to our current circumstance. As the assembled contributions show, we are making marked headway toward a more sophisticated concept of psychological health; toward a more precise grasp of pathogenic features of the social environment; toward the identification of sources of individual and community strength; and toward a much more clear-eyed appraisal of the value of mental health activities.

REFERENCES

1. Freud, S. *Civilization and its Discontents*. James Strachey, ed. & tr: New York: Norton, 1962.

2. Leighton, A. H. *My Name Is Legion*. Vol. I. The Stirling County Study of Psychiatric Disorder and Sociocultural Environment. New York: Basic Books, 1959. Chapter V, pp. 133–187.

3. Leighton, A. H.: Clausen, J.; and Wilson, R. N. *Explorations in Social Psychiatry*. New York: Basic Books, 1957.

Editorial Note

How can life be made better for more people? This question has guided both this book and its predecessor, Explorations in Social Psychiatry.

The issues of human survival and the quality of life are problems central to mental health. In our search for greater understanding in improving the quality of life, other problems of dominant concern come to the fore: What is mental illness, and how is it observed? What are the social "causes" of mental illness? With the realization of the high prevalence of mental distress and psychosomatic related illnesses, we are confronted with new challenges to defining and alleviating significant disturbance. What can be done?

In addition, these classic questions still confront us: What is the nature of society? What is the nature of the individual? What is the threshold for individual and group capacities to change? Where is the delicate balance between individual needs and social system needs found? How do we escape the stress of malfunctioning social systems?

B. H. K.

CHAPTER 2

Conceptual Perspectives

ALEXANDER H. LEIGHTON

Some General Assumptions

IT IS particularly important right now that any work dealing with mental health, mental illness, and societal process state its main assumptions. This is because we live in a period when there are many diverse and often incompatible assumptions held by thinking people. Passionate adherences to contradictory viewpoints about the nature of man are characteristic of our time.

The first assumptions we shall present pertain to the difference in circumstance of this book and its predecessor, *Explorations in Social Psychiatry*.[3] At the time of the first volume an imperative question in the minds of the authors, editors, and most of the readers was how to make life better for more people. The selection of frontiers of knowledge for exploration was guided by this goal.

At present, the guiding question is survival. This is because we realize more clearly that mental health and illness are interwoven with problems of poverty, minority status, counterculture trends, and political ideologies, and all of these with the control of population, with ecology, and with biological devastation.

Another difference is the fact that the concept of mental illness and the notion of what constitutes a mental patient have lost rather than gained in clarity. The phenomena have not changed, but perceptions and ideas about cause have, and numbers of definitions have drifted away like smoke. Among many professionals, of course, the core notions and traditional perceptions still exist, but the social support upon which the use of these ideas depends has become fluid and confused in a welter of competing ideas. Diagnostic entities are not wiped out, but are rather like a collection of wax images that have been exposed to heat and become partially and unevenly melted.

With the rise of doubt about mental illness, there has come a downgrading of psychiatry and clinical psychology, at least in their more scientific forms. Prestige has been replaced by hostility; and numerous competing offers of psychological help have arisen. The recent decline of federal support for mental health centers is in part symptomatic of underlying changes of sentiment by the public.

A third area of changed circumstance concerns the development of new knowledge. The two examples we shall note have not burst suddenly across the threshold between unknown and known since the previous book, but rather have become immensely developed. One of these consists of medications that affect moods and emotions. It is not an exaggeration to say that they have changed the face of psychiatry in hospitals, in outpatient clinics, and in private practice. They have also, in all probability, increased the treatment of emotional disturbances by many other types of physicians besides psychiatrists, and by nonphysicians. To the degree that such medication relieves distress, it seems likely that it also reduces incentives toward psychotherapy, and toward altering stressful conditions in the social environment, a matter of some profound significance that ties itself to the problem of drugs.

The second item consists in discovering the great frequency of those mental and emotional states which in the past were considered symptoms of psychiatric disorders, but which are probably now better labeled "behaviors of psychiatric interest." The reference is to states of depression, anxiety, apathy, suspiciousness, hostility, and delusions, and to an accompanying panoply of somatic disturbances, commonly cardiovascular or gastrointestinal, which sometimes result in serious organic outcomes.

There is clearly a paradox here: As the evidence for high prevalence rate has increased, so too has uncertainty about what constitutes such disturbances and whether, after all, there is such a thing as mental illness. We interpret this to mean that as the size of the problem has grown and more and more people are evidently involved, consensus regarding its nature and how to cope has decreased.

The Nature of Society

Our first assumption in this area is that every human society is an open system. This statement may seem nowadays both obvious and tautological, but it has implications that are not obvious, and so deserve some discussion. When we say

15

"system" we are speaking technically in terms of systems theory. The referent for the word "society" is community theory which embodies the notion of geographic location and some degree of semipermeable boundary. If the reader will imagine a town with rural surroundings, he will have in mind a model that illustrates what we shall say, but it should be remembered that many other kinds of groupings, such as a tribe, would serve as well.

The community as a system is continuously active. It is in fact a kind of living organism and, like any other organism, is engaged in performing functions. These have been called the "functional prerequisites of a society" [1,2] and consist in such activities as:

1. Family formation and perpetuation.
2. Indoctrination of new community members.
3. Patterns of leadership, fellowship, and association.
4. Meeting emotional needs in life's crises and in day-to-day living.
5. The maintenance of communication.
6. Protection against weather, disease, and disaster.
7. Systems of economic enterprise.

To exist at all, these functions have to be coordinated so that they can be transacted in time and space without collision and interference with each other. As an expression of this, the community system is divided into subsystems. Schools constitute one subsystem, the family is another, the government of the community is still another, and so on. Altogether, the subsystems make up "social structure."

The latter phrase has unfortunate static implications, and for this reason we prefer to think in terms of functions, systems, and subsystems. Overall, community system and component subsystems, with their various functions related to the ongoing processes of the whole, may be likened to an organism and its component organs. Essential to survival is coordination, and coordination implies predictability, transmission of signals, and regulation.

Just as the total system of the community is composed of subsystems, so too the subsystems have others within them. The basic unit out of which all the rest is built may be represented by "role." Roles are demonstrated in such words as father, wife, lawyer, storekeeper, community council member, and mayor. One can regard the total social system that is the community as composed of a network of interacting roles, with some roles more densely interconnected with each and thus constituting "social institutions" that have at least vaguely defined boundaries, thereby forming the subsystems of the community.

Roles are to be distinguished from the individuals who fill them. Characteristically, roles last longer than individuals, and this is particularly true of those most concerned in the functional prerequisites. On the other hand, a given individual fulfills many roles (e.g., father, lawyer, husband). Because this relationship holds for individuals and roles, it also obtains between individuals and the system and subsystems of the community. Individuals come and go, but the community system and its components ("structure") continue. Individuals often introduce modifications in roles, and sometimes these are handed on to successors as part of the role. A point to note with reference to contemporary thought is that individual freedom consists in the ability to modify roles, to move about among roles, or to avoid roles, but there are limits which, if exceeded, result in faltering or failure of functional prerequisites. This is because of the ramifying interconnections. It is characteristic of open systems that a change in one part has effects which spread more or less widely from the seat of the change.

The phenomena of interconnectedness may be conceptualized as *dynamic equilibrium*. The word "dynamic" is employed because energy is involved. The patterning of community systems and subsystems is maintained through the expenditure of energy. The principle can be illustrated by a whirlpool, a pattern that is maintained by the input and output of moving water. Unlike the whirlpool, but like all living systems, the community exerts control over its energy flow and utilizes part of it to maintain its continuing existence. This distinction is a major one between life and nonlife.

Dynamic equilibrium consists in this self-maintenance operating against a multitude of forces, both within and external to the system, which would otherwise dissolve and dissipate it. The label "steady state" has been applied to this kind of energy balance and encompasses the idea of an optimal point that is continuously being lost and regained. Any new event which alters and thereby impairs the functioning of the system is met with counteractions which restore equilibrium.

Inherent in the concept of dynamic equilibrium is the potential for growth and change. This is because restoration does not necessarily mean return to the status *quo ante*. On the contrary, change can be met by establishing a new pattern of equilibrium. While there is some resistance to changing patterns because of multiple interconnections that act like inertia, the central issue in dynamic equilibrium is maintaining the functional prerequisites upon which the group's continuity and survival depend. This is generally achieved through adjustments that involve modifications of roles, of subsystems, and eventually of the community as a whole. New action patterns emerge.

To illustrate with an oversimplification, the community can be regarded as composed of two major sets of forces, one centripetal, concerned with self-maintenance, and one centrifugal, tending toward dissolution—a struggle, in short, between pattern and dissipation.

The nature of the centrifugal force is not a mystery. It constitutes in part all those things which are recognized as dangerous to individuals, such as drought,

17

disease, war, famine, and poverty. There are others, however, which spring from disharmony between individual aspirations and the constraints of roles and the limitation of choice among roles. This disharmony is both a source of inventiveness, creativity, and development, and of destruction.

Dynamic equilibrium, then, involves a process of continually seeking adaptation in the face of continuing change. The capacity for adjustment is not, however, infinite, and this brings us to the phenomenon of threshold. Every community system can adjust easily to small changes, and even to large changes if they come about slowly enough to permit the time necessary for the transaction of interlinked chain reactions, and for the formation of new habits, establishment of relevant cues, and soon.

Changes can, however, be so great in magnitude, so widespread and simultaneous, or so abrupt, as to overwhelm adaptive capacity, with resultant failure of the functional prerequisites. This failure becomes a component of the centrifugal forces, and thus a trend toward self-destruction of the social system is established. Between this stage and ultimate destruction there are many degrees of chronic malfunction—conditions in which survival continues, but some or all of the functional prerequisites are badly performed. A first threshold, therefore, may be conceived as lying on a line between capacity for adjustment and lack of such a capacity, with resultant chronic malfunction. One can suppose that with special effort, particularly with help from some outside source, a community such as our town model can recover. A second threshold is postulated as one beyond which no recovery is possible, and the centrifugal forces win out.

The above outlines some of our main assumptions about social process and has been presented as a basis for understanding interrelationships with mental health and illness. These relationships must now be presented, but first there may be usefulness in trying to illustrate some of the implications inherent in this view of society. For one thing, the view is favorable to values that emphasize the importance of the individual, his protection, and his access to opportunity. At the same time it raises several questions about social values that stress individual rights without commensurate emphasis on individual obligations. Inasmuch as individuals are parts of social systems with roles to perform and can exist in no other way, there are necessarily limits to individual freedom. When issues of social reform, radical politics, or participant democracy are examined in terms of the frame of reference presented, interrelationships and functional consequences must be considered. This means that neither the individual nor "the State" can be considered paramount, and philosophies that insist on either extreme are at best impractical (in the long run), and at worst threats to survival. Or again, it is necessary to examine critically current enthusiasms for solving social problems through adversary tactics and confrontation, whether legal or illegal. Accepting that the goals are laudable and necessary, the question is still open as to whether the methods are the best for achievement, or whether they are destructive in the sense that they increase centrifugal forces and add considerably to the risk of social disintegration. This does not imply that goals concerned with relieving deprived people of their disadvantages should be abandoned, but it does suggest that the methods be questioned and that serious thought be given to finding better ways.

The Nature of the Individual

Like the community, the individual person is also an open system. This idea is inherent in most theories of personality, even though the terms employed may not be those of system theory. Inasmuch as the concept of personality as a state of dynamic equilibrium (molded in infancy but with inputs and outputs going on throughout life) is familiar to most readers, we shall not review it here, but move on to considering some of our assumptions about the relationship of individual processes to community processes.

The tension between the individual and the role repertoire made available to him by society has already been pointed out. We think that there is far too little known about this phenomenon and that it should be a focus for major investigation. Why is it that at times the tension appears to be dormant and at others becomes a matter of great agony? The answer to this surely lies not only in various patternings of social systems that limit individual freedom in diverse ways, but also in variations in individual perceptions and aspirations.

Be that as it may, the prime link between individual and social system is the interplay between constraints on the individual and the meeting of his needs through the functional prerequisites. Without reliable subsistence, protection from excessive fear, opportunities for love and for achieving self-esteem, and so on, the personality is in difficulties both in its development and in its adult functioning. In our view it is very apt to react with psychological and psychophysiological patterns of strain manifested as anxiety, depression, apathy, hostility, and delusion formation, often combined with organic disturbances.

One of the most vital processes in the interaction between personality systems and social systems is that which transpires when the capacity-for-change-threshold of a social system is exceeded, leading to social disintegration. Everyone is aware that human society is undergoing change at an unprecedented rate, but it is worth pausing to note some of the main trends.

Technological development is one, leading to weapons of gigantic power, the pill, mass forms of communication, and mood-altering drugs, to name but a few of the items that have confronted communities with major demands for adaptation.

Population increase is another, and this has at least two aspects. Size itself has an influence on what is feasible in terms of system and subsystems of a community. A town of fifty thousand that becomes a town of two hundred fifty thousand must change qualitatively as well as quantitatively. The other aspect of population change is age distribution: The present and the recent past exhibit an unusually high proportion of people in the years of transition from child to adulthood. The future will see a burgeoning of older people, and this change will doubtless raise a host of new problems for adjustment.

Population movement must also be mentioned as a problem confronting many communities. There is evidently an almost world-wide trend away from the country into urban areas that are ill prepared to handle the influx. There is also a circulating kind of migration in which people move from community to community in search of jobs, especially jobs that will constitute improvement in economic status. It is easy to see that if this turnover is great, considerable instability must be introduced into community systems.

Derived from both population increase and technology are the well-known problems of pollution, and communities must deal with the question of how long they can go on fouling their nests or the nests of other communities. At issue here is the relationship between long- and short-range requirements for the functional prerequisites.

As a final example of major and apparently accelerating change, there is the matter of ideologies and values. That these have changed drastically is a commonplace, and it is plausible to suppose that the roots are to be found in the products of technology and population configurations mingling and leading to various actions and reactions. Certainly mass war, rapid communication (including cross-cultural communication), ease of travel, large numbers of young people, and imbalances in the possession of the world's resources have all played a major part. The result at the present time is not so much a change from old to new values as a state approaching chaos. And yet a necessary condition for the existence of a community is a set of articulated values. These serve as a combination of chart, guidelines, and incentives whereby that coordination of roles and subsystems is attained upon which the functional prerequisites depend. One is tempted to suggest that what is needed today is a National Association for Better Human Relationships.

Having sketched some of the changes assaulting community systems today, we may now state that it is our assumption that these constitute a state of risk for many communities, the risk being that the capacity for adaptation will be exceeded. In other words, the first threshold has been crossed, centrifugal forces predominate, and the process of self-destruction has begun. For this we employ the term *social disintegration*. As we have already stated, it means that the functional prerequisites falter, thereby adding new secondary stresses to those present because of the changes that pushed the community beyond its threshold. As the social system fails, roles become punishing or inoperable. The increase in prevalence and intensity of stresses constitutes a state of risk for the emergence of manifest psychiatric disorders—that is, behaviors of the type already listed. These may be natural reactions to adverse circumstances, "not mental illness," as some would say. One can equally say that it is natural to have broken legs and severed arteries in an auto accident. Whichever way one chooses to look upon the psychological and somatic conditions, they are distinctly miserable for those who experience them, and they are not under voluntary control. They are nonrational, counterproductive, and compound the difficulties both for the sufferer and those around him. Of particular importance is that as the prevalence of people with such difficulties increases in the population, there is a corresponding further reduction in the coping ability and competence of the community. When prevalence rates of mental disorder become as high as those shown in various surveys—between 15 and 20 percent, with subgroups running much higher—this is not a trivial matter in the total question of community welfare. Nor, obviously, is it a minor matter for mental health. The model illustrates our assumptions about one important way in which mental health and illness are related to social process, a way which is inherent in regarding society as a functional system.

So What?

The framework that has been sketched is a basis for evaluation and making choices—choices with regard to one's own conduct and values, and choices with regard to what is to be preferred in numerous contemporary issues. From the point of view of this book, these pertain primarily to community mental health; examples will become evident in the course of many of the chapters. We can anticipate here, however, with two examples.

As previously noted, one of the recurrent themes of today is a tendency to advocate the rights of the individual above all else. Our framework would say that if this is pushed to extremes in practice, the results will be not only dangerous to social process, but also bad for mental health.

While we share very deeply concern for individuals, and recognize fully the assaults on individual freedom and integrity that stem from bureaucracies and traditional prejudices, nevertheless it seems clear to us that to give emphasis only to individual freedom is to push the social system of communities toward disintegration. One outcome of this can be the kind of reactive process that established Napoleon after the French Revolution—in other words, a highly restrictive system with centralization of power and vast reduction in individual choice with regard to role performance and role selection. Thus, the overpush for freedom results in its destruction.

Another alternative is that the social system is carried beyond the threshold of recovery and disintegrates—an outcome apparently wished by some proponents of a remade society. Our frame of reference would point to the great unlikelihood of their expectations of resurrection in a better, systemless society being realized. The concept of functional social systems in dynamic equilibrium would predict a failing of functional prerequisites, and a concomitant extinction not just of freedom, but of life itself. Given the postulated relationship of mental illness and social disintegration, one could regard this as fulfilling the dictum that those whom the gods would destroy they first make mad.

Another recurrent theme of today is to escape from the constraints of the mass society by the formation of groups to which individuals strongly adhere. To our way of thinking, this is an instance of "flocculation," an intermediary condition that appears as reaction to growing disintegration. In an effort to escape from the stress emanating from the malfunctioning of the social system, which reaches individuals largely in terms of role difficulties, people seek relief in small groups which can, at least for a time, meet their emotional needs. It is as if clumping occurred around nodal points in the social network, and hence the label *flocculation*. To the extent that the clumps are actually capable of being functional communities, or of contributing to the functioning of a larger system of which they are a part, they have a viable potential. One difficulty, however, is that many of the flocculants are actually subsystems, and their efforts to straighten out things for their component members can and often do result in failure to contribute to the larger system. They are like organs which have given up their interdependent position in the body and are acting as if they were whole organisms, and thus they become parasitic upon the larger society. This phenomenon is widespread at present, especially in large cities where one can see various organizations concentrating on the "rights" of their members with disregard for the effect on the whole. "Meet our demands or else" becomes the theme, which can have many resemblances to skyjacking. Examples are evident in the strikes of hospital workers, bridge tenders, garbage collectors, and others. Flocculation appears to contain two impulses: "Let's get together so we can wield power," and "Be small so we can cope."

The flocculation trend is pivotal in terms of outcome in a system that has begun to move toward disintegration. It can take the form either of parasitism, which is then part of the spiral of community self-destruction and disintegration, or of viable social systems which fulfill functional prerequisites for their component members *and for other systems with which they interact*. To the extent that the flocculants accomplish this latter task, they mitigate stress and promote mental health by counteracting disintegrative trends.

We conclude, then, that the trend toward reorganization in terms of new functional groups—a type of flocculation—in communes and "new towns" has great significance for the welfare of mankind, including reduction in the frequency of mental illness and promotion of mental health. The essential is that the flocculants be functional both for themselves and for other groups.

REFERENCES

1. Aberle, D. F.; Cohen, A. K.; Davis, A. K.; Levy, M. J.; and Sulton, F. X. "The Functional Prerequisites of a Society." *Ethics* 9 (January 1950):100–111.

2. Leighton, A. H. *My Name Is Legion*. New York: Basic Books, 1959, pp. 194–225, 254–256.

3. ———; Clausen, J.; and Wilson, R. N. *Explorations in Social Psychiatry*. New York: Basic Books, 1957.

Part II

Patient Care

IN ASSESSING the issue of patient care, it is clear that the magnitude of the number of persons at risk to psychiatric disorder and the number of sick persons who are not receiving care are crucial concerns. The table below, compiled by Morton Kramer, provides vivid data on the extent to which the requirements for psychiatric services would be met, varying as to assumptions of need. Kramer's table uses 1971 estimates of use rates, while giving 1975 and 1980 projections of need and unmet needs by age groupings.

In examining Kramer's data, it is important to focus on the last three columns, which present estimates (by age group) of the percentage of unmet need assuming 2 percent in need, 10 percent in need, and 20 percent in need.

The magnitude of unmet needs is large even under the most conservative 2 percent estimate. If 10 percent is used, the unmet need is staggering. Yet, in the rural setting of Nova Scotia, Leighton reports that, "Our conclusion from all the available information is that at least one half of the adults in Stirling County are currently suffering from some psychiatric disorder defined in the American Psychiatric Association *Diagnostic and Statistical Manual*" (p. 356).[2]

Realizing the problems of valid estimates, it is presently clear that an inverse relationship exists between socioeconomic status and psychological disorder. The low socioeconomic groups consistently have higher overall rates. If we use Kramer's 2 percent, 10 percent, or 20 percent estimates of need, the problem is overwhelming. Using Srole's Midtown New York results, in the lowest stratum the minimum estimate of psychological disorder is 12.5 percent, the maximum 47.3 percent (p. 17).[1] Consequently, the interest of Part II in the nature and effectiveness of the care system takes on added significance.

REFERENCES

1. Dohrenwend, Bruce, and Dohrenwend, Barbara. *Social Status and Psychological Disorder*. New York: Wiley Interscience, 1969.

2. Leighton, D. C.; Harding, J. S.; Macklin, D. B.; Macmillan, A. M.; and Leighton, A. H. *The Character of Danger*. New York: Basic Books, 1963.

Extent to Which Needs for Psychiatric Services Would Be Met in Relation to Various Assumptions of Need: Assuming 1971 Use Rates Only, by Age, United States, 1975 and 1980

AGE	ESTIMATED GEN. POP.[a] (IN 000s) (1)	ESTIMATED PT. CARE EPISODES (2)	ESTIMATED NO. PERSONS RECV'G CARE (3)	ESTIMATED NUMBER OF PERSONS NEEDING CARE, ASSUMING			NUMBER IN NEED NOT RECEIVING CARE, ASSUMING			PERCENT UNMET NEED, ASSUMING		
				2% IN NEED (4)	10% IN NEED (5)	20% IN NEED (6)	2% IN NEED (7)	10% IN NEED (8)	20% IN NEED (9)	2% IN NEED (10)	10% IN NEED (11)	20% IN NEED (12)
				1975								
Total, All ages	215,324	4,237,576	3,390,061	4,306,480	21,532,400	43,064,800	1,060,510	18,142,339	39,674,739	24.6	84.3	92.1
Under 18	68,109	809,377	647,502	1,362,180	6,810,900	13,621,800	714,678	6,163,398	12,974,298	52.5	90.5	95.2
18–24 ...	27,780	716,150	572,920	555,600	2,778,000	5,556,000	0	2,205,080	4,983,080	0.0	79.4	89.7
25–44 ...	53,835	1,504,340	1,203,471	1,076,700	5,383,500	10,767,000	0	4,180,029	9,563,529	0.0	77.6	88.8
45–64 ...	43,430	932,267	745,814	868,600	4,343,000	8,686,000	122,786	3,597,186	7,940,186	14.1	82.8	91.4
65+ ...	22,170	275,442	220,354	443,400	2,217,000	4,434,000	223,046	1,996,646	4,213,646	50.3	90.1	95.0
				1980								
Total, All ages	228,676	4,500,344	3,600,275	4,573,520	22,867,600	45,735,200	1,030,028	19,267,325	42,134,925	22.5	84.3	92.1
Under 18	69,646	859,566	687,653	1,392,920	6,964,600	13,929,200	705,267	6,276,947	13,241,547	50.6	90.1	95.1
18–24 ...	29,156	760,558	608,446	583,120	2,915,600	5,831,200	0	2,307,154	5,222,754	0.0	79.1	89.6
25–44 ...	62,332	1,597,622	1,278,097	1,246,640	6,233,200	12,466,400	0	4,955,103	11,188,303	0.0	79.5	89.7
45–64 ...	43,489	990,076	792,061	869,780	4,348,900	8,697,800	77,719	3,556,839	7,905,739	8.9	81.8	90.9
65+ ...	24,053	292,522	234,018	481,060	2,405,300	4,810,600	247,042	2,171,282	4,576,582	51.4	90.3	95.1

[a] U.S. Bureau of the Census, Series D projection of the U.S. population (Current Population Reports—Series P-25, No. 493).

Derivation of columns 2 through 12:

Col.2—Total patient care episodes obtained by applying 1971 patient care episode rate per 100,000 population (1,968 per 100,000) to the projected 1975 and 1980 total U.S. population. Age distributions of patient care episodes obtained by applying 1971 percentage distribution of patient care episodes by age to the 1975 and 1980 estimated total patient care episodes.

Col.3—Represents a conversion of patient care episodes into number of persons accounting for these episodes by multiplying patient care episodes by a factor of 80. This factor was derived from findings of the Maryland Psychiatric Case Register that every person in that register had an average of 1.2 episodes of care per year.

Col.4 = Col.1 × .02
Col.5 = Col.1 × .10
Col.6 = Col.1 × .20
Col.7 = Col.4 – Col.3 (NOTE: For this column negative values were assumed to be zero, i.e., the need for services would be met. Also the total is the sum of the parts.)
Col. 8 = Col.5 – Col.3
Col. 9 = Col.6 – Col.3
Col.10 = Col.7 ÷ Col.4
Col.11 = Col.8 ÷ Col.5
Col.12 = Col.9 ÷ Col.6

Source: Dr. M. Kramer, presented at World Psychiatric Association Symposium, University of Teheran, Iran.

Editorial Note

With this, the first of the contributed chapters to our volume, we plunge into a knot of key issues. The problem of the use and misuse of state hospitals, a matter vital to the lives of millions, makes apparent the need to understand better the relationships of mental illness to social and cultural environment; to restructure professional roles in the mental health field; to achieve coordination and continuity in care; and to clarify the respective roles of expert, layman, and community representative in policy formation and health planning. Also pertinent are problems created by conflicting views about the biomedical and psychogenetic nature of mental illness, and the relative importance of social processes such as labeling and stereotyping.

Dr. Greenblatt is a distinguished former commissioner of mental health for Massachusetts. Before that he was director of a state hospital, as well as a university professor of psychiatry. He therefore brings to his topic both the experience and viewpoint of a scholar and the results of practical experience. It should also be noted that he has for many years been particularly interested in behavioral science research and its application to the problems of mental health and mental illness.

Dr. Greenblatt gives a devastating picture of the state hospital. It is possible that some people who have worked or have been patients in a state hospital will consider this overdrawn. We might point out that even forty years ago there were good and bad state hospitals, and that Dr. Greenblatt is describing the latter.

A. H. L.

CHAPTER 3

The Evolution of State Mental Hospital Models of Treatment

MILTON GREENBLATT

IN LESS than four decades, state mental hospitals in the more progressive parts of our country have changed from punitive custodial institutions to comprehensive community mental health centers. This remarkable metamorphosis has occurred *pari passu* with major shifts in the public sense of responsibility for the sick, the poor, and the downtrodden; a gratifying change in basic public attitudes toward the mentally ill; a major revolution in the role of therapeutic institutions; and perhaps an even more revolutionary change in man's conception of himself and his environment.

These changes have not been painless; on the contrary, they have been fraught with turmoil and struggle. Now, looking back, we appreciate that a great new day has finally dawned for those hapless individuals afflicted with emotional disorder. We note also that not only have the alterations within the hospitals and the changes within society occurred in parallel, but there has been a most fascinating interpenetration and interaction between the two, most of which has not been fully recorded. For example, as the hospitals, formerly rejected institutions, gradually began to be accepted by society, so the patients, who were the rejected individuals within the hospital organization, began to be accepted by the professional and service staffs of the hospitals. It has been a complex mosaic of movement and interchanges deeply meaningful and powerfully motivated.

The Custodial Authoritarian Model

Before the 1930s state mental hospitals were often monuments of custodial stagnation and neglect. Overcrowding, understaffing, hierarchical social organization, and autocratic management were the rule. Communications were mostly downward from entrenched and often dictatorial administration. Freedom was limited for both patients and staff. As an almost necessary consequence, many patients stayed for long months and even years. The image of the hospital was of a remote, barren, and punitive institution. Prospective patients felt banished from society and frightened of possible incarceration. Once patients, they were forever stigmatized, even if they were fortunate enough to be discharged.

Remoteness of the state hospital from population concentrations was not an accident, but generally derived from the community's fear of the mentally ill, and the prevailing notion that treatment of the mentally ill was best carried out in a quiet, isolated environment, free from the stresses and strains of normal society. Unfortunately, this meant that many families found it expensive, difficult, and time consuming to visit their sick relatives. Moreover, the custodial hospital of this period compounded the problem by viewing the family as a noxious and irritating element. In fact, visits by family members were often followed by an increase in disturbed behavior in the patients. But this phenomenon was seen primarily in its negative aspects as an indication for greater separation rather than as an opportunity to bring the family into the treatment orbit and work through the basic interpersonal problems that plagued the patient. Most hospitals in this period restricted visitors and hours of visiting, and limited the actual visit physically to a well-kept visiting room to which the patient was transported, rather than permitting the family to see the ward, the beds, the day space, and other patients with whom their own relative was expected to find a way of life.

The same attitudes that applied to families applied even more forcibly to other community members. Visits by interested citizens, volunteers, students, clergy, lawyers, and even the patient's personal physician were not generally encouraged. People found it depressing to visit such hospitals, and once a patient was referred for admission, his ties to the community were broken. For example, the family doctor rarely continued to see the patient after referral. The hospital, short of a brief note of acknowledgment, rarely gave out further information even to the referring physician or agency. Indeed, the concept of confidentiality of patient information, exaggerated by fear of stigma, operated to make the hospital stay more of a jail sentence than a therapeutic experience.

By and large, the wards in those days were drab and the patients unkempt and apathetic, sitting in rows or lying on the floor. Activities were minimal, with most of the important daily functions carried out on a mass impersonal basis. For example, at mealtime the patients queued up at a food line or cafeteria, received their rations, and ate without sociality or even awareness of each other. Showers and bathing were carried out on a mass basis without regard for privacy. Toilet functions were nonprivate and toilet seats were often lacking. Poverty, empty hours, and lack of personal attention made the individual an inmate or a number rather than a true patient who received medical and psychiatric diagnosis and attention. He certainly was not a true citizen or living member of any social group.

The therapeutic staff was grossly inadequate in number and usually received considerably lower pay than their counterparts in general hospitals and private facilities. But more to the point, their roles were defined as primarily custodial, watchdogs of a group of individuals considered far different from themselves and, in fact, inferior. Most patient management rested with the least-trained, least-paid, least-esteemed, and lowest in the hospital hierarchy—the attendants, some of whom could hold no other job. Some were alcoholic; some were morbid, sadistic, and overcontrolling of others. Their training and supervision were usually limited to a few hours or weeks of orientation at the beginning of their employment. No continuing in-service education was offered, and opportunities for personal growth through education or promotion were limited. None of the preceding is meant to derogate the impressive dedication to job and patient manifested by a very large corps and often a very large majority of ward staff. But there was no defined path of upward mobility for this largest group of workers continuously in contact with patients. And few administrators were making any systematic attempt to cultivate and utilize the therapeutic potentials that we know now were latent in many of them.

The professional staff was too often inadequate in number and too often of inferior quality. Physicians who could not make it successfully on the outside, or who themselves wanted to retreat from society in a comfortable sinecure, drifted to these hospitals. Many institutions were manned wholly or in part by foreign physicians, often with inadequate training and frequently possessing minimal qualifications or certification above graduation from a medical school.

Nurses, social workers, and occupational therapists found themselves overwhelmed. Vacancies were frequent, recruitment difficult, job gratification limited. Many of these staff members lived in the hospital, where the room was either free or almost free, where laundry would be done for them, meals were furnished, and socialization was inbred. Thus the workers together formed an enclave, ill-equipped to meet the vicissitudes of life outside, and therefore uninterested in helping the patient to adapt to the world outside.

Patient management—we can hardly call it therapy—consisted of interview to ascertain mental status, physical examination and history taking, followed by diagnosis, the latter usually little more than a labeling process. Then came some attempt to understand the background and developmental process, more descriptive than psychodynamic, followed by classification and assignment to the appropriate ward—acute, disturbed, incontinent, chronic, alcoholic, or senile. And, of course, there was segregation by sexes. If patients assigned to the acute ward did not improve with the aid of drugs, work in hospital industry, occasional interviews, and some occupational activity, they were relegated to the chronic wards, where the staff complement was even poorer than on the acute wards and personal contacts therefore limited, and where a climate of failure, boredom, and loss of motivation prevailed. Here "institutionalitis" began to set in. Hospitalization was prolonged and the prognosis was regarded as unfavorable.

As a whole, the hospital was divided into acute and chronic divisions, the former about 10 to 15 percent of the total beds, the latter making up the rest. The average duration of stay in the acute wards might be up to six months; in the chronic, five to ten years. Many patients lived out their lives in these chronic wards.

Perhaps the worst features of hospitals prior to 1930 centered around a number of therapeutic procedures then regarded as necessary or even progressive, but which we now see as punitive, restrictive, rejecting of patients, and laced with routinization and impersonalization. We refer to the following:

Seclusion.   Certain dangerous, impulsive, disruptive, and belligerent patients were incarcerated in locked rooms or cells with little or no furniture, with interruptions only for food, for toileting, maybe for a physical examination, or for medication. This could go on for hours or for days.

Forced tube-feeding.   Patients who manifested their hostility fears and disorganization by refusing to eat were forcibly restrained and tube-fed. A severe and destructive indignity thus was visited upon a sick human soul, compounded by the danger of aspirational pneumonia if the fatty viscous mixture happened to lodge in the respiratory tract of the struggling patient.

Chemical restraint.   Heavy doses of medication, usually given parenterally, were administered to patients who, it was thought, could not otherwise be controlled.

Continuous tubs.   Agitated, depressed patients were left soaking in tubs of water, heated to body temperature, in which all eliminative functions would go on. Not a few such patients attempted to drown themselves.

Physical restraints.   Self- or otherwise destructive patients were spread-eagled on the bed, with thongs attached to hands and feet tied to bedposts. With occasional interruption to assure circulation to the extremities, this could go on for hours, even days.

Wet-sheet packs. The patient was wrapped in wet sheets to reduce body movements and to quiet agitation. The risk of hyperthermia and death was significant.

We now regard all of these procedures as punitive and outmoded. No specific or therapeutic gains are attributed to them. Instead, we see them as frightening to patients, drawing effort and attention away from an understanding of their inner life and needs, and, of course, entailing a total negation of the patient's opportunity for social interaction and social belonging. The fact that many patients got well under these circumstances we now attribute to their strong constitutions, their ability to take advantage of personal relationships with an understanding attendant, nurse, doctor, or other patient, or to the time-limiting nature of their basic psychiatric affliction.

The Therapeutic Egalitarian Model

In the 1930s, with the introduction of somatic therapies such as electric shock, insulin hypoglycemia, and lobotomy, a transformation began to take place in state mental hospitals. Electric shock gave dramatic relief to crippling depressions and involutional conditions. Insulin-coma therapy appeared to be of benefit to schizophrenic patients, and lobotomy was reported to relieve anxious agitation in a variety of disorders, aiding particularly in the improvement or recovery of many chronic "hopeless" individuals.

The dramatic effect of these new therapeutic devices was not so much on the patients whose disorders were alleviated, but on the revolutionary new attitude about the hopefulness of a field long regarded as therapeutically dead. Psychotherapeutic techniques began to be used with renewed vigor by proponents who felt that their approach could rival the effects of somatic methods even in chronic patients. A spirit of competition among therapeutic enthusiasts was added to the note of hope.

There followed vigorous explorations of the use of work rehabilitative programs for hospitalized patients. These, too, showed their worth beyond a doubt. The introduction in the 1950s of the tranquilizers, and then antidepressant medication, was a great boon to patients, altering their social environment to a startling degree in the direction of less overactivity, less agitation, less belligerence

33

and hostility, and less destructiveness. It was also a great boon to collaborative endeavors of hospital professionals with pharmacologists, biochemists, and behavioral scientists of all types, and gave rise to a great broadening of scientific and intellectual horizons in the mental hospitals. This was accompanied by collaboration between scientists from medical schools and institutions of higher learning with certain vanguard hospitals.

But more valuable than all else was the growth of interest in experimentation with the social milieu as a therapeutic force. The alliance of the profession of psychiatry with sociology, anthropology, social psychology, and behavioral science produced most substantial benefits in patient care and treatment. In addition, there were the benefits of expanded intellectual horizons and the appreciation of the remarkable influence on patient progress of such factors as set, expectation, social interaction, behavioral goals, rewards, the overt and covert ideological tenets and values in each ward unit, and, above all, the therapeutic climate or atmosphere that characterized and pervaded an institution.

We were beginning to deal with social concepts broad enough to embrace the total situation within which each new therapeutic modality or therapeutic trial could have its place. Scientists from many of the humanistic fields began to see the mental hospital as a place worthy of their work, even a place in which a career could be fashioned, and soon many of the subtle social variables of the therapeutic environment began to be identified and investigated.

It was during this time that the so-called evils of the "custodial authoritarian" period began to be mitigated or eliminated. Seen through social systems clinicians' eyes, what ailed the mental hospitals, beyond lack of staff, poor buildings, and general impoverishment, were barriers to communication, fear of patients and the need to control and isolate them, emphasis on hierarchy, and lack of upward flow of ideas, suggestions, and contributions to decision making. There was a need to reexamine roles, foster social and recreational work activities, open doors, intermingle men and women, promote discussions of hospital life for all kinds of groups, and release creativity in the ranks.

It was through the power of this great social revolution that routinized, restrictive measures such as seclusion, tube feedings, wet-sheet packs, and physical restraints were finally eliminated. In like manner, activity therapies were developed and incentive work programs instituted. Teamwork became the model of the day, and staff strove to make the patient's twenty-four hours meaningful, not simply to rely on an occasional hour of psychotherapeutic discussion with the doctor, if such were even possible in the average mental hospital.

The therapeutic relevance to the patient of every individual in the hospital system, and of every contact, began to be a proper concern. Role analysis and role change, social and physical environmental analysis and change, and analysis of leadership, together with changing of the roles of executive figures, became the accepted thing. Inevitably, the self-esteem of both patients and staff and their enthusiasm for the work they were doing rose significantly and, of course, added further to the hospital's therapeutic potential.

The Mental Health Center Model

During the 1950s and the 1960s the concept of a state hospital serving as a mental health center was popularized. This followed logically from the reduction of restraints of patients, the freeing of communication, the opening of doors, the beginning of merging of hospital and community, and the development of hospital-community liaisons and collaborations on behalf of the patient.

The barriers were broken down in many ways. The open-door policy allowed family members and friends in. Volunteering in mental hospitals increased greatly. One of the major developments was the college student volunteer. Some of these students came to the hospital out of curiosity, some to search out career opportunities in a field that was of increasing interest, and some to render service to the less fortunate. They paved the way to what has become a massive mental health volunteer movement in America, and brought to the scene optimism, enthusiasm, and the natural therapeutic makeup of the young.

This was the phase in the history of the mental hospital in which the greatest strides were made in collaboration with institutions of learning. Colleges and universities made use of the hospital not only as a place for volunteering, but also as a field placement for training of social workers, psychologists, occupational therapists, and nurses. Clergymen and work rehabilitation counselors were soon added to the expanding treatment team. With the growing awareness of the potential of the mental hospital as a laboratory for social-behavioral studies, a small but influential number of social scientists adopted the mental hospital as the subject of their research. A rather special but important change was the adoption of the open staff system so that physicians from the community could visit and treat patients they had referred, similar to the way they functioned in relation to patients in general hospitals. This added the possibility of continuity of medical care for their patients when discharged.

The greatly increased access to the mental hospital by community caretakers was accompanied by a significant movement of staff and patients out of the hospital. Employees who formerly used the institution as a retreat from the stresses of the world found it desirable to establish living arrangements on the outside when administrators began to seek intramural space for new patient and staff activities, and recognized the desirability of getting out of the hotel business.

35

The commuting of staff from community to hospital helped bridge the gap for the employees, and eventually for the friends and relatives who followed their careers. The employee could then exploit his opportunity to become an ambassador of good will for the institution he served, to teach people about the hospital, to tell them about its realities, and to diminish prejudice and superstition about life in the mental institution.

Most remarkable was the patient movement into the community as hospital barriers broke down. First, professional staff and administrators began to experiment with earlier discharge, testing the hypothesis that for many more patients than previously realized life in the community was a great therapeutic experience. The planning for discharge, which had formerly taken place only after the symptoms abated, was continually moved earlier in the clinical course until finally discharge planning began on admission. When first interviewed, relatives were informed that the illness was in all probability time-limited, and that they should plan not only for active visiting during hospitalization, but also to preserve a place in the family hearth and heart for the patient's return. Employers, too, were contacted, and they agreed, in most instances, to take back the person whose work performance had been satisfactory before his illness. And schools and colleges began to be more lenient about the return of a student who had had an emotional breakdown during the course of his studies.

But now it became necessary to make more vigorous efforts to prepare the patient for discharge. This led to the burgeoning of work programs with community relevance. Emphasis was put on training of skills involved in "social competence" (a measure especially applicable to backward patients who had long forgotten how to get along in public), on "practice trips" into the community, and on searching for suitable living arrangements in the community and proper social groups with which the patient could identify. New educational opportunities were continually being explored.

A number of formal therapeutic modalities typify the efforts of this period: for example, the day hospital as a stepping stone to the community, or an option against hospitalization; the night hospital for those who could work during the day, returning for treatment in the evening; the halfway house or community home for those not quite ready for full discharge, and requiring a semi-sheltered supervised setting before venturing forth; or an apartment dwelling in which a group of patients making common cause could live together, working in the community and receiving psychological and social work assistance from the outreach staff of the hospital.

Outpatient departments and walk-in clinics became thriving services for patients with a will to remain in the community, and a home treatment service evolved out of the attempt of the hospital staff to treat patients in their home settings as soon as an emotional upset threatened, without moving them physically to an often remote mental institution. The staff, in other words, brought treatment to the patient instead of demanding that the patient be brought to the treatment—a radical change in philosophy compared to the days of custody and authority.

Part of the effort of this period was to render educational services for a large variety of potential and actual caretakers in the community—social agencies, clergymen, general practitioners, teachers, and police officers (who so often in former days brought the patient to the hospital frightened, worried, and in handcuffs). Thus, seminars and conferences were developed for clergymen and for general practitioners, and lectures and case demonstrations for police officers, both in the barracks and in the field or on the beat.

The image of the mental hospital was changing in the public mind from a place of horror to a haven or refuge. Patients and families came earlier in the course of illness to seek help. Patients already helped were able to continue to lean on the hospital during their postdischarge period, and many of them profited greatly from the aftercare network into which they settled. These aftercare networks spelled the critical difference for many borderline patients between remaining in the community and being rehospitalized.

During this period, hospital admissions rose sharply, partly as a function of better care and treatment, and partly as a function of earlier case finding. Readmissions, too, rose sharply. The latter was a signal of two sorts: one, that patients were allowed out before full symptomatic recovery; and two, that patients were less fearful of the hospital and thus more inclined to use its resources. The "revolving door" became the slogan of this period just as the "open door" was the slogan of the earlier phase.

This period was also characterized by the emergence of public relations as a recognized part of hospital administration (a subspecialty which still does not have the status it deserves), and some important experimentations took place in this field, mainly with federal support. These explored ways of communicating a more positive and realistic image of the work of the hospital to the public, with the dual aim of increasing financial support and making it easier for society to accept patients released from the institution.

The Comprehensive Community Health Center Model

Once the success of the mental health center model had been demonstrated, the federal government, following publication of the report of the Joint Commission on Mental Illness and Health in 1961 and the proclamation of John Fitzgerald Kennedy on mental health in 1963, determined to get into the mental health business in a big way. The federal government formalized and legitimized the model of the community mental health center which according to its specifications, should have five essential services: inpatient, outpatient, transitional care, twenty-four-hour emergency care, and community consultation and education. An enormous spur to the development of these centers was federal financial aid, both in construction grants and staffing grants; over a period of approximately five years some four hundred fifty such centers were spawned with federal assistance.

The great impact of the comprehensive community mental health center model was due to the insistence of the federal government that these centers serve defined geographic areas, or catchment areas, whose population would include from seventy-five thousand to two hundred thousand citizens. Federal aid is based on priority ratings of these areas, based in turn on an analysis of need in relation to resources. Each area must plan comprehensive centers for total care and treatment of mentally ill persons without regard to race, sex, age, ethnic membership, or diagnostic category.

These centers may be planned as a variety of services related to one physical setting, that is, under one roof, or as affiliated services in several physical structures or systems, public or private—provided they are properly linked under one clear administrative auspice, and provided continuity of services is guaranteed by a smooth flow of patients, records, responsibility, and, hopefully, therapeutic personnel from one system to another. Further, community participation must be satisfactory and the poverty areas must be served first. After the initial grants, later special dispensations were allowed by the federal government for children's services, drug rehabilitation programs, and programs for minority groups.

Most of the new centers developed under federal guidelines are small facilities with relatively few inpatient beds, and relatively large outpatient and aftercare activities. They are located by design in or near centers of population. The large state mental hospitals do not necessarily lose out in these changes—though for many the new emphasis on small centers as primary caretakers of acute disorders constituted a downgrading of their functioning. Establishment of a community mental health center meant that the state hospital would no longer receive new admissions, but only long-term cases or chronic problems discarded by the comprehensive centers. This was seen as a blow to their esteem; they were to become wastebaskets for disposal of undesirable patients who failed to improve in the comprehensive facility. Though many state hospitals were actually improved by an increase in specific resources as a result of federal aid, they nevertheless often did suffer downgrading in relation to new intensive care centers which enjoyed the limelight, as well as the lion's share of the new money.

On the other hand, many state hospitals were actually upgraded insofar as they, too, adopted a specific catchment area to serve, and thus could apply for federal largesse to enrich and extend their activities and render more comprehensive services. Thus, in many places, the state hospital came into its own, sharing the advantages of the new federal inspiration, and involving itself in all of the new and fascinating challenges related to delivering services to a defined community. Some state hospitals, in fact, took on two roles: one, to serve the catchment area as a comprehensive community mental health center; the other, to serve as a backup for centers and areas other than their own.

When we look back ten years from now, I think we will find the idea of responsibility for a catchment area to be the most significant development of this period. From it flowed a new coalition between the citizens of a community and the hospital; renewed interest in public health psychiatry; restimulation of the sciences of epidemiology and preventive medicine; deeper concern for the way of life of the people and a study of life styles that contribute to unhappiness and disease; a further attempt to identify and treat high-risk groups; concern for minority and disenfranchised people; greater use of crisis and emergency intervention techniques; more interest in mobile treatment teams; and, finally, mobilization of paraprofessionals and volunteers in order to try to meet the needs of a defined population. All of this is, of course, modern community psychiatry, which could not have come of age without the delineation, definition, and description of the community itself.

Definition of a catchment area brought the citizen movement to its greatest height of involvement and participation, including actual management functions. Citizens earlier had involved themselves as volunteers, either working directly with individual patients on wards, or in broader recreation or socialization activities. Later citizen involvement took the form of assisting the patient in adjusting to society by finding a living situation for him; connecting him with church, school, or social club; helping him find a job; and eventually organizing community homes, halfway houses, and apartment dwellings as transitional residences.

The other major form of citizen involvement is serving on boards of trustees or boards of directors of state facilities. Here they advise on policy, approve critical appointments, or scrutinize budgets. Mostly they are appointed by state governors. In some states, however, they are appointed by county authorities, themselves appointed or elected by the people.

Most characteristic of the comprehensive community mental health center era is the citizen area board representing the area, and essentially responsible to citizens of the area. These boards vary in origin, function, and authority, but virtually all have the following characteristics in common: they form a sort of unstable partnership with professional mental health authorities; they move toward greater and greater involvement in policy making, budgetary functions, and control; they challenge and compete, therefore, with professionals who formerly had it their own way. Inevitably, they press strongly for better care for the mentally ill and retarded, impatient of delay, bureaucratic complexities, or administrative defensiveness.

In addition to involvement with citizen boards, many new questions are being raised in relation to the social causes of mental disorder, and in relation to the role of psychiatrists and mental health workers as social activists or political change agents. What part do poor housing, rat infestation, poor diet, lack of privacy, disenfranchisement, environmental pollution, unemployment, family dismemberment, one-parent families, an intellectually and conceptually impoverished life, and a hopeless attitude toward the future, play in the evolution of mental illness and retardation? And what is the responsibility of a psychiatrist or mental health worker, either as a professional or as a citizen and taxpayer, to seek the negation of these evils? How far does the psychiatrist's expertise extend in the development of a more satisfactory society? And how does he work best with various community groups, and with the increasing number of city planners, housing experts, lawyers, legislators, political scientists, and social revolutionaries interested in effecting change?

One of the essential skills of this period, then, for the administrator of mental health organizations, is his ability to gain confidence and continued support from citizen boards and the community. This is a time-consuming problem, requiring patience, skill in producing consensus among disparate groups, and ability to subordinate one's expertise to the group mind.

Total Health Care Model

Administrators recognize that the job is too big to be done well within prevailing budget limitations. We are aware of the duplication and overlapping of functions of various agencies. We know of the need to plan for the health and welfare of all of the people within a catchment area, and are aware that health, education, and welfare are in reality all part of one life fabric. All this knowledge serves to motivate us strongly as we stand on the threshold of planning and implementing total health care delivery systems, the fundamental target being the catchment area defined and legitimated during the comprehensive mental health center period.

Although few can claim they know how to do the job, there are still signs of progress everywhere. For example, with federal government assistance, both in conceptualization and implementation, comprehensive health councils are being formed for defined regions all over the country. Notably, these councils contain a high percentage of nonprofessionals, the so-called consumers of the region. The councils develop plans, review applications for funds, and encourage innovative projects leading to the goal of total health care. Many states, too, are moving toward a cabinet system which includes at least one cabinet officer representing human services or human resources in the generic sense. This individual is charged with facilitating cooperation between departments and fashioning master plans for total care through optimal economies.

Within this context it becomes necessary for mental health and retardation administrators to rethink the goals and functions of their institutions. For example, can a large state hospital now serving a given catchment area expand its medical and surgical services to include total health care, and not only mental treatment, for the area? Or can an area information and referral center be set up that will successfully screen and assign patients to the proper facilities, having previously organized these facilities under one system, using the greatest strengths of each? Would this then involve a gradual phasing out of all duplication and overlap? Can the institutions involved begin to delimit their services to the catchment area in question, gradually phasing out services to adjacent areas without serious damage to their image, loss of citizen support, or fiscal strain?

In planning new facilities and construction, how will the new structures include the variety of services under one roof that are subsumed under total health? What will be the space allotment, the flow of traffic and communications, and how will the patient ultimately benefit? Finally, will the various departments and agencies, within their entrenched traditions and power bases, be able to collaborate with each other, even to the point of giving up power, jealously guarded functions, and perhaps even money?

Several final considerations are obvious from the above. First, total health care will require cooperation and collaboration among public and private sectors and university health resources wherever possible and feasible. Second, citizens who have been thinking narrowly in terms of specific interests in mental health or retardation will soon find themselves rubbing elbows with citizens planning total health services. Area boards will then either have to expand into total health boards, or contribute as one of many to a total health and welfare council. Citizens who have come to power in the old systems, like the professionals, will find it difficult to adapt when shaken or loosened from their entrenched foundations.

Along with all of this is the ultimate question of financing. Judging only by the multiplicity of plans for health insurance before Congress today, one could venture the prediction that a final total health insurance plan, such as in England and other European countries, will not be long in the making. Not only will it cost a great deal of money, but its implementation will also involve increasing control over the providers of health care—their pay, their services, their geographic distribution—and gross inroads will be made into the autonomy of

visit their patients after hospitalization, attend staff meetings at which such patients were presented, and participate in the discussions regarding plans for treatment and return to community.

A. H. L.

REFERENCE

1. Winters, E. E. ed. *The Collected Papers of Adolf Meyer*, vol. 4. Baltimore: Johns Hopkins Press, 1952. Original paper, entitled "Where Should We Attack the Problem of the Prevention of Mental Defect and Mental Disorder?" was presented at the National Conference of Charities and Correction, May, 1915.

Editorial Note

In this chapter Christopher Perry begins by looking back some fifty years and reviewing the antecedents of the mental health movement—the mental hygiene movement. He then looks further at some of the roots and problems of the mental health movement itself, and at the end turns to a consideration of the human services model now emerging as a focus of attention.

A. H. L.

CHAPTER 4

Four Twentieth-Century Themes in Community Mental Health Programs

J. CHRISTOPHER PERRY

THIS CHAPTER identifies four models or themes in the twentiety century of community mental health programs, specifically:

1. The child guidance clinic and the mental hygiene movement.
2. Hospital-centered mental health programs.
3. The community mental health center model.
4. The community mental health and human services model.

Following is a description of these themes or models and an explication of some of the features and problems associated with them.

The Child Guidance Clinic and the Mental Hygiene Movement

THE ZEITGEIST

From its inception the mental hygiene movement oriented itself toward affecting the mental welfare of a large population in the context of the community. State mental hospitals were available for the severely disordered, but by and large there existed little else to offer formal mental health services. The child guidance clinic, however, soon became the exemplar of the application of mental hygiene principles both in dealing with incipient behavioral problems in the community and by extending its effect to the larger population, mainly via education.

Clinics dealing with children and their mental health concerns had existed since the Juvenile Court of Cook County, Illinois, established a clinic in 1909 (p. 46).[35] In 1921, however, the Commonwealth Fund, in cooperation with the National Committee for Mental Hygiene, began a five-year demonstration of child guidance clinics. The demonstrations—lasting from six months to two years in seven different cities—easily became the models for other private and public agencies interested in offering child guidance services. Development of the technique in the United States owes its origin largely to these early clinics.[23] The ultimate mission was to prevent delinquency and the later development of severe mental disturbances in children with present problems—an idea now called "secondary prevention." If successful, it was planned that the demonstrations would be taken over by community agencies—public or private—and run on a permanent basis.

THE MODEL

The child guidance clinic team originally consisted of a psychiatrist, a psychologist, psychiatric social workers, and a pediatrician (pp. 48–65).[14] This team provided investigation and treatment. From the outset, however, more was planned than just dealing with individual families and children. According to the Annual Report of the Commonwealth Fund for 1924 (pp. 24–32),[10] the major objectives and activities were as follows. First priority was demonstration of methods of study and treatment of childhood behavioral problems. Second came the educational concerns, specifically to provide:

1. Lectures and publicity to groups in the community at large to inform and arouse their interest in backing the efforts of the clinic.
2. Lectures and discussions for social workers employing mental hygiene principles.

3. For parents, lectures on the part they played in producing childhood disorders.
4. For school teachers, lectures and direct contact with them regarding the effects of school in producing behavioral problems.
5. Training and contact with the medical profession over mental hygiene concerns.
6. For students in colleges and professional schools, courses in psychiatry, abnormal psychology, and psychiatric social work.

The third overall objective was the analysis and further development of both the study and treatment of behavioral problems.

The three groups most active in referring children to the clinics were social agencies, schools, and parents or relatives. Early in the clinics' operation the problem of caseload was encountered. This was partially solved by a functional division of clinic activities into three parts. The first was, of course, investigation and treatment of individual cases. The second was a "cooperative service" in which clinic personnel supervised the general methods of investigation and treatment methods used by other social agencies which had referred cases. The aim was to increase such an agency's understanding of various techniques and principles in handling cases. The third service was "consultant," and assisted other agencies directly in handling of certain of their difficult cases (p. 36).[11] When further data had been gathered on the operations of the clinics at the four and one-half year point on the project, the services rendered were roughly consultation 12 percent, cooperative service 30 percent, and actual clinic work 58 percent (pp. 30–49).[12] At this point, six of the clinics had been made permanent.

Early in the demonstration period it was decided that it was unrealistic to limit the scope of the clinics to dealing with only one diagnostic group of behavioral difficulties (p. 50).[35] Problems most often cited for referral were disobedience, stealing, temper, nervousness, lying, disturbing behavior in school, truancy, running away from home, retardation in school, failure in school, enuresis, bad sex habits, and quarrelsomeness.[14] Witmer described the behavioral problems encountered as amenable to treatment by the clinics, and said they had the aim of helping the patients adjust to the requirements of social living either "in working through their conflicts or in adjusting the environment to fit their needs . . . (p. 38)." [35] This latter method of having the clinic interact therapeutically with the environment of the individual "problem" child perhaps best distinguishes it from the alternative of institutionalization. In terms of actual patient treatment, however, the clinics offered mostly diagnostic service in the course of one, two, or three visits and advice or directive guidance rather than psychotherapy (p. 253).[35,27] This was the most common pattern, although private clinics were oriented toward more long-term treatment (p. xvi).[35]

In July 1927 the Bureau of Children's Guidance of the Fund officially ended its participation in the project, but the now broadened activities were to be carried further by the new Institute for Child Guidance of the Commonwealth Fund. A study of the results of the clinics' effectiveness showed that children receiving service directly or from a cooperating agency apparently did quite well: 73.5 percent met with partial or complete success in one city, and 62 percent in another,[13] although the criteria of "success" are left unstated, and the concept of control groups had not yet arisen. This did not reflect the totality of the clinics' effect, of course, since many lectures on mental hygiene principles were delivered to women's groups, PTA's, and so on. Since child guidance was thought not to be remedial so much as preventive, those directly treated were not thought to be the only beneficiaries:

> The welfare of the child is paramount, but the by-products in education are of tremendous importance indirectly to many parents and children who never become known to the clinic.[12]

By virtue of the clinics' commitment to dealing with children's problems by dealing with the child's social system, solid community support for the efforts of the clinics was essential. Witmer noted three reasons why (pp. 35–36): [35]

1. Families needing help required the support and understanding of the community at large to facilitate their use of the clinics.
2. Since the clinics often involved agents in the community—such as teachers, ministers, nurses, and so on—their conscious participation in a treatment program would be worthless unless they were in sympathy with the assumptions of mental hygiene, either through knowledge or intuition.
3. The clinics needed the cooperation of the community in the form of social institutions and social attitudes to foster healthy mental growth.

The clinics lived in symbiosis with state or local mental hygiene societies and gained much of their sanction through these ad hoc community organizations. The societies were constituted of both professionals and representatives of many functional groups in the community. The mental hygiene societies provided:

> an agency through which the special mental health needs of the community may be carefully studied and evaluated as to their importance and urgency and makes possible the development of concerted plans on a community-wide scale to meet such pressing needs, instead of the promotion by isolated individuals of sporadic, competing and uncorrelated plans which do not visualize the needs of the community as a whole.[3]

From the beginning of the demonstration clinics, the cosponsorship with the National Committee for Mental Hygiene reflected this willingness to have the clinics responsive to local needs and to evolve services taking the peculiarities of the community into account.[11]

49

Fiscal support of the clinics came from a mixture of fee for service, private—e.g. the Commonwealth Fund—and public sources, although some clinics, notably those in schools or attached to courts, were supported through tax monies. Witmer noted several reasons for disputing the notion that the clinics should be private and self-supporting. First, mental hygiene services were too expensive and only the rich could afford to pay for them. Second, inasmuch as child guidance benefits not only the child but the many persons and agencies dealt with as well, the family of the child should not bear responsibility for the total cost (pp. 36–37).[35]

EFFECTS AND PROBLEMS WITH THE MODEL

No doubt due to the utility and visible presence of the clinics in the community—unlike state hospitals—the mental hygiene societies rapidly established many child guidance clinics. One source noted that in the 1928 *Directory of Psychiatric Clinics for Children* four hundred seventy separate agencies were listed, serving more than forty thousand children that year. More than three hundred of these agencies had come into existence since the inception of the Fund's demonstration projects in 1922, and more than one hundred of the agencies might properly be classified as child guidance clinics.[14] Later data collected in 1935 by the National Committee for Mental Hygiene reported six hundred seventeen community clinics which accepted children. Of these, two hundred thirty-five had a threefold staff of psychiatrists, psychologists, and social workers. Approximately 30 percent relied on private funds (fee for service, gifts, and so on) and 60 percent were supported by the state governments. New York, the most populous state, also had the largest number of agencies, two hundred nine; the rest of the services were very unevenly divided among the other states (p. 57).[35]

Although the mental hygiene movement was certainly successful in establishing the acceptability of the child guidance clinic among much of the citizenry, it is still worth asking why the result has not been the establishment of adequate child guidance services everywhere. This is a complex question involving professional, political, and historical considerations, but even if one focuses on the professional perspective alone, several points arise.

First, one might ask how effective in preventing delinquency and severe behavioral disturbances did child guidance prove? Succinctly put, was the original zeal favoring the clinics later bolstered by convincing evidence? While evaluative research has traditionally been of spotty quality in the mental health field, one can do no better than refer to the Cambridge-Somerville Youth Study completed in 1948 as an excellent test of the efficacy of certain aspects of the child guidance clinic. Briefly, all boys aged six to ten adjudged likely to become delinquent in Cambridge and Somerville, Massachusetts, were included in either a treatment or control group. The study ran from 1937 to 1948 and encompassed at least a three-year follow-up on each boy well into adolescence. The treatment group received from two to eight years of individual "psychotherapy," while the control group received none. Although results in the treatment group appeared impressive when taken alone—in terms of later court appearances and correctional sentences—when compared to the control group there was essentially no difference in outcomes.[33] This can hardly be said to have confirmed professional faith in the worth of the thirty-year-old movement.

As Gerald Caplan pointed out (pp. 319–348),[8] mental health movements lose their general persuasiveness—as did the moral treatment movement in nineteenth-century America—when they have been oversold. People find themselves discouraged when such a movement does not produce millennial results. Learning from this example, one sees that it is better to distinguish the humanistic reasons behind a mental health movement—i.e., to help suffering people—from the alleged scientific evidence concerning what professionals actually can accomplish, rather than allow the two to fuse in the same aura of social concern.

Hospital-Centered Community Mental Health Programs

THE ZEITGEIST

The child guidance clinic existed as the major model of a community mental health program until the close of World War II, when citizens and professionals took stock of the mental health findings which the war inadvertantly turned up. By the war's end over one million, one hundred thousand men in their prime years had been rejected by the selective service for mental and neurological conditions. Approximately 40 percent of the inductees who were later discharged on medical grounds were found unsuitable for psychiatric reasons.[5] Never previously was there a greater awareness of the prevalence of psychiatric problems in the population, especially that portion of it which had been presumed the healthiest. At the same time there was growing dissatisfaction with the state mental hospitals, partially in response to the experience of conscientious objectors who had worked in them during the war.

The concept of the mental hospital as isolated from the community received a notable blow when Duncan Macmillan and T. P. Rees, superintendents of mental hospitals in England, and G. M. Bell, a superintendent in Scotland, unlocked their wards. According to Dr. Macmillan:

> The hospital assumes its correct role of providing the patient with the opportunity to redevelop social relationships in an environment which is more tolerant and understanding than the outside world.[25]

Robert C. Hunt, superintendent of the Hudson River State Hospital in New York, noted that much of the aggressive, disturbed, suicidal, and regressive behaviors hitherto the hallmark of mental hospitals abated as contact with the outside world was reestablished.[19]

Maxwell Jones, director of the Social Rehabilitation Unit of Belmont Hospital—later renamed Henderson Hospital—in England initiated the "therapeutic community." Although working largely with persons with antisocial behavioral problems, he ran his wards with intent to maximize the patients' learning social behavior in preparation for reentry into the community.[16]

In viewing the models of community mental health care in Northern Europe, Furman identified five types (pp. 4–5),[16] four of which are hospital-centered:

1. "Mental hospital dominated," in which the services flow primarily from a central mental hospital.
2. "Mental hospital-local health authority partnership, in which responsibility for the community services is shared by the two branches of a tripartite health system.
3. "General hospital comprehensive psychiatric unit," in which the responsibilities for community services is also shared with the local authorities.
4. "Mixed or transitional types," in which the programs may be shifting from the large central hospital base to general hospital psychiatric units and the local health authority.

The fifth type, "public health department controlled," exists largely in Holland, where admissions to hospitals and some of the community programs are not controlled by the hospitals. In fact, however, some of the programs are still hospital-centered. For the purposes of this chapter, however, the similarities among all five types of programs under the broad category of hospital-centered are of more significance than are their differences.

SERVICES FOR THE ACUTELY DISORDERED

Crisis theory, the doctrine that rapid and directive intervention during crises may obviate hospitalization, may itself have been born out of crisis. Dr. Arie Querido, the psychiatrist and director of the public mental health program in Amsterdam, Holland, found it necessary as a result of the 1929–1930 world economic crisis to reduce admissions to Amsterdam's already crowded and no longer economically viable mental hospitals. He saw the patient at home in time of emergency and gave whatever aid he could to avert hospitalization and to reestablish the patient's equilibrium.[4]

Querido had perfected his emergency psychiatric service by about 1936, and it evidently has needed little changing since. A psychiatric social worker or psychiatrist is available on twenty-four-hour call every day. Most of their visits are at patients' homes in order to understand the patients' environments as they relate to the disorders encountered. The next morning the service meets as a whole to determine the disposition for each patient seen the previous day. The patients may be visited at home again, or referrals made to other agencies or to general practitioners with whom the service works closely as consultants, or a patient may be admitted to hospital (pp. 99ff).[16] Reflecting on the decades since the crisis service was introduced, Dr. Gravstein, director of the Bureau of Mental Hygiene after Dr. Querido, said that the availability of beds "simply creates more patients to fill the beds (p. 108)."[16]

Dr. Duncan Macmillan has characterized the value of making domiciliary visits in Britain as being that of preventing the rejection of the patient from the family. By using preadmission domiciliary visits, especially to geriatric patients, it is easier to determine whether or not the patient can be maintained outside of the hospital. Macmillan noted the difficulty of working with relatives once an attitude of rejection had formed. To avert this, patients are taken away from the family for short periods of time during periods of stress to the family, thus preserving the long-range ability—both psychological and otherwise—of the family to care for the patient (p. 32).[25] This is, in a sense, treatment of the family's acute strain for the long-range benefit of the patient.

AMBULATORY AND REHABILITATION SERVICES

More and more hospitals began to establish outpatient facilities for the treatment of those not requiring hospitalization and for follow-up of patients previously discharged. Aftercare may have actually gotten its start in 1898 when Adolf Meyer convinced the State Charities Aid Association to divert one of its planned activities toward the counseling of patients' families when the patient was ready to return home. He noted that "Those families that are poor in experience and poor in mind are most in need of help," and that such concern on the part of the hospital might reduce the relapse rate (p. 19).[35] Dr. Meyer also proposed extramural clinics within hospital-centered districts which utilized part of the time of the hospital psychiatrists.

In certain British programs domiciliary visits have been part of the aftercare procedure. Social workers visit the discharged patients until they claim they feel well. If the social worker isn't convinced, then she or he continues visiting in the attempt to build up a relationship with the patient.[28]

Dr. Anthony May, successor to T. P. Rees at Warlingham Park Hospital in England, noted a very broad involvement by staff in community programs, including outpatient clinics, rehabilitation and industrial therapy, and follow-up clinics. While superintendent he envisioned, as well, a set of day hospitals (as satellites of the central hospital) placed in the various subcommunities, each with a team and a certain section of beds in the main hospital. He felt such outreach work would counteract the tendency for the hospital, rather than the patient and his needs, to become the center of the system (pp. 40ff).[16]

In 1944, partially as a result of the war, a rehabilitation law was passed in Great Britain. Labor was very scarce and so industrial rehabilitation was considered important. Employers were required to employ 3 percent of their work force from lists of the disabled (including epileptic and psychiatric cases), and the government set the example by employing at 5.5 percent in its labor force. As a result hospital-centered or -run sheltered workshops and industrial rehabilitation units were started in order to train these patients.[24] These were originally fashioned after the British borstal system in which work therapy was considered as part of the treatment of delinquent youths.

Furman noted (pp. 7–9) [16] that the British, as well as other Europeans, pay great attention to the social consequences of psychiatric disorders and the ensuing disabilities incurred. Work therapy is a vital part of the therapeutic regime, for instance, at Glenside Hospital in Bristol, England. An industrial therapy organization was created through a community-hospital partnership. Inside the hospital patients progress through a graded series of work projects done as contract work from industry.

The feeling, as expressed by Dr. John K. Wing, was that there should be a ladder of economic, as well as domestic, rehabilitation, leading by progressive but easy steps from the wards to the community.[1]

PREVENTIVE AND CONSULTATIVE SERVICES

Dr. Duncan Macmillan noted that at his hospital in Nottingham, England, many preventive and consultative services have developed, and that hospital staff were heavily committed to these programs:

> We have also evolved a number of preventive clinics, such as marriage guidance, juvenile delinquency in relation to the Probation Department, a clinic for the treatment of epilepsy in the community, a session at the local rehabilitation unit of the Ministry of Labor, and so on. There are now thirty-four such clinics and the senior members of the Hospital's medical staff spend over 50% of their time at these clinics.[25]

The pattern of consultation seems to have been divided between social workers and psychiatrists. Social workers do consultation with various social agencies, perhaps mostly in relation to their own casework (p. 17).[16] Psychiatrists perform most of their consultations with general practitioners and other physicians. Both of these efforts being aimed somewhat at increasing the skill of the consulted person or agency in dealing with problems with psychiatric implications, thus averting poorer levels of coping on the patients' part.

At the 1955 Milbank Memorial Fund conference a document was presented that outlined the purposes of mental health personnel offering consultative services to various agencies in the community. The consultant was seen as an advisor to various community agencies and leaders on technical issues of mental health: how the agencies could better help people in crisis, and how they might help the needs of certain groups not in crisis. But clear admonition was given that this did not represent an effort to instill a "psychiatrocracy" into the community. The consultant was not going to be an advisor or decision maker who subverted the normal community decision process regarding any community issues.

CONSIDERATION AND PROBLEMS

The mental hospital-centered model of community mental health programs developed in Great Britain much more fully than in the United States. There may be many reasons for this. Foremost may be that with the creation of the National Health Service in 1946, the British made a sizable financial commitment to all areas of health care. This may have allowed for new growth in types of programs, as well as in the quantity of services available. Second, the hospitals were controlled by local or regional hospital boards which had citizen representation, thus allowing the sharing of power between professionals and nonprofessional citizens. This was unlike the situation in the United States, where most public mental hospitals are controlled exclusively by governmental agencies. The British arrangement may have led the mental health care system to be more responsive to suggestions of change because of the decentralized control involving participation of citizens from the service regions of the hospitals. Third, given the relative density of Britain's population and the hospitals' relative proximity to population centers, basing both programs and personnel in the hospitals may have been more feasible. Fourth, the interests of psychiatrists may have been different in the two countries. According to Richard Anderson, British psychiatry was overall more psychosis-oriented and hospital-employed, devoting little time to such things as psychotherapy with neurotics, and other activities carried on more in private practice and not necessitating a mental hospital.[1]

Professionals examining the hospital-centered community mental health program, with its emphasis on nonhospitalization, have aired several criticisms, including the observation that a patient can deteriorate in the community just as he can in the hospital. Certain community programs in Britain, for instance, have been staffed with persons not trained in the hospital. As Richard Titmuss of the London School of Economics has observed of some of the hostels for mental patients, they are staffed with untrained personnel, uncertain of what functions to perform; the result is, in his opinion, care which is often more limited than that given on the back wards.[21] There is no magic in the community. As Furman also noted, a frequent criticism in Britain is that "keeping a sick person at home is not necessarily good for him, and a mental hospital is not an evil thing per se (p. 10)." [16]

The Community Mental Health Center Model

THE ZEITGEIST

Interest in keeping psychiatric care in the community accelerated after the close of World War II. As noted earlier, there was great surprise in the finding of a hitherto unsuspected high level of psychiatric impairment in draft-age men. Partly as a result of this, the government began to promote basic, applied, and program research in the mental health field. The National Mental Health Act of 1946 allowed the creation of the National Institute of Mental Health in 1949, which has since played a crucial role in nourishing the community mental health movement.

In 1954 New York State passed the first state community mental health services act in order to stimulate the development and operation of community services in conjunction with county or municipal governments. Congress in 1955 passed the Mental Health Study Act, which directed the creation of the Joint Commission on Mental Illness and Health. The charge of the act [20] was, first, to make a thorough analysis and evaluation of the needs of the mentally ill, and the resources, practices, and methods of diagnosing, treating, and caring for them. Then the Joint Commission was to make comprehensive recommendations, the implementation of which would lead, it was hoped, to a marked reduction of the incidence or duration of mental illness, and a reduction in its effects.

In 1956 Title V of Public Law 911, the Health Amendment Act, was passed. This allowed the surgeon general, as Glasscote noted (p. 35),[17] to make "Mental Health Project Grants" for pilot projects in improved methods of care and treatment. This amounted to two million dollars in 1957, and 5.7 million dollars by 1961.

Over this same period action was taking place in another area which further documented the need for new approaches to the problems of mental health in the community. The field of psychiatric epidemiology, in which disorder in the community was a prime concern, began to emerge. Studies of the prevalence of psychiatric symptoms and disorders were begun most notably in Sweden, Nova Scotia, Connecticut, and New York. Hollingshead and Redlich [18] documented the rather unequal distribution of diagnosed psychiatric disorders by type among social classes, and the inegalitarian distribution of types and durations of treatment by social class. Later publications [22,31] documented the shockingly high prevalence of behaviors of psychiatric interest and psychiatric impairment in the community. An important finding in these prevalence studies was that the great majority of symptomatic persons were not getting any kind of psychiatric treatment.

The Joint Commission[20] published its final report in 1961 and, by its multidisciplinary representation, provided a broad impetus to the development of community programs. It also served as the beginning of a mandate for additional federal support. The commission recommended that no further building of mental hospitals with more than one thousand beds take place, and that the larger ones be gradually converted to chronic disease hospitals for both mental and physical disorders. Mental hospitals should be regionalized within each state, the commission felt. One full-time, fully staffed psychiatric clinic should be set up on an outpatient basis for every fifty thousand persons, to prevent the prolonged or repeated hospitalization of patients. These could exist as part of mental hospitals, general hospitals, or as part of a state-wide network of community clinics. The Joint Commission stated very clearly the purpose:

> The objective of modern treatment of persons with major mental illness is to enable the patient to maintain himself in the community in a normal manner. To do so, it is necessary (1) to save the patient from the debilitating effects of institutionalization as much as possible, (2) if the patient requires hospitalization, to return him to home and community life as soon as possible, and (3) thereafter to maintain him in the community as long as possible (p. xvii).[20]

Perhaps as important as the substantive recommendations themselves, the commission urged that the federal government assume more and more of the costs for the development of such programs, since there existed no other source with as adequate a financial base to cover such an expensive, albeit necessary, venture as the one proposed.

The Joint Commission was constituted as a task force representing many of the professional and lay groups and interests which would have concerns in the field of mental health. Its tolerance of a multifaceted approach to meeting the needs of the mentally disturbed reflects this diverse makeup; for example, it advocated the involvement of both private resources and public agencies operated at all levels of government. Canada approached the same problems as those faced by the joint commission, and it is of interest to note that despite overall similarities, there are differences in the solutions suggested.

According to Marshall,[26] the fact that only the discipline of psychiatry was represented on the Canadian committee reflected itself in the orientation evidenced by their report, *More for the Mind*.

Marshall noted five major recommendations in *More for the Mind*. First, there should be better medical integration of psychiatric services with medical services in general, and the psychiatric patient should be seen as a medical patient. Second, there should be a regionalization of psychiatric services, with each large community having a clinic offering a full range of services. Third, the mental health care system should be decentralized, with administration and management occurring at the local and regional levels, and with the provincial responsibilities being largely that of consulting and financing. There is great emphasis on the functioning of well-organized and efficient local boards, a recommendation unlike any parallel in *Action for Mental Health*.[20] Fourth, there should be an emphasis on continuity of care for the mental patient. Fifth, regional mental health councils should be created to coordinate local general hospital services, mental hospitals, and clinics in order to provide maximum efficiency. On the issue of private versus public participation in community programs, *Action for Mental Health*[20] recommended that private psychiatrists devote some portion of their time to public concerns. As Marshall further noted,[26] however, *More for the Mind* expressed much skepticism about the utility of private psychiatrists. Mental disorder was seen as multifactorial in its causes and, hence, its treatment should involve a multifaceted effort in the community. This implies a public effort.

Several years after the Joint Commission's work had been publicly received, in February 1963, President Kennedy sent a message to Congress urging that it take action to establish a heavy federal commitment to community mental health centers. The legislation which ensued in October of that year, Public Law 88–164, The Mental Retardation Facilities and Community Mental Health Centers Act of 1963, formalized the model around which community mental health centers would be formed.

THE MODEL

In May 1964 the federal regulations appeared which outlined what an agency would have to do to qualify for federal matching funds for mental health center construction. As Glasscote noted (p. 66),[17] services to be offered by a community mental health center were divided into two classes: five essential services and five additional services. The five essential services:

1. Inpatient.
2. Outpatient.
3. Partial hospitalization, including at least daycare.
4. Emergency services on a twenty-four-hour basis.
5. Consultation and education to community agencies and professional personnel.

The five additional services:

1. Diagnostic.
2. Rehabilitation, including vocational and educational.
3. Precare and aftercare in the community, including foster placement, home visiting, and halfway houses.
4. Training.
5. Research and evaluation.

Together the five essential and five additional services were designated as "adequate" services for a community mental health center. Glasscote observed in the regulations the expectation that there would be adequate coordination among the divers service elements of any one center (p. 8).[17] The program as a whole was to consider the needs of all age groups, thus assuring continuity of care for patients within the program.

Though this legislation and the ensuing regulations formalized the concept of the community mental health center, it was hardly the most detailed or conceptual exposition of the model even for the time. Dr. Gerald Caplan, then head of the Community Mental Health Program of the Harvard School of Public Health, presented a very thorough model of a community mental health program in 1961.[7] He stated what he felt the principles of community care should be and, as well, he delineated the specific elements of such a comprehensive program. His eleven principles which define the purpose, scope, and limitations of community mental health care are summarized here:

1. The patient is the focus of the program, with all services and institutions functioning as interlocking parts.
2. The program is comprehensive, including primary, secondary, and tertiary prevention, case finding, screening, investigation, diagnosis, treatment, and rehabilitation.
3. The patient is seen as constantly being affected by his interpersonal and social environment.
4. Mental disorder is seen as an episode in a patient's life.
5. The purpose of psychiatric intervention is to return the patient as soon as possible to his ordinary life situation.
6. Psychiatric intervention is an artifact in the patient's life.
7. Psychiatric programs should, therefore, focus on continuous movement of the patient as rapidly as possible through a variety of successive treatment stages to eventual return to the community.
8. Continuity of therapeutic relationship should be provided from beginning to end of intervention, and if possible in successive interventions.
9. Treatment should be segmented and not global, that is, psychiatric intervention should deal with the current presenting problem.
10. Active communication must be maintained among all levels of the program, barriers between services must be lowered, and good coordination must exist.

59

11. Psychiatric responsibility should extend unit boundaries and administrators should make themselves aware of how the patient fares in other agencies.

The model which Caplan outlined was made up of sixteen "basic units" which, taken together, defined a comprehensive program of community psychiatry. Since Caplan's presentation was both seminal and clearly stated, it, too, is summarized:

1. The program starts and finishes with the patient at home, whenever possible.
2. Domiciliary Psychiatric Service: This is an emergency team consisting of a psychiatrist, psychiatric social worker, psychiatric nurse, and possibly a psychologist, which undertakes initial screening and arranges the initial disposition. The team also receives the patient back for follow-up after termination of treatment by visiting the patient at home, or keeping in contact with other agencies with which the patient might be in contact.
3. Central Record Room: Patients' records are kept in a family file. At the termination of treatment the record remains open in a "for follow-up" category.
4. Local Mental Health Center: This is a small inpatient short-term unit for two- to four-week hospitalizations. It has an outpatient clinic for children and adults and a day and night hospital as well. It may be associated with the domiciliary service.
5. Psychiatric Outpatient Clinic: It may be associated with any type of inpatient unit or with a community mental health center.
6. Community Mental Health Center: This has extramural services as its focus. There will be primary preventive services for groups in life crises or at risk, and there will be consultation to other caretakers and agencies. This may be associated with an outpatient clinic, local mental health center, or domiciliary service.
7. General Hospital Psychiatric Inpatient Service: This would function similarly to the local mental health center but give liaison consultation to the hospital physicians as well.
8. Mental Hospital Admission and Treatment Service: Patients would be accepted for prolonged periods of observation and diagnostic treatment from one to four months in time.
9. Day Hospital and Night Hospital.
10. Rehabilitation Service: Primarily part of the mental hospital, it would be activated upon admission of the patient. It would include occupational, recreational, and vocational services and work closely with vocational rehabilitation services in the community.
11. Services for Patients with Residual Defects: This would include hostels and villages for those who need chronic care.
12. Transitional Institutions: By this is meant the halfway house which helps the patient make the step back into the community.

13. Foster Homes: These would help those with residual symptoms which proved intolerable to their families.
14. Sheltered Workshops and Supervised Industry: Patients and expatients would be served by these. Consultation would be available to industries participating when trouble arises with any patient.
15. Psychiatric Social Clubs: These are primarily social and recreational to help combat the problems of social alienation.
16. Community Organization: This includes several functions. First, public relations to inform the public about the program's work. Second, public education to alter attitudes to facilitate the program's mission. Third is the organization of volunteers. Fourth is the stimulation of citizen action through working with voluntary organizations to feel out the current needs for new programs.

Caplan insisted that his model was adequate for dealing with the mental health needs of a community and that its being short-term, crisis-oriented, and based in the community would be assets in meeting such a challenge. He recommended that the community mental health system be decentralized down to the level of fifty thousand to one hundred thousand population units, with the domiciliary service being the fundamental arm of the program, thus avoiding the drawback of isolated distant hospitals. As mentioned above, Caplan's presentation is perhaps the most thorough of any single contribution.

Taking virtually the same service units that Caplan and others have sketched, Herzl Spiro [30] proposed a regionalized system of community mental health services based on primary, secondary, and tertiary levels of treatment resources. In this view, the primary level of care should originate in a comprehensive neighborhood health center or satellite clinic for a district of fifteen thousand to thirty thousand persons. Primary service should include functions best carried out at the local level: general intake, early case finding, outpatient care, day care, home visiting and care, as well as consultations to primary health care physicians and neighborhood programs and agencies. Obviously, with only one, two, or three mental health personnel per district, many functions would need to be left to a more centralized facility dealing with a larger population base.

The secondary level of care would be the community mental health center serving the federally defined catchment population of from seventy thousand to two hundred thousand persons. More costly and specific services would be offered, namely:

1. Emergency services.
2. Inpatient services.
3. Partial hospitalization.
4. Intensive rehabilitation.

5. Training, research, evaluation.
6. Consultation to:
    a. superordinate agencies (e.g., school or social welfare systems).
    b. general hospitals.
    c. primary level facilities.

More specialized personnel could be efficiently utilized at this level.

The tertiary level of services would encompass several catchment areas and deliver highly specialized services requiring a population base of from one hundred forty thousand to one million persons. This would include categorical programs of specialized care—e.g., drug abuse, mental retardation—specialized inpatient care—e.g., operant wards, residential child care—and, as well, consultations to primary and secondary level facilities and agencies relevant to categorical programs. Tertiary level facilities could exist in a special wing of a community mental health center, a state hospital, or nursing home meeting the highly specialized needs of several catchment areas. Again, Spiro's concept aims at the most efficient and effective deployment of mental health resources using the community mental health model and taking both local and regional needs and resources into account.

PROBLEMS AND VIEWPOINTS

One of the fundamental intentions in the original legislation was to ensure care to many heretofore ignored groups of patients. By creating a comprehensive system of care, no mental health need would go unrecognized or without at least some attempt to mitigate its effects. Glasscote (p. 10),[17] in his review of eleven of the best community mental health programs in existence at the time of the 1963 legislation, says that certain groups—children, geriatric patients, delinquents, alcoholics, and other deviants—were still given short shrift.

Glasscote also noted various lacunae in the programs of the eleven community mental health centers he examined (pp. 22–28).[17] Five of the centers offered no inpatient facilities for children, and children's services in general were slighted. Emergency services were generally of the general hospital emergency room type or an emergency telephone service which would ultimately connect with the psychiatrist on call. Only one of the eleven centers had a twenty-four-hour emergency walk-in service. Some centers also made emergency house calls, but in general this was seen as a waste of time. Programs for alcoholics were highly structured at some centers, but others neglected all but the psychotic alcoholics. No center at the time had specific programs for drug addicts. Several centers had diagnostic services for the mentally retarded, and most would accept them as patients if they were psychotic. Only one center had facilities to care for chronic patients in the geriatric age group.

Regarding rehabilitation, there was less emphasis on vocational retraining than at state and Veterans Administration hospitals. Three of the centers did have work-for-pay programs, however. Transitional and placement services existed in several centers with, for example, several using halfway houses in the community, and two making foster home placements. All of the programs offered some form of consultation, with one center having its own full-time consultation staff. These were mostly case-centered consultations to other agencies, although educational and training consultations were made. Training of psychiatric residents took place at seven centers, with slightly fewer centers training other graduate students. There was much research taking place at the university-affiliated centers, but there were two centers, as well, which undertook none. Evaluation of program effectiveness was severely limited at all centers. Several had launched ambitious programs to determine effectiveness and results, but many limited such ventures to staff discussions, and two centers made no effort at all in this direction.

Perhaps one of the reasons for these program lacunae is that, although the treatment services were ostensibly of varied kinds, the actual types of treatment rendered still did not adequately meet the needs of these outcast groups. Saying that a center will meet everyone's mental health needs does not mean that it can or that it actually will try. As Glasscote said later, there were many indications in his review that most centers considered individual psychotherapy the treatment of choice (p. 22).[17]

In addition to offering a complete range of mental health services, another intention of the original legislation was to facilitate coordination of the divers agencies or units of a community mental health program. Glasscote pointed out that this was one of the stiffest challenges of the whole movement (p. 10).[17] Bertram Brown noted that in 1967 there were close to three hundred community mental health centers funded under the federal legislation. More than 75 percent of the centers were cooperative efforts involving two or more agencies, with a significant number involving four or five (p. 23).[6] Stanley Yolles, director of the National Institute of Mental Health, stated that in 1969, of the three hundred fifty-one centers which had received federal construction or staffing grants, 84 percent involved two or more agencies. Yolles noted further that 51 percent of the agencies involved were private nonprofit in sponsorship, the remaining 49 percent being publicly sponsored by local, county, municipal, or state government.[36] Coordination of services—and making certain that no patient needs are systematically overlooked, ignored, or scorned—must certainly be a major concern in a system of such pluralism.

One aspect of the community mental health center model which should be made very explicit is that it is a professionally controlled model. Although professionals in a center commit themselves to serving the mental health needs of their catchment area, and although they may be employed or funded in part or in whole by some governmental body, the professionals themselves determine the policy and the program content within the very broad bounds of any sanctions they may be granted by their funding source. The lines of accountability run away from the population of the catchment area as a rule, and usually remain within the domain of other professionals' judgments and decisions. Since evaluation is one form that accountability may take, one needs to delineate very carefully by whom evaluations are made, for whom they are meant, and to what end. The model itself does not reveal clear answers to these questions, although evaluation does seem to be meant to serve as information to professionals at some level. It should also be clear, however, that this was largely true for the other two models described prior to this one.

Attitudes toward the utility of the community mental health center model vary. Clearly a spirit of humanism pervades the intentions of many community mental health center enthusiasts. As Bowen pointed out:

> Innovators are inspired by moral and by humanitarian feelings, rather than by those of any scientific process. The same arguments of persuasion, assertion, and dramatic illustration have been as true in the field of community mental health as they have been true in moral treatment.[4]

Robert Jones, when speaking of such principles which the community mental health center model proposes, said:

> Early and comprehensive treatment readily available and close to the patients' homes; minimal hospitalization or none at all; a wide spectrum of community services; continuity of medical care. . . . Even though most of these principles are appealing on humanitarian grounds, we have little proof that programs based on those principles do indeed lead to improving the mental health of the people.[21]

But as Glasscote points out (p. 10),[17] it is the consensus of those in the center movement that unless it can be demonstrated that more traditional services away from the community—and often very fragmented—are more efficacious than the community mental health center model, then it is unsuitable to postpone implementation of this model.

The Community Mental Health And Human Services Model

PROBLEMS WITH PREVIOUS MODELS

Several problems exist with previous models of community mental health programs which seem to have spurred the evolution of a conceptually new approach in the delivery of mental health services at the community level. One problem has to do with the role—or lack of role—to be played by the consumer of services in determination of program policy. Another problem relates to the difficulties encountered in coordinating the various mental health services and other human services to join together in helping meet those needs of any patient or client which require crossing service boundaries. This latter difficulty is a problem of professional roles and domains.

Some kind of consumer representation in the form of mental health volunteer agencies, advisory boards to mental health agencies, and so on, has existed for a long time. For instance, the 1966 legislation in Massachusetts, which created the present state-wide network of area and regional mental health services, called for citizen participation in the form of advisory boards at many levels of the system. Their power, however, is minimal, and that which does exist is largely limited to merely approving professionally initiated plans. It is questionable to what degree and how significantly this represents citizen participation.

Catharine Stepanek [32] has encapsulated many of the problems which supervene when a mental health agency has lost its citizen support as the price paid to increase the autonomy of the agency. In the city she describes, various citizen mental health groups finally succeeded in establishing a mental health clinic for adults in addition to the child guidance clinic already in existence. The county governing body appointed a mental health board which controlled the program policy of the clinic and received funding from the county as well. Over several years a bad relationship developed between the professionals in the clinic and the county governing body. All of the citizen groups originally involved gradually disappeared as the clinic board, which allegedly represented the citizens, lost contact with them. In a series of fiscal arguments between the clinic board and the county governing body, an unworkable relationship grew.

Crippled by resignations, unable to attract new persons at low salaries, and bereft of community support, many of the clinic's activities were drastically curtailed. Only after new citizens were appointed to step in and work with the clinic board did the struggle subside. Stepanek summed up as follows:

> With reference to citizen initiative in governmental affairs, this case study demonstrates the folly of setting up semi-official boards as representatives of the community and then leaving them without constant community surveillance and support. . . . Also, responsibility evolves upon official or semi-official governmental units to seek out and cultivate citizen interest in public affairs. [32]

Perhaps this is no different from other problems of democracy in other sectors of society.

The second problem mentioned concerning previous models of mental health programs was that of professional relationships between various helping agencies and mental health. Very often poor coordination of the services offered by social agencies has left many areas of individuals' needs unmet. Professionals sometimes retreat into a rigid domain of agency responsibility and fail to define authority and responsibility for areas that may be shared or common to several agencies. As Rafferty has said, not all of the personnel who affect mental health are to be found in the mental health hierarchy. This is further complicated by the fact that even within the mental health domain, professionals have not agreed upon a common mission, nor have they a consensus about what responsibilities obtain under the banner of "comprehensive care." [29] All of the existing community mental health models have evolved very little that is effective in moving toward resolution of these professional problems.

INTIMATIONS OF A COMMUNITY HUMAN SERVICES MODEL

Properly speaking, it can hardly be said that a community human services model has yet been reified. Rather, it is evolving as a hybrid of the community mental health center model. The essential difference from the latter, however, is that this model includes in its scope a unified or highly coordinated system for dispensing all of the human services—health, welfare, rehabilitation, and so on—at the community level. Furthermore, it would perform these activities in ways which transcend the rigid boundaries that presently characterize each human services specialty system. As Raquel Cohen has described the purpose of such an approach:

> The goal of the human services model is to organize multi-level delivery of services to troubled individuals and their families through the coordination of many agencies and professional workers. The focus is on a unified multi-agency approach based on the expectation that the agency criteria can be modified or adapted to match the objectives of servicing individuals and their specific needs in a non-divisive manner, as is currently practiced. [9]

The model implies an exquisite effort on the part of professionals in defining their roles and responsibilities so that all human services personnel fully understand the role each person has as a specialist—e.g., psychiatrist—with a certain expertise to offer. With a process allowing for such a continual defining and redefining of roles, suspiciousness, ignorance, and lack of continuity of care are much less likely to prove themselves major problems as patients or clients traverse specialty system boundaries.

Bernard Bandler [2] has conceptualized successive models or themes of prevention in the mental health field in a way that aptly characterizes the progression toward the total human services approach. These can be considered as a series of concentric circles, with the innermost model or theme at the core, and each successive one encompassing the activities of the preceding ones. The core is the medical-diagnostic-treatment model which views disorder dynamically in full awareness of the relevance of social and family phenomena to individual problems. The second model is a developmental one which focuses on primary prevention of disorder at the population level. It is concerned with the normal and full development of personality and prevention of pathology by ensuring the proper supplies needed for growth. The third model is the organizational model:

> The model states that the nature of organization, the participation of all members of it in the decision-making process, plays a major therapeutic role in the community. . . . It involves a redefinition of leadership rather than a leveling and repudiation of it. . . . The milieu is the community and the well-being of each individual depends on the health of the community. . . . Our patients' lives are inextricably involved with education, housing, jobs, welfare, church, police, city, county, state, and federal bureaucracies, and the complex shifting structures of their communities.[2]

This theme is concerned with the participation of the members of the community in the leadership and design of all of the human services, rather than the present system wherein the governance of each human services specialty resides within its own ranks. The fourth and outermost model is the ecological model.

> [This model] states that the health of the total system depends upon the appropriate interactions and balance of all elements and components of that system. Mental health is one system. . . . The citizens in our communities, however, may be much more concerned, for example, with issues of garbage collection and rat control, street lighting and police protection than with mental health.[2]

This perspective places great importance upon balancing the various service elements in a system of human services to ensure that they function in response to the overall needs and limited resources of the community, rather than as specialty systems concerned only with their own domains and responsibilities.

While Bandler has illuminated the importance of systems in the emerging human services model, Robert Curtis [15] has delineated the elements which such an approach might include. There are three dimensions to human service networks, as Curtis has noted. First is the dimension of the state-wide specialties such as welfare, corrections, and mental health. These services tend to be deployed on a regional or state-wide basis, rather than in the community per se. Second are the "community care-givers"—such as teachers, clergy, local social agencies, and so on—who work in the community itself and are known in it. Third, there are citizens of the community frequently found working in voluntary capacities in social agencies, societies, and clubs. They are unpaid and usually nonprofessional human service personnel. Curtis points out that the citizens of a community serve two very important functions. First, they donate manhours to human services, as big brothers or sisters, foster parents, day-care workers, members of a "problem-solving" team, and so on. Second, they serve as a network in the community which can identify problems, unearth new resources, and give sanctions for the delivery and planning of new community programs, as well as take part in planning unique programs for the community on their own initiative. This latter function is very important in preventing the estrangement of services from the actual needs of the community. Curtis is correct in his emphasis on the citizen dimension.

Curtis further identifies five elements which he says would lead to the integration of the human services into a viable network. The first element is decentralization. Many services are best delivered at the community or neighborhood level, especially those which focus on a person in a particular social environment. Consumer boards would participate in the design of the human services network at the local level, assuring that local needs are given mindful consideration. The second element is coordination. A human services coordinator would be responsible for bridging the various specialty service systems at the local level. He would help build working relationships across the systems and, as an employee of the local human services board, would be directly accountable to it. A third element is community organization. Volunteer citizens would work through the human services board and in other capacities, not only to help shape the network of services but also to organize the community and to give sanctions and fiscal support when needed for improvement of the system and community as a whole. The fourth element requires that the three dimensions of the human services be trained to work in complementary ways. Much work will be required to forge unity among these three groups of personnel. The fifth element entails the development of new models or types of services which will more effectively meet human needs in the community. Curtis gives one example of such an innovative service: "team problem solving in a social network." This consists of a small team of three or four members from the three different groups of personnel coming together with a segment of a social network that is experiencing a problem. In a small number of meetings the team applies its specialty expertise, knowledge of the problem, and knowledge of available resources for solution and mitigation.

Considering the emphasis on flexibility of professional boundaries, it is obvious that professionals in mental health will need to enlarge their repertoire. Raquel Cohen has identified sixteen roles which the "collaborative coprofessional" must be able to play as a member of a human services system. These are:

68

negotiator, planner, advocate, convener, consultant, educator, linking agent, coordinating agent, catalyst, information disseminator, conflict resolver, leader of small groups, resource member, advisor-specialist, generalist, and change agent.[9]

Cohen also outlines four problem areas which will require continuing effort to resolve or minimize.[9] First, the multidisciplinary team will have a continuous need to reshape the goals of service through a dialectic among the goals that each specialty system may now have. Second, there is the need to resolve problems arising in a shared domain. Working with professionals in other systems requires that specialty boundaries dovetail and that boundaries be understood by all. Third is the requirement of collaboration among personnel at many levels of expertise, something which necessitates working without being arrogant, authoritarian, or otherwise hurtful to tenuous relationships. The fourth issue is that of determination of degrees of responsibility for patients' problems. The degree of responsibility that any one professional takes in any patient's case should be harmonious with the overall goals of the system. Again, an exquisite effort at coordination and communication will be required to make this viable.

PROBLEMS NEW AND OLD

When a new model is examined, it is tempting to anticipate problems that will arise from the aspects of the model that are new, while failing to recognize problems that will arise from old and familiar elements. Both types, however, are worthy of inspection.

No civil libertarian will fail to recognize the perils that may present themselves whenever government social service agencies work with people "for their own benefit." Given the novelty of personnel from state and local agencies uniting with the local citizenry to solve many human services problems, the dangers may be magnified. What will happen to issues of confidentiality? Will the police function of the agencies be facilitated and then enlarged by the human services networks? Will these networks become instruments of oppression, wherein the surveillance of individual needs for human services becomes the harassment of individuals in moral and social situations that human services personnel dislike? Will certain of the citizenry become involved in human services networks with a fanatic desire to "reform" others? The fact that the human services model exists to facilitate the satisfaction of real human needs no more prevents it from abusing personal liberties than have the noble intentions of many zealots kept them from perpetrating human suffering in the name of good. These concerns over the preservation of individuals' privacy and freedom will require more than a moment's attention while the human services model is implemented.

69

In addition to the above, several other difficulties exist, difficulties which are familiar to many as general problems with democracy. The first of these resides in the inertia that often characterizes communities. One of the reasons that mental health programs were originally taken over by the state was the abominable level of care that patients had been receiving in their locales. The jails and poorhouses were filled with the criminal, the poor, and the insane; these were groups of people that many were inclined to ignore or even punish, and few were inclined to help or rehabilitate.

The human services model will require much on the part of the local citizenry. Is there anything in the history of social welfare programs which would indicate that each locality functioning as an independent, democratic realm will evolve a successful and well-supported network of human services? It is questionable whether many communities would consider human services to be worthy of adequate attention and initiative. This, like certain other problems of democracy, may require guidance and incentives from more central state or federal sources in order to counteract local inaction. It may be, as some have suggested, that democratic localities can only be expected to act effectively when they are prodded by a national or state social welfare or human services policy which is designed to reward local initiative. Even then, special effort would be needed to organize disintegrated or disorganized communities wherein the greatest levels of need for services are to be found.

One other nexus of problems familiar to all communities revolves around the personal tensions which democracy creates. These are the tensions felt by any person who has a private life which will be affected by his public actions, e.g., as a school board member. As a representative of a community elected to further some community purpose, one may often be in a situation in which the best course may be to propose, support, or enact measures which will offend or even enrage some members of the community. Will an individual risk supporting measures which may reflect back unfavorably on his business or employment? A long-term natural experiment has been going on in the United States which could provide a specific answer to this question for each locale. One need only examine the character of the decision-making process of the local school boards to gauge how the exigencies of private life will affect the public decisions of future human services board members.

In viewing the four themes described here, many similarities are apparent in the hopes which the proponents have or had for them. It may also be evident that these themes do not represent competing models of community mental health care so much as they appear like a theme and variations. This is particularly true when the problems associated with each model are considered.

Description of these themes can facilitate and stimulate efforts to evaluate actual systems of community mental health programs which are in operation. Perhaps drawing out these pardigms from the words of those supporting each theme will add a perspective, one that will allow easier recognition of the model or models which implicitly underlie a particular system of community mental health programing. It is certainly easier to evaluate something in which one can see sensible patterns, and description of a program and its goals are prerequisites of any evaluative effort. The need to evaluate is clear. Without evaluation of utility, these models will no doubt eventually wither, like their predecessors, for want of public trust and support.

Editorial Discussion

Perry's analysis and account of recent history raises with insistence the question of why proposals that have enormous face value have not been more adequately implemented. That a model of community psychiatry has been before us for half a century is indicated by the following quotation from a paper by Adolf Meyer, originally published in 1915 (pp. 195–197) [34] *under the title "Where Should We Attack the Problem of the Prevention of Mental Defect and Mental Disease?"*

> *The districting of our cities is at present carried out in different ways for different purposes. As far as I know, the political wards and the police and fire department districts, the school districts, the criminal and juvenile court districts, the districts of charity organizations, all are apt to follow different lines of division. The ideal will have to be an organization so made that as many districts as possible may form reasonable complete households within themselves. Such an arrangement would make it possible for more people actually to realize what the community has to make itself responsible for; and it might become practicable to have district problems, district committees, and district meetings, such as the political parties have long been shrewd enough to maintain in their wards.*
>
> *However much of a dreamer I may be, I pride myself on having seen a good many of my dreams come true. Can you see the ward or district organization—with a district building instead of a police station? With policemen as constructive workers rather than as the watchdogs of their beats? A district center with reasonably accurate records of the facts needed for orderly work? Among the officers a district health officer, and a district school committee and a district improvement and recreation committee, a district tax committee, a district charity or civic work committee—a tangible expression of what the district stands for?*

71

With a system of helpfulness and fairness and true democracy, avoiding bureaucracy as well as militarism and its primitive residual, the boss system, this country can safely go on developing methods tolerant of individuality and yet effective in its essential purposes. . . . There is plenty of room on this globe for many kinds of people. The art of community building begins with the cultivation of community centers and community ideals, for the small as well as the big units.

Clearly something more than exhortation, policy formation, politicking, and financing are required. The core of the problem gives every evidence of lying somewhere in implementation. If this is so, then this particular frontier in social psychiatry is one that calls for comparative empirical studies of models that have built into them provision for objective evaluation of impact on the client population.

A. H. L.

REFERENCES

1. Anderson, R. W. "British Community Psychiatry and Its Implications for American Planning." *Community Mental Health Journal* 1 (1965):223–232.
2. Bandler, B. "Community Mental Health and the Educational Dilemmas of the Mental Health Professions." *Education for Social Work*, Fall 1972.
3. Bassett, C. *Mental Hygiene in the Community*. New York: Macmillan, 1934.
4. Bowen, W. A. L. "The Community Mental Health Center." In *Third Annual Meeting, Western Conference on the Uses of Mental Health Data: Social and Economic Values in Mental Health Program Development*. Boulder, Colorado: Western Interstate Commission for Higher Education, 1969.
5. Brand, J. L. "The United States: A Historical Perspective." In *Community Mental Health: An International Perspective*, edited by R. H. Williams and L. D. Ozarin, pp. 18–43. San Francisco: Jossey-Bass, 1968.
6. Brown, B., and Lons, S. E. "Psychology and Community Mental Health: The Medical Muddle." Washington, D.C.: Pamphlet, American Psychological Association, September 5, 1967.
7. Caplan, G. "Comprehensive Community Psychiatry." In *An Approach to Community Mental Health*, pp. 231–255. New York: Grune & Stratton, 1961.
8. Caplan, R. B. *Psychiatry and Community in Nineteenth-Century America*. New York: Basic Books, 1969.
9. Cohen, R. E. "Models in Search of Community Mental Health Programs—The Function of Psychiatrists as a Variable." Paper presented at 126th Annual Meeting of American Psychiatric Association, May 1973, Honolulu, Hawaii.
10. Commonwealth Fund. *Annual Report, 1924*. New York: Commonwealth Fund, 1925.
11. ———. *Annual Report, 1925*. New York: Commonwealth Fund, 1926.
12. ———. *Annual Report, 1926*. New York: Commonwealth Fund, 1927.
13. ———. *Annual Report, 1927*. New York: Commonwealth Fund, 1928.
14. ———. *Annual Report, 1928*. New York: Commonwealth Fund, 1929.
15. Curtis, W. R. "Community Human Service Networks: New Roles for the Mental Health

Worker." Paper read at the Annual Meeting of Psychiatric Outpatient Clinics of America, March 15, 1973, New York.

16. Furman, S. S. *Community Mental Health Services in Northern Europe.* Washington, D.C.: U.S. Department of Health, Education, and Welfare, P.H.S.P. no. 1407, 1965.

17. Glasscote, R., et al. *The Community Mental Health Center: An Analysis of Existing Models.* Washington, D.C.: Joint Information Service of the American Psychiatric Association, 1964.

18. Hollingshead, A., and Radlich, F. *Social Class and Mental Illness.* New York: Wiley, 1958.

19. Hunt, R. C. "The Ingredients of a Rehabilitation Program." In *An Approach to the Prevention of Disability from Chronic Psychoses: The Open Mental Hospital Within the Community.* New York: Milbank Memorial Fund, 1958.

20. Joint Commission on Mental Illness and Health. *Action for Mental Health: Final Report of the Joint Commission on Mental Illness and Health.* New York: Wiley, Science Editions, 1961.

21. Jones, R. O. "Appraising the Total Network of Services." *Hospital and Community Psychiatry,* January 1967, pp. 6–11.

22. Leighton, D. C.; Harding, J. S.; Macklin, D. B.; et al. *The Character of Danger: Psychiatric Symptoms in Selected Communities.* New York: Basic Books, 1963.

23. Lemakau, P. V. *Mental Hygiene in Public Health.* New York: McGraw-Hill, 1955.

24. Lewis, A. "Rehabilitation Programs in England." In *Elements of a Community Mental Health Program,* pp. 196–205. New York: Milbank Memorial Fund, 1956.

25. Macmillan, D. "Hospital-Community Relationships." In *An Approach to the Prevention of Disability from Chronic Psychoses: The Open Mental Hospital Within the Community.* New York: Milbank Memorial Fund, 1958.

26. Marshall, C. "Nova Scotia's Expanding Mental Health Program." *Nova Scotia Medical Bulletin,* July 1962.

27. Milbank Memorial Fund. "Services for People with Personality Disorders: Early Diagnosis and Treatment Services." In *Elements of a Community Mental Health Program,* pp. 151–157. New York: Milbank Memorial Fund, 1956.

28. ———. *An Approach to the Prevention of Disability from Chronic Psychoses: the Open Mental Hospital Within the Community.* New York: Milbank Memorial Fund, 1958.

29. Rafferty, F. T. "The Community is Becoming." *American Journal of Psychiatry* 36(1966):102–110.

30. Spiro, H. "On Beyond Mental Health Centers: A Planning Model for Psychiatric Care." *Archives of General Psychiatry* 21(1969):646–654.

31. Srole, L.; Langner, T. S.; Michael, T.; et al. "Mental Health in the Metropolis." In *The Thomas A. C. Rennie Series in Social Psychiatry,* vol. 1. New York: McGraw-Hill, 1961.

32. Stepanek, C. G., and Willie, C. V. "A Community Mental Health Program: Its Rise and Fall." In *A Seminar for Directors of Mental Health Centers: Special Report No. 114,* edited by W. Cape. Lawrence, Kansas: Government Research Center, University of Kansas, 1962.

33. Teuber, N. L., and Powers, E. "Evaluating Therapy in a Delinquency Prevention Program." *Proceedings of the Association for Research in Nervous and Mental Diseases* 31(1953):138–147.

34. Winters, E. E., ed. "Where Should We Attack the Problem of the Prevention of Mental Defect and Mental Disease?" in *The Collected Papers of Adolf Meyer.* Baltimore: Johns Hopkins Press, 1952. Original paper presented at 42nd Annual Session of the National Conference of Charities and Correction, held in Baltimore, Maryland, May, 1915.

35. Witmer, H. L. *Psychiatric Clinics for Children.* New York: Commonwealth Fund, 1940.

36. Yolles, S. F. "The Community Mental Health Center in National Perspective." In *The Practice of Community Mental Health,* edited by H. Grunebaum. Boston: Little, Brown, 1970, pp. 787–806.

Editorial Note

Dean is concerned with the meaning and definition of social deviance. That is, how does the social labeling of mental illness take place? Who gets into treatment? Why? How are patients labeled by relatives and friends? These questions become decisive if one is interested in facilitating early treatment. Dean cites a number of factors that contribute to a person's being defined as a patient: life failures, unpredictability of behavior, and the limits of tolerance that exist in any social system. He examines the behaviors that define individuals as disturbed, the cognitive struggles of patients and significant others to label psychiatric disorder, the impact of the patient's behavior on friends and family, the adjustive process that is brought into action when labeling takes place, the identifying of treatment and treatment resources, and the ways in which the social system may be a source for the patient disturbance.

In my opinion these critical questions need further assessment: (1) Are there limits of tolerance of deviance in all societies? (2) Is mental illness really relative? (3) How can the treatment system make better use of the knowledge of the limits of tolerance, the labeling of mental illness, and the ways in which social situations help "produce" mental illness?

B. H. K.

CHAPTER 5

The Social System, Deviance, and Treatment Efforts

ALFRED DEAN

IT WOULD SEEM obvious that psychiatric treatment depends upon contact between the disturbed person and the professional helper, an effective relationship and a viable social contract. Yet there is distressingly ample evidence that these elemental conditions are often lacking.

Severely disturbed individuals and the families to whom they are linked frequently struggle with their problems without seeking the possible benefits of professional help. Treatment contacts, belatedly established, are experienced as frustrating and incomprehensible. Treatment relationships are broken and discontinuous. A history of social problems and limited treatment efforts is evidenced by a meandering trail of help seeking, punctuated by the records of multiple institutions. For many of the most seriously disturbed, those who experience hospitalization, yesteryear's one-way trips or extended institutionalizations have been replaced with a revolving door leading to and from the community. Such facts imply the need for more knowledge about the factors which facilitate or undermine earlier and more effective treatment relationships.

My attempt here is to offer a sociological perspective of help seeking. That the public's reaction to psychiatric disturbances depends upon complex social, cultural, and psychological factors had scarcely been recognized less than twenty years ago. In 1955 John Clausen and his colleagues published a set of pioneering papers richly suggesting both the practical and scientific implications of needed research.[5] Their work presaged a wide variety of relevant studies published over the past two decades. Where there had been a desert of inattention, there now exists a profusion of unintegrated, sometimes conflicting observations and concepts.*

Improved services to patients and families, as well as advances in this area of inquiry, require a more refined perspective of the *social systems* and *social processes* which appear to be implicated in the quest for help and in the service of helping. This chapter thus considers a framework of key concepts within which the dynamics of treatment efforts may be more systematically comprehended.

There are several major sociological facets to the public's confrontation with psychiatric disturbances and the responses which they make or fail to make to it:

1. The actual behavior of disturbed individuals.
2. The cognitive struggle of patients and significant persons to identify, under-stand, and cope with psychiatric disturbance.
3. The impact of the behavior of disturbed individuals on the social systems to which they belong.
4. The adaptive and adjustive responses which the social system is pressed to effect.
5. The social processes which are directly implicated in identifying appropriate treatment resources and effecting treatment relationships.

While each of these dimensions is analytically separable, they are actually inter-dependent and exhibit complex interactions. All of these aspects and their implications for treatment will be considered. I will give most attention to the impact upon the family as a social system and to the types of responses which are elicited.

The Social Stimulus for Treatment

It would seem impossible to enumerate the ways in which man is dependent upon various human groupings (such as family, community, and society) for his biological, psychological, and social well-being. It is an elementary sociological principle that such groups are not simply aggregates of individuals, but systems of

* See references 1, 7, 12, 18, 23, 30, 33, 34, 38, and 40.

interdependent parts including roles, values, beliefs, norms, and so on. It does not require adherence to a utopian view of social systems to recognize that they tend to serve both individual and collective needs.

However, as man's anatomical and physiological features enable him to function, so do they have requisites for sustenance, protection, maintenance, and integration. Disturbances to parts have multiple consequences, and some parts and processes are more vital than others. It goes beyond metaphor to indicate that social systems have analogous processes.

The so-called structural-functional approach in sociology, despite empirical-theoretical limitations, contradictions, and dilemmas, has much explanatory power and heuristic value. The public's confrontation with mental illness may be powerfully understood as a confrontation with socially problematic behavior—with events which disrupt the structures and functions of the social systems in which they occur.

The concept of *deviant behavior* is central to an understanding of the public's reactions to psychiatric disturbances. Deviant behavior is a generic term which, most clearly and traditionally defined, refers to any *rule-breaking* behavior. The rules of a particular group are most effectively conceived as attached to specific statuses, roles, and social situations. An example might be that Americans are expected to wear clothes in public, or that men and women should wear specific and different attire.

It is a normal, but remarkable, observation that breaking such rules typically elicits powerful social reactions which in effect constitute punitive sanctions. Undoubtedly these phenomena serve to explain a great deal about the ways in which family, community, and society have reacted to and dealt with the mentally ill or emotionally disturbed. However, their explanatory power has significant limitations which must also be considered.

A more adequate, empirically grounded theory of deviant behavior and social response must encompass the following facts: *

1. Deviant behavior does not always elicit negative sanctions.
2. Even when deviance does elicit social sanctions, existing data and theory are often inadequate to explain why it does so.
3. No groups have rules which govern the full range of behavior which individuals may exhibit.
4. Changing circumstances may arise for which rules may not exist, or may be ambiguous, conflicting, or inappropriate.
5. Not all types of deviance are equally significant.
6. Like illness, deviance is not simply inherent in any given behavior, but involves a process of labeling.

* "Labeling theorists" have called attention to the limitations of the deviance-as-rule-breaking concept. See references 3 (esp. pp. 1–40), 9, 19, and 32.

This chapter thus attempts further to specify: (1) factors which influence the labeling of deviance; (2) illness as deviance; (3) forms and functional consequences of deviance; and (4) mechanisms of social control. By looking at the *role-sets* of patients, and at who in them defines what behavior as a problem, it is possible to achieve a more detailed understanding of the *processes* involved.* The following case material will serve to illustrate our examination of several major types of deviance associated with severe psychiatric disturbances:

> Mr. Alan Ace, Jr. is a twenty-eight-year-old advertising salesman from Battle Creek, N.C. At the time of his admission to the Alcoholic Rehabilitation Center (ARC), he is separated from his wife, Ann, and living with his mother. The wife continues to live in the same community with her parents, Mr. and Mrs. King.
>
> On the basis of occupation, income, education, and residence, Mr. Ace's family of procreation would be described as middle class. They have been married eight years and have three children: a six-year-old boy, a three-year-old girl, and another son, twenty months. They belong to a Presbyterian church in their local community.
>
> Members of this family describe remarkably variant definitions of the nature and duration of problematic behavior and explanations for it. Mrs. Ace describes a five-and-a-half-year history which began shortly after the patient's brother committed suicide and he exhibited a "marked change in personality." From a quiet, unassuming, amiable person he began acting like his deceased brother: cocky, loud, and aggressive. From this point on, Mr. Ace showed a progressive, elaborate, and provocative history of deviance.
>
> Included in his repertoire of deviance were: atypical drinking (frequent and inappropriate), but not associated with drunks or binges (wife); expressions of suicidal thoughts on two occasions; extreme hostility and verbal abuse toward his mother-in-law; coming home at all hours; threats to kill his wife and children; threats to kill his in-laws; squandering of money; excessive drinking on the job; and failure to work his sales territory.

Instrumental Role Failure. Instrumental roles are those which are oriented to the fulfillment of *tasks* associated with the group's adaptation to the environment. Basically, they refer to the *division of labor*. In a money economy and a nation of largely hired employees, the husband's occupation is a key instrumental role. Moreover, family structure in the U.S. is critically shaped by

---

* For clinical as well as research purposes, this approach leads to some conclusions very different from those drawn by survey approaches to the study of factors prompting psychiatric hospitalization. Generally stated, I believe such studies [1,12,30] tend to underestimate and undercharacterize the role of sociological factors. Although these studies should invite examination by basic social scientists, particularly those interested in deviant behavior, they have largely not done so.

the husband's occupation.[27] Depending on the family's cultural characteristics, occupations not only serve critical economic functions, but also serve strivings for status, mobility, and life styles which are defined as desirable or "necessary."

By the time Mr. Ace reached the ARC, he had been deviant in his occupational role in a number of ways, including failure to work his territory, excessive drinking on the job, and writing abusive letters to his boss. He had already been transferred to a new territory in an effort to cope with his behavior, and had been warned that he was close to losing his job.* These events had been a source of worry for his wife, and later for himself and his mother as well. Mrs. Ace confronted her husband with these problems, accused him of squandering his money, and complained about the unpredictability of their income.

The division of labor in a family is partly an effort to increase the efficiency and effectiveness of mutual goal attainment. The distribution of tasks also occurs along lines which are defined as appropriate and equitable. Instrumental role failure violates these principles and imposes *the burden of displaced roles upon others*. Noting, for example, that they "were in debt over their heads," Mrs. Ace reluctantly made arrangements for the care of her children so that she could work part-time.

Many new tasks were imposed upon the Ace family. These *coping functions* included financing treatment; monitoring the deviant's behavior; bailing him out of difficulties; pressing for behavioral revision; and attempting to get him to comply with treatment.

In viewing role relationships as "transactions," Goode suggests that the "role-bargain" may be of greater importance than normative consensus in maintaining social relationships.[14] He also proposes that the family acts as a "role budget center" in the allocation of its members' roles to the other groups. Other sociologists have noted that role interdependence serves as a mechanism of cohesion, social control, and the allocation of power.† Thus, in a social body of interdependent parts and processes, instrumental role failure can threaten the whole system.

Expressive Role Failure. Recognized as the prototype of a *primary group*, the family is arranged to serve such functions as providing love, security, response, and other profound social psychological needs. It has been proposed that urbanization and the breakdown of the extended family have led to the need for an intensive personal relationship in depth which is satisfied within the nuclear family. Romantic love has been viewed as an exaggerated expression of this need. The "companionship marriage" and permissive attitudes toward divorce reflect the cultural emphasis on the "pursuit of happiness" in the con-

* Mr. Ace "voluntarily" entered the alcoholic treatment center, despite denial that he was an alcoholic, in an effort to persuade both his boss and his wife that he deserved another chance.

† For example, see references 17, 25 (pp. 36–45), 29 (pp. 190–243), and 39.

jugal family. Pitts maintains that the conjugal family is the major institutional form of tension reduction in modern society.[31]

Disruption of expressive functions may result directly from failure to fulfill expressive role expectations, or indirectly from other sources of conflict. The psychiatrically disturbed individual may tend to withdraw, be uncommunicative, argumentative, moody, and ambivalent about close relationships. Such behavior violates the performance of primary roles. The significance of Mrs. Ace's characterization of her husband's "change of personality" and her statement that he was "not like the man I married" may be partly understood if one considers them as implying a breach in primary relationships.

Tension and conflict are often symptoms of deviance arising in a social system when there is a lack of *compatibility*. This occurs when someone behaves in a manner objectionable to other members of the system; or when there are different goals (lack of consensus). Gouldner and Gouldner state:

> When an individual desires things different from those commonly desired by others in his group (lack of consensus), or when he behaves toward others in ways that differ from what is desired (lack of compatibility), his actions and his person become particularly noticeable because they are frustrating, threatening, or disliked. Commonly, some kind of an appraisal is made of these actions and persons; it is a negative appraisal that expresses and communicates the frustration and resentment of the others and, in effect, also serves to inhibit further displays of such behavior. This negative appraisal is commonly expressed by labelling the resented behavior or persons in some opprobrious way; some term of reproach is assigned to such actions and persons. We shall speak of persons treated in this way as "deviants" and of such actions as "deviance" (p. 569; see also pp. 546–603).[15]

While serving the function of identifying and communicating unacceptable behavior, conflict is a source of stress and tends to rupture social relationships, particularly if defiance and dissent persist.

In the Ace family there was enormous tension, conflict, and argumentation, leading Mrs. Ace to numerous episodes of avoidance and distance from her husband. He prevailed upon a local clergyman to attempt to restore his relationship with his wife.* On two occasions she separated from him and threatened him with divorce.†

---

* Mr. Ace's recourse to a clergyman was consistent with his tendency to reject psychiatric explanations. When the clergyman eventually recommended psychiatric treatment, the patient and other family members rejected him. The roles of clergymen, police, and others as *care givers*, *defining agents*, and *gatekeepers* to medical and psychiatric treatment require substantially more research.

† Despite the singular importance of expressive roles in the family, the study of expressive role failure has been virtually ignored in surveys of the dynamics of hospitalization. By contrast, the pa-

It should be noted that Mrs. Ace's withdrawal *imposes expressive deprivation upon herself as well as her husband*. In such terms, deviance may be regarded as *triply problematic*: (1) implying a loss of function; (2) imposing the stress of conflict; and (3) introducing the problematics of social persuasion.*

Avoidance—decreased interaction—is a common result of deviance. We tend not to communicate or associate with people of whose behavior we disapprove. [16] This may be simply a "natural response" on the part of the "injured" party. Since role systems are systems of exchange, avoidance may also be a deliberate "tit-for-tat" response in which the "plaintiff" withdraws his "consideration" from the role-bargain. [17] In some groups avoidance is a culturally prescribed response to deviance and a deliberate mechanism of social persuasion, as is "shunning" among the Amish.

Representational Role Failure. Bank clerks are typically expected to dress conservatively and otherwise project an image of competence, efficiency, and stability. An executive trainee in a large bank told me that even the newspapers he carried to the office were governed by norms of propriety. I refer to such expectations as *representational roles* because they *oblige the individual to behave in ways which appropriately represent the group and his social position in it.* Goggman touches upon this aspect of roles as follows:

> It is important to note that in performing in a role the individual must see to it that the impressions which he conveys in the situation are compatible with role-appropriate personal qualities effectively imputed to him: a judge is supposed to be deliberate and sober; a pilot, in a cockpit, to be cool; a bookkeeper to be accurate and neat in doing his work . . . (p. 87). [13]

Representational role failure also reflects unfavorably on the group and implies role failure on the part of others.

Thus, Mr. Ace's excessive drinking on the job and other socially inappropriate behavior was regarded by his boss as a problem largely because it "reflected poorly on the company. It might also imply to his customers that he couldn't do his job competently." His behavior was also a source of considerable embarrassment to his wife, and one relative was vehemently opposed to his being in a State Hospital—"None of *his* family had ever been *there!*" The implication of culpability, imagined or real, may be a distinctly threatening aspect of both "mental illness" and "deviance." Blame, guilt, and stigma can be contagious.

---

tients' participation in social activities has been typically measured. I would submit that an adequate theory of the utilization of psychiatric services would also substantially apply to the family's struggle with other types of problems and the dynamics of divorce.

* Surveys of the families of psychiatric patients have barely described these processes. Similarly, these processes are insufficiently examined in theories of deviant behavior and social control.

Unpredictable Role Performance. Social order and social functioning depend upon *predictability*. It has been forcefully argued that the need for predictability is basic to the development of culture and social organization. Predictable role performances are the intended function of clearly defined and socially shared role expectations (p. 26).[24] An individual charged with a particular role must be able to "rely upon" others to perform complementary roles. W. I. Thomas long ago recognized that social unpredictability constitutes a *crisis* tantamount to *social disorganization.* It may also lead to personal crisis and disorganization (pp. 10–15).[36]

Unpredictable behavior is thus a distinct problem experienced by significant persons in our own studies. Periods of satisfactory behavior are reported as inexplicably broken, and problematic behavior just as enigmatically abates. Unusual or dangerous behavior also appears to symbolize the unpredictability of the "patient." Complaints about disruption of family routines may be partly understood in these terms.

The concern about unpredictability is also reflected in states of vigilance assumed by significant persons—in their concern to know how he will do today or what he will do next. The significance of a particular deviant act may not be its present consequences, but the uncertainty which it implies about the future. One of the most threatening connotations of "mental illness" may be unpredictability.

Significant persons, including employers, often continue to charge the "patient" or deviant with his usual roles in an effort to determine his "reliability." Similarly, job loss, separation, divorce, and involuntary hospitalization sometimes reflect the conclusion of these persons that he is too unreliable, rather than some decisively new precipitating event.

How much of what kind of deviance will be tolerated? The client of an investment firm expects his broker to be honest without fail, but not always to be a successful investor. With what level of expectation, and under what conditions, does a woman expect her husband to be a good companion or faithful? Social scientific data and theory is not sufficiently developed to answer these questions. Our studies document considerably more tolerance of role failure than theory suggests.

Corrective Role Failure. By *corrective role* we refer to a number of observations which indicate that individuals labeled as either "sick" or "deviant" are assigned to a new status and role. The most essential requirement of the role is the obligation to do everything possible to "correct" the behavior or conditions which render them deviant. Parsons has recognized that role failure associated with illness is the foundation of the *sick role.* [26,28]

The usual roles incumbent upon the sick person are tentatively modified. However, in an apparent effort to restore the functions of the group, the sick person is charged with a new set of role expectations. He is obliged to do everything necessary for him to get well and resume optional role functions. Analogous expectations are made of the deviant. We may regard the *sick role* and the *deviant role* as simply variant forms of a *corrective role*, since they reflect common principles of social behavior.

To illustrate, when Mrs. Ace denied her husband's plea that she come back to live with him, she said she would do so only when "he proved he could do right." Mr. Ace is thus placed in a new status and role. She regarded his refusal to comply with treatment efforts as a particularly crucial form of deviance. Similarly, Mr. Ace's employer shifted him to a new territory where he was explicitly on trial to establish that he could perform his role properly or be subject to dismissal.

An interesting aspect of the corrective role is the responsibility of the deviant to acknowledge "guilt," express remorse, and pledge intentions of future propriety. This is tantamount to acceptance of the "sick" or "deviant" label and the corrective role, and may be regarded as the first stage of the role which serves to "undo" stored-up grievances and repair relationships. We have warned that the development of social consensus regarding the *existence* of illness and deviance may be quite problematic. Patients and family members may dispute both and offer counteraccusations.

Failure to accept the role of patient or alternatively modify deviant behavior is a distinct problem. Disturbed persons are often unwilling or "unable" to comply with treatment efforts. Severe psychiatric disturbances are often long term, implying chronic or episodic deviance. Denial of illness or deviance is frequent if not characteristic, making "motivation for treatment" a special problem in the psychiatric field. For those involved with disturbed persons, corrective role failure sabotages their most traditional, familiar, and preferred mechanisms of restoring social functioning.

Dangerous Behavior as Limits of Tolerance. The capacity of many families to *tolerate* acutely disturbed individuals for remarkably long periods of time without recourse to treatment or rejection from the group has been repeatedly observed. Whitmer and Conover state: "The impression was that many patients were admitted following long, severe mental illness and, according to available information, the need for hospitalization had been as great in years past as it was at the time of hospitalization" (p. 89).[38,*] In a study of the help-seeking behavior of wives of alcoholics, no relationship was observed between the duration of al-

---

* The nature and role of differential tolerance in deferring or prompting hospitalization is subject to debate. Freeman and Simmons (pp. 6–14 and passim),[12] for example, reversed their early formulations. There has been a tendency to measure tolerance by essentially asking families if they would tolerate certain behavior rather than by what they did tolerate. This is a little bit like asking somebody what he would do if there were a fire (pp. 308 and passim).[1]

coholism and recourse to treatment agencies, or between duration and the incidence of divorce (pp. 459, 463).[18]

Dangerous behavior precipitates more forceful social responses. Jackson and Kogan found that physical violence toward family members served as a decisive factor in the decision of wives to divorce their alcoholic husbands (p. 468).[18] Lowenthal concluded that "potentially harmful behavior" and actually harmful behavior precipitated the hospitalization of elderly patients to a psychiatric ward in 54 percent of 507 cases (pp. 55–77).[23] Yarrow, Schwartz, Murphy, and Deasy indicate that sixteen out of thirty-three wives of acutely disturbed husbands described aggressive, assaultive, or suicidal behavior upon admission to the hospital (p. 17).[41] Whitmer and Conover report the case of a man who had apparently been psychotic for ten years but had not been brought to treatment until he attempted to kill his father (pp. 90–92).[38]

Mr. Ace's first referral did not occur until one year after his wife noted his marked personality change. It was precipitated by his expression of suicidal thoughts. *Perceived danger* precipitated eight of thirteen referrals to various treatment agents and both occasions when his wife separated from him. *Perceived danger poses an urgent need for social control,* and *signifies the unpredictability of the deviant's behavior.*

The Struggle for Definition

The public is faced with the struggle of identifying and understanding the manifestations of psychiatric illness. That this fact has been recognized by health professionals and by social scientists is reflected in health education programs and studies of the public's conception of mental illness.* Existing research has only begun to suggest the complex psychobiological, cultural, and social processes which are implicated in the recognition or labeling of mental illness.

It is clear that what is regarded as illness, like other aspects of experience, observation, or "reality," is partly a matter of cultural definition. This fact is as applicable to the professional subcultures of medicine and psychiatry as it is to the dominant or variant cultures of the lay American public. This point is aptly illustrated in the mental health field today by serious debates regarding the validity of the very concept of mental illness.† Various social classes, for example,

---

* Among the parameters implicated in help-seeking behavior, the cognitive dimension received early attention.[4,41]

† "Alcoholism" is also a revealing example of a problem which has been subjected to a variety of nonillness and illness conceptions in American medicine as well as in the public's views.[2]

hold different conceptions of mental illness and mental retardation. There are cross-cultural variations in conceptions of physical illness as well as conceptions of mental normality. The early studies of Clausen and associates indicated that behavior which professionals would regard as exotic and severe symptoms of mental illness were normalized by intelligent and educated American women (pp. 8–24).[5]

Perhaps the least-examined aspect of this struggle is the interpersonal processes involved in achieving consensus regarding the nature of the problem, the need for outside help, and appropriate helpers. This is inherently a process of social persuasion involving such issues as legitimate participation, authority, and power. The general neglect of this area is probably partly due to the attempt to conduct verificational surveys of the dynamics of hospitalization without sufficient in-depth, exploratory case studies of process. Undoubtedly, it is difficult to design quantitative studies of these interpersonal processes.

When we look closely at the circumstances surrounding admission to mental hospitals, we find that *hospitalization does not necessarily imply the recognition of illness by patients or family members.* Conflicting definitions, uncertainty, and even denial of illness regularly accompany the "treatment efforts" of patients and their families.* Conversely, they may *neglect* to seek treatment *despite their recognition* of illness.† One is pressed to conclude, with only apparent simplicity, that people do not go to "physicians" because they are sick but because they are in critical difficulty. (The nature of those difficulties is decisively determined by their specific role systems.) The appearance, persistence, or exacerbation of symptoms are frequently not the events which precipitate recourse to treatment. There are interesting parallels to this process in the use of medical services.[42]

Of course, nonillness conceptions, uncertainty, denial, and *preferred definitions* particularly, do serve to defer treatment contacts and undermine treatment relationships.‡ In turn, there are compelling factors which contribute to those untoward definitions, including the vicissitudes of symptoms or problematic behavior; the complexity of psychiatric disorders; the "availability" of alternative nonillness explanations; variant conditions of observation; the stigma of mental

---

* The denial of physical disorders has also been well documented.[37] The denial of myocardial infarction is an interesting parallel.[6] These findings are consistent with other data which emphasize the role of deviance and social control processes in prompting hospitalization or other help-seeking activity.[7,41]

† Such a circumstance exposes other factors which condition help seeking, including: (1) the problem of achieving consensus about the nature and source of problematic events and appropriate "helpers"; (2) the degree of help provided by prior treatment efforts; (3) the actual or perceived sources of help available; and (4) cost.

‡ I have found that individuals exhibit an emotional attachment to particular definitions of the situation. For example, in the Ace family, the patient's mother, when no longer able to deny his deviance entirely, preferred to regard him as an alcoholic than as mentally ill (pp. 517–533).[7]

illness; and the threatening implication of profound changes in social arrangements and "life organization."

Under these conditions, it is not surprising that we find many manifestations of severe shock in such families, including personal disorganization, impulsive behavior, selective perception, and disturbances of communication. In the face of conflicting studies, it is my present conclusion that families tend to offer a number of nonillness explanations for problematic behavior; that there is a "definitional crisis" marked by a lack of consensus. Yet both psychiatry and medicine evidence a failure to examine the conceptions which patients and families hold, or to respond to their quest for information.*

Parsons and Fox recognized illness as a special case of deviant behavior to the extent that the sick person is unable to fulfill his normal social roles.[28] This view emphasizes that regardless of its cause, role failure has a serious impact on the social system. Illness illustrates that social reactions to behavior ordinarily regarded as deviant depend upon the circumstances in which it occurs and the ways it is "explained."

In American society we do not regard the role failure of sick persons as deviance precisely because we consider these people "disabled." Recognizing illness *legitimates* role failure and redeems the otherwise deviant person. We must thus distinguish between behavior which, *in effect*, constitutes role failure (*de facto deviance*); and role failure for which the individual is held responsible (*perceived deviance*).

Existing theory and data neglect the uncertainty and disagreement which may surround the existence of illness.[20] Psychiatric disturbances highlight this problem. When, for example, Mr. Ace assaulted his father-in-law and threatened to kill him, his wife regarded this behavior as undeniably dangerous and "sick," but other family members did not. The forms of problematic behavior and the terms by which "illness" and "nonillness" are explained require further documentation, as do the conditions under which such behavior and explanations are elicited.

To the extent that the psychiatrically disturbed are held responsible for role failure, their behavior represents problems of perceived deviance for all concerned. Regardless of perceived legitimacy, role failure has serious consequences for group members and processes. The Eskimo practice of leaving elderly or infirm individuals to die, and the altruistic suicides of such persons, are social responses to the problem of role failure, apart from cause. While this example may be exotic, it has its parallels in Western society.

---

* In studies of psychiatric patients and their families, this has been a matter of recurrent observation.[8,11] I have examined the relationship of family members and treatment agents (pp. 542–553).[7] Studies of the doctor-patient relationship have also documented this problem.[20,21,22]

Types of Coping Responses

The family makes a variety of responses in an effort to cope with the disturbances associated with problematic behavior. *Remedially oriented responses* refers to those which attempt to define given forms of behavior as unacceptable and to bring behavior in line with expectations. Most notably, these include *sanctioning mechanisms*, such as argumentation, threats, and rejection, and *treatment efforts*—coerced, "voluntary," or "involuntary." The basic intended function of remedially oriented efforts is to effect preferred social arrangements, whether it be the system prior to crisis or an alternative structure.

It is extremely important to regard treatment contacts as a special form of remedial effort for several reasons:

1. They seem to occur only when other remedially oriented efforts have failed.
2. The events which precipitate recourse to specialized community agents appear to reflect the limiting conditions of tolerance being exceeded by cumulative stress or particularly threatening situations, rather than the full range of disturbances which actually serve as incentives for treatment efforts.
3. It serves to explain the participation of various parties in referral despite uncertainty, denial, or conflicting conceptions of the basis of problematic behavior.
4. Treatment efforts represent an invitation to therapists to play fundamentally social roles in a system in which they may not ordinarily function; the invitation is issued despite many forces which militate against it.

Accommodation refers to responses which serve to enable the group to reduce the impact of problematic behavior.* This can be achieved by a number of mechanisms: (1) *revising expectations of the deviants*; (2) *a reallocation of functions*; and (3) *denial of deviance*—the creation of "myths" of satisfactory performance.†

Total rejection of the deviant and social reorganization, while an obvious option of the group, is not an easy alternative. The deviant may continue to serve some highly valued functions, particularly if his deviance is low-keyed and episodic rather than chronic. Rejection may be difficult to achieve or may imply other problems. Two prosaic examples may suffice: the tenured professor and the alienated couple with children. Of course, such rejections do occur. Persons

---

* The processes of accommodation to psychiatric disturbances by the family have been seriously neglected. This has probably been due to the limitations of theoretical formulations brought to research and methodological difficulties inherent in their investigation.

† Several studies have noted that recourse to treatment results from the breakdown of accommodation. The concept and its empirical referents, however, are developed differently by researchers.[7,10,33]

with known psychiatric histories are less likely to be married and more likely to be separated or divorced.

The above types of responses are not mutually exclusive. They can exist simultaneously. Similarly, a single response may serve several of these functions. Separation, for example, may communicate the seriousness of the situation, serve as a persuasive sanction, reduce the impact of deviance, and set the stage for divorce.

Treatment Issues

Definitive knowledge about the nature of most psychiatric disturbances is lacking. However, it has long been recognized in principle that they implicate biological, psychological, and sociological factors in complex interaction. There can be little doubt that the sociological and social psychological correlates of psychiatric disturbances, whether contributors or consequences, constitute the most neglected dimension of psychiatric education, perspective, and practice.

The family's encounter with treatment agents may be hardly less problem-: than its encounter with deviance. It is often characterized by: (1) failure to sustain treatment relationships; (2) failure of treatment agents to involve the family adequately as sources or objects of information; (3) a generally limited relationship to family members; (4) discontinuities in care; (5) an incoherent and uncoordinated delivery system; (6) conflicting evaluations; and (7) an unfortunate tendency on the part of treaters to assign culpability. The study of the dynamics of help-seeking points up the need for furthering the development and application of several functions: (1) life-situational analysis and social diagnosis; (2) social therapy; and (3) definitional functions.*

Social Diagnosis. Despite signs of growing dissatisfaction with the limitations of the "medical model," there is evidence that the adaptational strivings, contingencies, and problems of patients and families—so decisively shaped by sociological factors—are insufficiently documented or conceptualized in clinical work. Biological or personality models continue to dominate diagnosis and treatment. The increasingly compelling data point to the significance of satisfactory human relationships and social roles for physical and mental well-being, and suggest the need for a more sophisticated social science base and improved techniques of social observation and analysis.

Regardless of the multiple possibilities in form, sequence of cause and ef-

* American psychiatry has long recognized the importance of these functions, as exemplified in the work of Adolf Meyer.

fect, or varied origins of psychiatric disturbances, the social situations of disturbed individuals are marked by deviance, conflict, and problematic role relationships. If some resolution of this disorganization is essential to the psychosocial well-being of the patient, a more advanced understanding of the properties of social systems and of individual-group relationships will be required.

Social Therapy. As the pathways to treatment are marked by social conflict and directed by social crisis, the task of repairing and restoring social relationships becomes a priority therapeutic task. The clinician's failure to recognize or deal with social disorganization may represent a significant explanation for the failure of patients and family members to sustain treatment efforts. The clinician's attempt to restore role relationships may serve to ventilate the stored-up grievances which constitute obstacles to the restoration of patient and family alike. While family members may have conflicting motives, they may hold a common investment born of interdependence. The clinician may capitalize upon this investment in his attempt to effect higher levels of adaptation and adjustment.

Certainly the therapist charged with the task of after-hospitalization care faces a problem of social rehabilitation. He is confronted with the task of assessing the therapeutic assets and liabilities of the family (and other social systems) and the obstacles and dangers involved in the restoration of role relationships.

In many respects, psychiatry and the family may look toward but past one another, partly because they don't share a frame of reference to their mutual understanding or their relations. As Smith has suggested, it remains for psychiatry to consider whether a discrepancy between its own conception of treatment "needs" and the family's "wants" does not serve as an important explanation for the failure to sustain treatment.[35]

Before the patient opens the door to a treatment institution, there has been a complex social and psychosocial struggle. To operate effectively, the clinician must consider the nature of that struggle and by whom and for what reason he has been given what mandate. Eventually, probably fairly quickly, he will be placing the patient back into a specific sociocultural context of family, community, and society. The therapeutic or antitherapeutic potentials of those social systems must be considered. If he is to consider the interests of his client, he must not only identify clearly what these potentials are, but see beyond them to the interlocking interests of others in the social system.

Definitional Functions. An important task for the clinician is that of providing meaningful and workable definitions of the situation to the patient and family members. In this effort he must recognize the personal and social barriers to effective communication, and penetrate or manipulate the preferential cognitive patterns of significant persons. He should recognize that from a technical point of view, the public may be expected to confront a situation of definitional uncertainty; that the family probably exhibits conflicting definitions; and that he must attempt to comprehend the nature and implications of their explanatory definitions. He should be particularly alert to *ad hominem* definitions.*

The terms of his definitions ideally should provide the family with some understanding of the patient's behavior and how to respond to it. The definitional task is of central concern if the milieu of the family is to be favorable to the recovery of the patient and to the movement of the family as a unit to higher levels of role enactment. It would appear that the definitional task will be a continuing one and will probably require changing definitions over relatively long periods of time. Enactment of this function may serve as an important bond between the clinician and significant persons, permit the family to carry on its everyday functions, and bolster the probability of continuity of care.

The definitional function is relevant to a broad range of family concerns associated with illness, including technical knowledge, an understanding of the emotional correlates of illness, and the implications of illness for the patient's roles.

Summary

With its many facets, social psychiatry is like a patchwork quilt whose common thread and identifying pattern is an examination of the role of sociological factors in health, illness, and treatment. The study of the dynamics of help seeking is a late addition to that fabric. This area of inquiry requires a perspective of the sociological manifestations, impact, and response to what might professionally be defined as "psychiatric disorders."

The past two decades have witnessed the emergence of a variety of studies bearing on those processes. The developing literature has been the product of multiple disciplines and professions—e.g., sociologists, social psychologists, social workers, psychiatrists, and physicians—indicating that despite varied theo-

---

* *Ad hominem* definitions explain problematic behavior in terms of interpersonal conflicts. For example, when Mr. Ace broke into his in-laws' home and threatened to kill his mother-in-law, his uncle and mother denied his deviance and minimized his dangerousness. Instead, they blamed his mother-in-law for interfering with his marriage. Similarly, when Mrs. Ace complained about her husband coming home "at any and all hours," he countered with the accusation that she was incapable of being an "executive's wife." These types of explanations prominently reveal the patterns of problematic social relationships which may bear complex antecedent or consequent relationships to the patient's behavior.

retical and applied concerns, there has been a congruence of recognition that the "pathways" to treatment are curious avenues for serious exploration.

The data and concepts which have been generated possess double-edged significance, that is, relevance to both basic behavioral science and treatment efforts. The literature has implications for our understanding of such phenomena as the processes by which illness and deviance are defined and dealt with; the group structures and functions which are disrupted by illness and deviance; and processes of disorganization, reorganization, and change.

Similarly, these studies serve to inform us about such applied concerns as the factors which defer the recognition of illness and its treatment; the social motives which prompt treatment contacts; the social problems of patients and families; factors which may be responsible for ineffective treatment relationships; and factors which may be associated with the ability of formerly hospitalized patients to remain in the community. So rich a vein surely deserves to be further mined.

Nonetheless, as a young area, it is not surprising that it has not adequately fulfilled its promise. Neither social scientists nor the mental health professions have sufficiently assessed the value and limitations of its current status or its requirements for future growth. Like other areas of social psychiatry, it not only requires the critical evaluation and continuing efforts of those who are committed to it, but the attention of the basic scientists and mental health professionals who may be scarcely aware of its existence.

The concepts considered here represent an attempt to bring the sociology of treatment efforts into a sharper and more detailed perspective. I have also tried to highlight the value and limitations of the field. Finally, if not foremost, I hope that this chapter may serve to invite further attention from the various audiences upon whom the growth of knowledge and its application so vitally depends. Everyone should be granted three wishes.

REFERENCES

1. Angrist, S. S.; Lefton, M.; Dinitz, S.; and Pasamanick, B. *Women After Treatment*. New York: Appleton-Century-Crofts, 1968.

2. Bacon, S. D., issue ed. "Understanding Alcoholism." *Annals of the American Academy of Political and Social Science* 315, January 1958.

3. Becker, H. S. *Outsiders*. New York: Free Press, 1963.

4. Clausen, J. *Sociology and the Field of Mental Health*. New York: Russell Sage Foundation, 1956.

5. ———, and Yarrow, M. R., issue eds. "The Impact of Mental Illness on the Family." *Journal of Social Issues* 11, Spring 1955.

6. Croog, S. H., and Levine, S. "Social Status and Subjective Perceptions of 250 Men After Myocardial Infarction." *Public Health Reports* 84(1969):989–997.

7. Dean, A. "Alcoholism and Social Structure: A Sociological Study of Illness, Deviance and Social Response." Ph.D. dissertation, University of North Carolina, Chapel Hill, 1965.

8. Deasy, L., and Quinn, O. L. "The Wife of the Mental Patient and the Hospital Psychiatrist." *Journal of Social Issues* 11, Spring 1955:49–60.

9. Erikson, K. "Notes on the Sociology of Deviance." *Social Problems* 9(1962):307–314.

10. Ferreira, A. J. "Family Myth and Homeostasis." *Archives of General Psychiatry* 9(1963):55–61.

11. Freeman, H. E., and Simmons, O. G. "Treatment Experiences of Mental Patients and Their Families." *American Journal of Public Health* 51(1961):1266–1277.

12. ———. *The Mental Patient Comes Home.* New York: Wiley, 1963.

13. Goffman, E. *Encounters.* Indianapolis: Bobbs-Merrill, 1961.

14. Goode, W. J. "A Theory of Role Strain." *American Sociological Review* 25(1960):493–496.

15. Gouldner, A. W., and Gouldner, H. P. *Modern Sociology.* New York: Harcourt, Brace, 1963.

16. Homans, G. C. *The Human Group.* New York: Harcourt, Brace, 1950.

17. ———. "Social Behavior as Exchange." *American Journal of Sociology* 63(1958):597–606.

18. Jackson, J. K., and Kogan, K. L. "The Search for Solutions: Help-Seeking Patterns of Families of Active and Inactive Alcoholics." *Quarterly Journal of Studies on Alcohol* 24(1963):449–472.

19. Kitsuse, J. I. "Societal Reaction to Deviant Behavior: Problems of Theory and Method." In *The Other Side*, edited by H. S. Becker, pp. 87–102. New York: Free Press, 1964.

20. Klein, R. F.; Dean, A.; Wilson, M.; and Bogdonoff, M. D. "The Physician and Postmyocardial Infarction Invalidism." *Journal of the American Medical Association* 194(1965):143–148.

21. Korsch, B., and Negrette, V. F. "Doctor-Patient Communication." *Scientific American* 227(1972):66–74.

22. Korsch, B.; Gozzi, E.; and Negrette, V. F. "Gaps in Doctor-Patient Communication." *Pediatrics* 42(1968):855–871.

23. Lowenthal, M. F. *Lives in Distress: The Paths of the Elderly to the Psychiatric Ward.* New York: Basic Books, 1964.

24. Olmsted, D. W. *Social Groups, Roles and Leadership.* East Lansing: Michigan State University Press, 1961.

25. Parsons, T. *The Social System.* New York: Free Press, 1951.

26. ———. "Illness and the Role of the Physician: A Sociological Perspective." In *Personality in Nature, Society and Culture*, 2nd ed., edited by C. Kluckhohn and H. A. Murray, pp. 609–617. New York: Knopf, 1954.

27. ———. "Age and Sex in the Social Structure of the United States." In *Selected Studies in Marriage and the Family*, edited by R. F. Winch et al., pp. 68–82. New York: Holt, Rinehart, 1962.

28. ———, and Fox, R. C. "Illness, Therapy and the Urban American Family." In *A Modern Introduction to the Family*, edited by N. W. Bell and E. T. Vogel, pp. 347–360. New York: Free Press, 1960.

29. Parsons, T., and Shills, E. A., eds. *Toward a General Theory of Action.* New York: Harper Torchbook, 1962.

30. Pasamanick, B.; Scarpitti, F. R.; and Dinitz, S. *Schizophrenics in the Community: An Experimental Study in the Prevention of Hospitalization.* New York: Appleton-Century-Crofts, 1967.

31. Pitts, J. R. "The Structural-Functional Approach." In *Handbook of Marriage and the Family*, edited by Harold T. Christensen, pp. 51–124. Chicago: Rand McNally, 1964.

32. Rubington, E., and Weinberg, M. S., eds. *Deviance: The Interactionist Perspective.* London: Macmillan, 1968.

33. Sampson, H.; Messinger, S. L.; and Towne, R. D. "Family Processes and Becoming a Mental Patient." *American Journal of Sociology* 68(1962):88–96.

34. Schwartz, C. G. "Perspectives on Deviance—Wives' Definitions of Their Husbands' Mental Illness." *Psychiatry* 20(1957):275–291.

35. Smith, H. L. *New Roles for Psychiatry.* Unpublished monograph. Chapel Hill: University of North Carolina, 1952.

36. Volkart, E. H., ed. *Social Behavior and Personality: Contributions of W. I. Thomas to Theory and Social Research.* New York: Social Science Research Council, 1951.

37. Weinstein, E. A., and Kahn, R. L. *Denial of Illness.* Springfield, Ill.: Charles C. Thomas, 1955.

38. Whitmer, C. A., and Conover, G. C. "A Study of Critical Incidents in the Hospitalization of the Mentally Ill." *Journal of the National Association of Social Work* 4(1959):89–94.

39. Wolfe, D. M. "Power and Authority in the Family." In *Studies in Social Power,* edited by D. Cartwright, pp. 99–117. Ann Arbor: University of Michigan Press, 1959.

40. Wood, E. C.; Rakusin, J. M.; and Morse, E. "Interpersonal Aspects of Psychiatric Hospitalization." *Archives of General Psychiatry* 3(1960):443–454.

41. Yarrow, M. R.; Schwartz, C. G.; Murphy, H. S.; and Deasy, L. C. "The Psychological Meaning of Mental Illness in the Family." *Journal of Social Issues* 11(1955):12–24.

42. Zola, I. K. "Pathways to the Doctor-from Person to Patient." Revision of paper delivered at McGill University, 1966. Mimeographed.

Editorial Note

Susser uses the psychiatric register to provide examples of one point of view in look-
ing at a treatment population and its epidemiologic characteristics. In so doing,
he shows the psychiatric register to be an assessment device for describing: (1) the
recognized mental sickness in a defined population; (2) the monitoring of commu-
nity agencies; (3) evaluation of the effectiveness of such agencies; and (4) sugges-
tions for the determinants of mental illness. Consequently, solutions to the
problems of planning, coordination, innovation, manpower, and evaluation can
be approached through this device.

There are two implications in the use of the psychiatric register that promise
interesting future applications. First, the psychiatric register is a general in-
strument for assessing risk factors in the functioning of the care system which also
raises fundamental questions about the key issues of treatment system effectiveness
and patient compliance. Second, the register is a useful device for developing hy-
potheses on the relationship between a person's environment (past and present)
and the development of mental disorder.

B. H. K.

CHAPTER 6

Psychiatric Registers and Community Mental Health Services

MERVYN SUSSER

IN THIS CHAPTER I approach the question of psychiatric registers primarily from the point of view of community psychiatric services. Psychiatric registers have scientific shortcomings. They are selective in identifying psychiatric disturbance only among service users, and the routine psychiatric diagnoses on which the data are founded are noticeable. These problems, in different guises, beset all psychiatric epidemiologic studies. They are special only to the extent that registers aim to exploit and link service records, and are, therefore, subject to the constraints of services. Essentially, however, the problems are research problems.

I will argue that a register can be set up without an effective community service, but the converse does not hold. A community psychiatric service without a register cannot show that it is a community service, nor whether it is helping or harming the target population. The psychiatric register is a basic instrument in the development of a community service in any full sense.

By "community," I mean the people in an area that has been defined administratively to coincide, however crudely, with the social organization of those people; that is, it comprises population, area, and organization. By definition, a service of the community must aim to be comprehensive in terms of that population. To be effective in the community as a whole, it must also aim to be comprehensive in its range of services. It should include prevention, first contact care, general therapeutic services, specialized short-term and long-term therapeutic services, rehabilitation, follow-up, and even custody.

The psychiatric register is an instrument which makes visible the structure, function, and interplay of the array of services, and also the extent to which the services reach into the community. By a psychiatric register, I mean a comprehensive ongoing statistical system, founded on items of service, that aims to link and analyze systematically recorded data about patients from all the elements of the psychiatric services in a defined administrative area.

It is no accident that most work on psychiatric registers began in the late 1950s, just as the movement for the community care of mental disorder was gathering momentum in the United Kingdom and in North America. The trickle of patients in and out of mental hospitals during the custodial era grew into a steady flow; a substantial part of the mental hospital population was shifted out into the community; and outpatient clinics and social services grew, if haphazardly, and absorbed some of the shifts out of the mental hospitals.

What was happening inside the hospitals was clear, but no one could be sure what was happening outside. For a century and more, mental hospital statistics had given an adequate description of how many people psychiatric services provided for and in what form, but these informative data, simply obtained and facilitated by the legalized custodial functions and autonomy of psychiatric institutions, now dealt with a decreasing segment of psychiatric operations.

The need for an information base on which to approach the rational care of mental disorder in the community stimulated the development of registers. If there is to be an effective program of community care, there will have to be a continuing interaction between services and registers.

An effective program of community care requires that attention be given to at least five important objectives:

1. *Planning:* To discover need and demand, and to select priorities.
2. *Coordination:* To coordinate existing psychiatric services facilitates continuity of care for individual patients through all stages of sickness, provides ready access to a wide range of facilities according to the needs of patients, and avoids duplication and competition for scarce resources.
3. *Innovation:* To experiment with a variety of new services suited to the needs of mentally sick people in the community, and to maintain the ones that prove useful.
4. *Manpower development:* To train a body of professional workers in commu-

nity psychiatry; this involves their socialization to community aims, as well as equipping them with new knowledge and skills.

5. *Evaluation:* to discover the effects of the community program.

A psychiatric register has a part to play in every one of these five objectives. The patent uses of a register can be listed under four heads:

1. Description of recognized mental sickness in a defined population.
2. Monitoring of flow and process between community and agencies, and between agencies.
3. Evaluation of programs, and of their overall accomplishment.
4. Study of the determinants of mental sickness.

I shall consider in turn the contributions of each of these uses to the objects of a community program.

In its *descriptive* function a register is invaluable in planning. The information contributes to understanding of needs and demands. It tells who is being served—rich or poor, old or young, male or female, single or married or parents—and by implication it indicates their needs for service. These demographic data, combined with clinical data, enable the planner to construct profiles of the patient population in terms of their social roles, obligations, and dependency and supportive networks, and so to infer their social needs. The register also shows where people are being served, and what they are being served, whether in mental hospitals, general hospitals, clinics, general practice, hostels, day-care centers, clubs, or homes. Again by implication, these data can indicate what gaps exist in the services provided, what new services are needed, and how extensive the need is.

It fell to me to develop the community mental health service in Salford, a Northern English industrial town of about 150,000 people. We took care to develop extramural facilities on the basis of estimates made from needs known and recognized through the register. In the matter of residential hostels, this procedure saved us from the chagrin of many places across the country which built hostels and could not fill them with patients. Problems enter into such estimates, especially the problem of translating need into demand, or as it could be put, the problem of getting those in need to see their needs as professionals do, and to use the services provided. Nor is any planner safe against unpredictable events, like the discoveries of streptomycin and isoniazid that so quickly emptied the tuberculosis sanatoria.*

In its second *monitoring* function, the register helps predict trends and

* In Britain these untoward events saved the faces of the health administrators, who by default had failed to build any new sanatoria at all after World War II; retrospectively they could claim foresight.

consequent changes in needs and demands. In Salford we were at first undercon-
fident of our data and slow to react to what we found. For instance, it took time
to convince ourselves that data suggesting a substantial growth of the severely
mentally retarded population were sound, and that a matching increase in
provision of care was needed. In retrospect it is easy to see that the population
growth was the result of the steady increase in the life expectation of affected
individuals.

The register, as a monitoring instrument, also becomes an instrument of
coordination. The flow between agencies is made evident; the degree of interdependence between them becomes apparent; and the degree to which they
complement, or simply duplicate, one another in the patients they serve and the
services offered becomes visible.

Figure 6.1 shows all the agencies that had a special concern in the psychiatric care of Salford patients. At the outset of the program for community care,
each of these agencies operated almost autonomously under their separate ad-
ministrations. The general hospital, the mental hospital, and the mental health
service each had their own psychiatrists, social workers, and psychologists. The
main gatekeepers to service were the general practitioners, and they referred independently either to outpatient services or to the mental health service of the
public health department. The mental health service arranged either for social
work support and day facilities with home care or, in about half the cases, for admissions to the mental hospital.

The continuity of patient care was interrupted by each of the many referrals
between agencies, and the disruptive effects of discontinuity were readily apparent. I shall give two examples of discontinuity and poor coordination picked up
through the register.

1. Between general practitioners and the mental health service: One-third of
the sixty-nine general practioners made virtually no referrals to the mental health
service. A substantial number of the patients of these general practitioners, however, were referred to the mental health service by other routes, presumably at a
late state of illness.

2. Between the mental hospital and the mental health service of the public
health authority: The mental health service had the formal responsibility for aftercare, i.e., social work after patients were discharged from the mental hospital.
Over a three-month period, only 8 percent of the patients discharged from the
mental hospital were referred for aftercare. Within three months of their discharge, another 40 percent of those discharged had been referred to the mental
health service from other sources, because of the problems that had developed in
the interim.

At the outset of the community care program, none of these agencies could

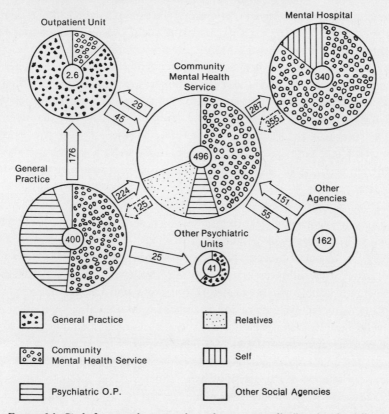

FIGURE 6.1. Circle for general practice shows the proportion distributed *to* the different psychiatric services; all other circles show the proportions of referrals received *from* different services. Actual numbers of referrals are shown by the figures in arrows. *Source:* M. Susser, *Community Psychiatry: Epidemiologic and Social Themes* (1968), Random House, New York, p. 247

know anything about the flow of patients from one to another. Agencies had vague notions of the services provided by each of the other agencies, and whom they were serving. They knew little of the characteristics, and even of the bare numbers, of the populations they themselves served. Consequently, they did not perceive the fragmented and fragmentary nature of the care they offered, nor could they perceive the extent of interdependence needed were they to provide a full range of services for their patients. They were largely unaware of the disruptive effects on patients of discontinuity of care, and each professional tended to see and assess the needs of his patient from his own isolated vantage point. Each autonomous organization put constraints on the perception of the professionals working within it, in terms of its own functions and aims.

In this situation, the knowledge culled from the register became power. The information conveyed in Figure 6.1 revealed the incoordination. It also pointed to strategic targets from which to achieve coordination, and helped persuade key members of the isolated agencies of the need for coordination.

In its third *evaluative* function, the register can be used at two levels: (1) the evaluation of technique; and (2) the evaluation of accomplishment. Evaluation of technique involves the monitoring of the actual input of a program, or so to speak, the delivery of the treatment. Too often a program, well described on paper, exists only in the mind of the writer. There are not a few examples of attempts to evaluate paper programs, just as there are not a few clinical trials that have tried to evaluate the effect of drugs that remained on the bathroom shelves of the patients.

Use of the register for the evaluation of technique is a specialization of its use for monitoring generally. Three examples will serve to illustrate the function of monitoring the treatment program.

An early object of program policy was to bring the work of the sixty-nine general practitioners into closer coordination with the work of mental welfare officers. Mental welfare officers were social workers who had legally designated powers in dealing with the admission and aftercare of mental patients. The general practitioners were the gatekeepers to services, and the program looked to the mental welfare officers as the vehicle by which general practice habits might be changed. The input of this program could be measured by the pattern of general practitioners' referrals to the mental welfare officers. In a period of five years, the number of general practitioners who made less than one referral per annum fell precipitously from twenty-three to only three of sixty-nine. The number who made more than eight referrals had been only three, and rose to include over half the general practitioners.

Another object of policy was to alter the mode of the mental welfare officers' relationship with patients. The dominant mode was that of bureaucratic officer/client, in which the mental welfare officers served chiefly to arrange, under legal constraint, admissions to a mental hospital. The desired mode was a therapeutic one between professional and patient, in which the mental welfare officer would serve to support the patient socially and psychologically, and to guide him through the maze of social services in an industrial state. This program technique could be evaluated by the trend in compulsory and voluntary mental hospital admissions. Over a period of five years, the register showed that compulsory admissions were halved. At the same time, the mental welfare officers also halved the total number of admissions among patients referred to them by general practitioners, and among those not admitted they did much more social work than before. The proportion of patients referred to whom no service at all was given fell, by a factor of five, to a negligible number. The mental welfare officers were clearly using their professional skills more than before, and using their legal powers less.

A third object of policy was to make more use of facilities outside the hospital wards, thereby to enable patients in treatment better to maintain everyday social relationships. In this instance the register showed a sharp reduction in length of hospital stay, without any compensatory rise in admissions and bed occupancy, while there was a concomitant rise in the use of extramural facilities.

Evaluation of accomplishment is the measurement of the sought-after or ultimate effects that must justify a program in terms of its objectives. These effects can be sought at the level of the psychological and social function of individual patients, at the level of the family, and at the level of the community, the whole target population. They may be conceived as short- or long-term, desirable or harmful, and anticipated or unanticipated by the innovators.

For example, the shift of patients out of the mental hospitals is now apparent in several developed countries. Yet there is no good evidence to show that this shift is not merely a transfer of patients with chronic disability from hospital into community locations. In Salford, the register helped establish a baseline from which to answer this question. We used the device of taking a census of patients, both in the hospital and out, who had been disabled for more than a year following mental sickness.

This census was readily possible because the register was kept in a manner that allowed a census to be superimposed at any time on the going statistical system. A 1966 census found almost as many chronic patients outside the mental hospital as were inside. The hospital patients, however, were predominantly long-term residents of earlier cohorts of patients; the extramural patients were predominantly drawn from recent cohorts. This pattern could have portended a build-up of chronically disabled patients in the community. At the least the distribution indicated that substantial services were needed for chronically disabled patients outside the mental hospitals. A report of such a census will reveal whether the rate of chronic disability was rising, falling, or stable, and thus provide one measure for evaluating the accomplishment of the program.

Studies needed to measure the accomplishment of social experiments in a virgin situation are usually difficult and elaborate. Where there is a register, they can often be simplified. The register can be augmented by special follow-up studies, by sample population studies, and by other opportune devices. In the matter of social work, sample studies were made. As noted above, in one sample the proportion of patients discharged from the mental hospital and notified to the mental health service for social work at any time was only 8 percent. Two years later, because of the response to this observation, well over half the discharged patients were notified to the social workers within one week of their discharge.

Among those not notified to social workers after discharge, however, the proportion readmitted within six months was almost twice as high as among those who were notified. The difference was even greater when account was taken of which patients had actually had the early aftercare that notification made possible. Not all patients notified were selected by the social workers to be visited within a month of their discharge. The lowest proportion of readmissions occurred among those patients notified to social workers and visited within one month, despite the fact that the increased attention they received also increased their exposure to the risk of admission.

This sample study of social work was based on the manual matching and linking of precoded records of service. Later, a computer program that automatically linked all records relating to a single individual gave a considerable fillip to the potential of the register for evaluating accomplishment. For instance, the program extended greatly the power to construct life tables for analyzing prognosis. Outcomes could be examined in relation to whatever antecedent conditions were included in the record. It became possible to follow the development of recurrences, chronic disability, admissions and discharges, and deaths, and to relate all these to previous experiences of the patient, either before or after he entered psychiatric care.

This extended capacity adds also to the potential of the psychiatric register in its fourth function of studying the *determinants* of mental sickness and of its outcome. Before we proceed, some problems of selecting a unit of observation for the register should be noted. The unit of observation recorded in Salford was the onset of an episode of entry to psychiatric care. The onset of every episode is marked by the mobilization of services. The total number of episodes over a period of time therefore gives a good index of the call on services during that time.

But unqualified episodes do not serve to tell us which individuals in the population, and what proportions of various groups, are being served. Total episodes include recurrences distributed unequally among individuals. Some individuals have many episodes, some have none, and some can have none because they remain sick. For these purposes, an unduplicated count of individuals receiving care, as well as of episodes of care, is wanted. Use of the individual as unit of observation, linked with episodes, can reveal which kinds of people have many recurrences, and which have few.

It is essential to follow individuals, moreover, to study outcome through the years. An account of individual experience can be derived from episodes, as long as care is taken to identify the first episode of all individuals who enter the services during the period of study. The first appearance of individuals in a service is, therefore, a unit used by some registers. For many purposes it is an unsatisfactory unit, because the count of individuals during the first years of study include the carry-over of past patients who are having recurrences, or whose illness is continuing through the period of study. These cases, which dwindle over several years, inflate initial rates and create an artificial declining trend of first episodes.

The decline continues until the reservoir of the past is exhausted. In some registers this problem is circumvented by using the *first annual* appearance of an individual in the register as the unit. This unit can also be derived from recorded episodes. The measurement is stable and does not decline from year to year. It serves to identify in each calendar year the size and characteristics of the service population. But this annual count of individuals does not give a clear measure of the number and characteristics of the *new* people coming into the service each year.

In order to get a clear view of both trends and determinants in mental sickness, one needs a measure of the onset of new sickness. A measure of *inceptions* of sickness tells what is happening at the time of concern; no overlay from the past is included in the trend to diminish its sensitivity to the present. The inception, that is, the patient's first episode ever, is also the best unit of measurement that a register can provide for the study of determinants of sickness. As time passes experience intervenes and changes the nature of the case. A study of determinants after the event, therefore, requires observations made as soon as possible after the first manifestation of the event, in order to exclude the intrusion of irrelevant confounding factors in the interim between onset and observation.

Three questions about inceptions arise: (1) how to measure duration; (2) the clinical identity and diagnostic reliability between inceptions and recurrences; and (3) the degree to which inception of service is a valid indication of inception of mental disorder.

The measurement of duration is difficult because episodes of mental sickness among ambulant patients do not end in the abrupt way that they begin. The simple measure of duration of stay used for mental hospitals has no equivalent for outpatient care. Episodes of care trail off into visits at increasing intervals, or patients themselves discontinue their visits, and the end of care is seldom definitely noted. To obtain an approximate measure of duration among outpatients thus requires regular review of all patient files in the relevant facilities, and some registers have deployed the relatively large resources needed for this task. In Salford, with minimal resources, the register made do with two inexpensive and clearcut measures related to duration. One was the frequency of recurrent episodes. The other was the prevalence at an annual census of chronic disability persisting for at least one year. A good estimate of overall duration of episodes could in fact have been obtained from a record of duration of care for all patients at each annual census.

The problem of diagnostic reliability and validity arises because a proportion of diagnoses are found to change between inception and recurrence. Reliability between diagnosticians, or of the same diagnostician at different times, is never complete. Training overcomes some but not the whole of this problem. Mental disorders unfold with time and new manifestations appear. Recurrences lead to new diagnoses: cases are more likely to be labelled as neuroses at the outset, and as schizophrenic after many recurrences. Recurrences may also be provoked by a new set of symptoms; for example, anxiety states may be followed or accompanied by depression. These shifts and turns create problems for the analyst of register data, but they can be turned to account as subjects for study in their own right.

The relationship of inception of service to inception of mental disorder is basic, and has created endless confusion and conflict among researchers. Each inception of an episode of service is an end point as much as a beginning. It is the end point of a process that turns a person into a psychiatric patient. The data on inceptions of service measure precisely a point of transformation, the individual's assumption of the role of psychiatric patient. This is a sick role, and therefore the unit of observation is designated as an episode of *sickness*. These episodes are a measure of the dysfunction of the individual's relation with others, a social phenomenon that has meaning in itself.

Mental *illness* is a term that conveniently describes the individual's subjective perception of his dysfunction, a process confined to the individual at the conscious psychological level. These are the conditions elicited, in the main, by the questionnaires and symptom-inventories of prevalence surveys. Mental *disease* or *impairment* are terms that conveniently describe pathology, a process confined to the individual at the organic, physiological, or psychic level. These are the conditions that traditional clinical methods are designed to elicit.

Organic, psychological, and social criteria yield different frequencies of mental disorder in populations. Each unit of observation measures something different, and makes separate contributions to our understanding of disorders. The fact that the criteria do not have a one-to-one relationship with each other is not a matter for despair. The use of different units of observation for the manifestations of each level of individual organization, if clearly conceptualized, well-defined, and applied with discrimination, brings new understanding as the relationships between the different units are examined.

Discrepancies among these three levels of observation are common to all types of health disorders, but with mental disorders the discrepancies are more obvious. Innumerable persons are affected by pathology without perceiving their dysfunction and being ill. Innumerable other persons perceive themselves as being ill without adopting the sick role. The converse also holds, if in lesser degree. Malingerers are sick without illness or pathology. Individuals of normal intelligence with a history of social deviance are often classed as sick and given the label of mild mental retardation, merely because they can thereby be incarcerated in institutions.

The degree to which inceptions of service correlate with inceptions of psychopathology varies with social circumstances and with the type of pathology. On the one hand, values and attitudes about mental disorders, available social support, and existing facilities for care influence entry to psychiatric services. The type of psychopathology is no less influential. Undoubtedly, many cases of psychoneurosis never reach psychiatric services. More severe derangements may bring people to psychiatric services only after some delay. This was surely the situation in Salford, but an intimate knowledge of the city led us to believe that the great majority of persons whose performance of social roles was entirely disrupted by mental disorder did reach psychiatric services.

Epidemiology, in its approach to the determinants of health disorders, generally begins with a description of the natural history of the disorder through the systematic study of its evolution, its distribution in the population, and its outcome. Service records provide a convenient checkpoint where sizable collections of cases can be gathered. Analysis of episodes gathered in this way by diagnosis and by basic demographic variables—age, sex, marital state, and social class—yields a great deal of descriptive information. For instance, the analysis tells what characteristics put people at high risk of an inception, or at high risk of repeated episodes. It can also tell what characteristics of an inception episode point to a high risk of recurrent episodes.

For example, Figure 6.2 shows inception rates and total episode rates for men, women, and total population by age. Both inceptions and episodes have bimodal curves, so that mental sickness, we can be sure, is not a simple deteriorative process of aging. Inceptions have one peak in the thirties, and another and

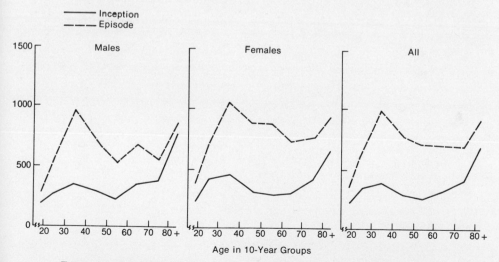

FIGURE 6.2. Salford mental illness, 1959–1963 (adults), all cases, inception and episode rates per 100,000 by age and ses. *Source:* M. Susser, *Community Psychiatry: Epidemiologic and Social Themes* (1968), Random House, New York p. 177

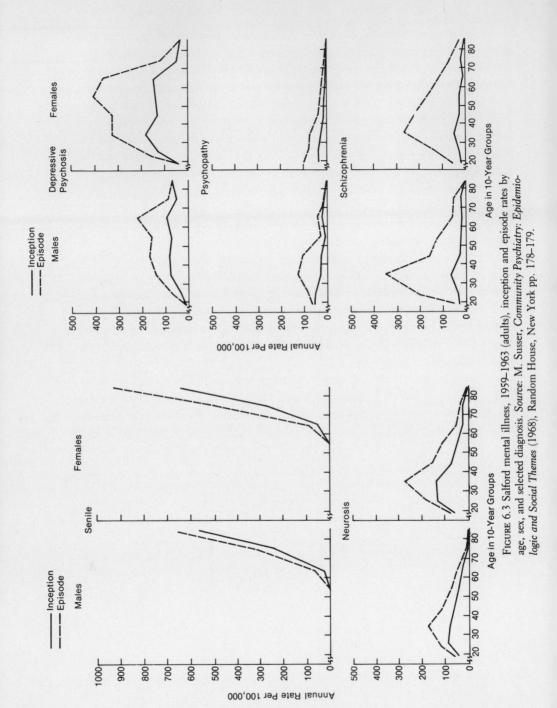

FIGURE 6.3 Salford mental illness, 1959–1963 (adults), inception and episode rates by age, sex, and selected diagnosis. *Source:* M. Susser, *Community Psychiatry: Epidemiologic and Social Themes* (1968), Random House, New York pp. 178–179.

higher peak in old age. The highest episode/inception ratio, however, the age group with the greatest number of recurrent episodes, is generated in the thirties age group. In old age there is a low ratio of episodes to inceptions, indicating that at this stage the high rate of inceptions tends to occur once and for all, with infrequent recoveries.

Figure 6.3 shows inceptions and episodes for selected diagnoses. The rate of senile dementia rises very sharply with increasing age. Psychopathy reaches a peak before twenty years of age, neurosis before thirty, schizophrenia before forty. Together these three diagnoses create the first peak of the bimodal curve for all diagnoses. A high episode/inception ratio, which suggests chronicity and a heavy use of services, is especially noticeable in schizophrenia, but the high frequency of recurrent episodes does not continue at the same rate throughout life. Even allowing for schizophrenic patients in long-term care, who could contribute no further episodes of schizophrenia, the sharp decline in the episode/inception ratio suggests that the sickness burned itself out. The same is true of psychoneurosis and psychopathy.

The curve for psychotic depression among women provides a good illustration of the function of descriptive epidemiology in generating hypotheses. The inception curve is bimodal, with a drop at the forty- to fifty-year age group following a peak in the thirties. This lowering of the rate at the time of the menopause reduces the tenability of a specific syndrome of "involutional melancholia." But the curve for total episodes at the time of the menopause indicates a very high rate of recurrent episodes, chronicity, and service usage. It seems likely that clinical impressions about involutional syndromes were generated more by the chronicity and cumulative recurrences of depressive illness at the time of involution than by its onset. The bimodal inception curves suggest two alternative hypotheses: (1) the determinants of depressive sickness are different among young and old people; or (2) the syndromes of depressive sickness are different among young and old people.

Figure 6.4 again illustrates the hypothesis-generating function of the descriptive epidemiology derived from a psychiatric register. The diagram shows the standardized distributions of each marital state in three Salford populations: (1) the 1961 census population; (2) among inceptions; and (3) among the chronically disabled. If the census is taken as the standard, the married have lower rates of inception and chronic disability than expected from the census, and the single have much higher rates.

But the widowed had higher rates only of inceptions, and they had a lower rate than expected of chronic disability. These distributions suggest that the state of widowhood was associated with an increase in mental sickness of short duration. These distributions alone, however, do not indicate whether widowhood is a causal factor in mental sickness, or even whether it is a factor antecedent to the inception of mental sickness.

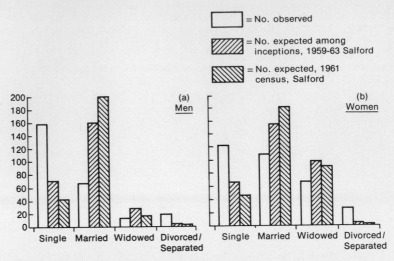

FIGURE 6.4. Numbers observed in each marital status among patients with chronic disability compared with the numbers expected, given the same age-sex distribution as the population and chronic disability; (1) among inceptions and (2) in the 1961 census. *Source:* Z. Stein and M. Susser, "Widowhood and Mental Illness," *British Journal of Preventive and Social Medicine* 23(1969):106–110.

The hypothesis was tested in an explanatory study based on other register data. This analytical hypothesis-testing study showed that transition into the widowed role, defined as the period shortly after bereavement, did in fact generate a high rate of inceptions of mental sickness. The register facilitated one of the all-too-few studies that demonstrate a clear-cut precipitating causal factor in mental sickness.

These examples have not illustrated the interaction of psychiatric register and community psychiatric service in full for every phase of development of such a service. They may perhaps be enough to establish their symbiosis. Even if register and community service might exist independently, each is bound to be poorer without the other.

SELECTED BIBLIOGRAPHY

Acheson, E. D., *Medical Record Linkage*. New York: Oxford University Press, 1967.

Adelstein, A. M., Downham, D.Y., Stein, Zena, Susser, M. W., "The Epidemiology of Mental Illness in an English City." *Social Psychiatry* 3 (1968): 47–59.

Bahn, A. K. "A New Psychiatric Epidemiology." *The Israel Annals of Psychiatry and Related Disciplines* 2 (1964): 11–18.

Bahn, A. K., Gardner, E. A., Alltop, L., Knatterud, G. L., Solomon, M. "Admission and Prevalence Rates for Psychiatric Facilities in Four Register Areas." *Amer. J. Publ. Hlth.* 56 (1966): 2033–2051.

Baldwin, J. A. *The Mental Hospital in the Psychiatric Service: A Case Register Study.* New York: Oxford University Press for the Nuffield Provincial Hospitals Trust, 1971.

Gardner, E. A., Miles, H. C., Iker, H. P., Romano, J. "A Cumulative Register of Psychiatric Services in a Community." *Amer. J. Publ. Hlth.* 53 (1963): 1269–1277.

Richman, A., 1970. "The use of case-registers of psychiatric care in epidemiological research of mental disorders," in *Psychiatric Epidemiology*, E. H. Hare, J. K. Wing, eds. New York: Oxford University Press for the Nuffield Provincial Hospitals Trust, pp. 257–272.

Susser, M. *Community Psychiatry: Epidemiologic and Social Themes.* New York: Random House, 1968.

Vanweerd, J., Giel, R. "Central Patient Registers." *Tijd. Psych.* 16 (1974): 543.

Wing, J., Bransby, R., eds. 1970. "Psychiatric Case Registers." *DHSS Statis. Rep. Ser.* No. 8 London HMSO.

Wing, J. K. and Hailey, A. M., eds. 1972.: *Evaluating a Community Psychiatric Service: The Camberwell Register 1964–1971.* New York: Oxford University Press for the Nuffield Provincial Hospitals Trust.

Wing, L. "Use of Psychiatric Services in 3 Urban Areas: An International Case Register Study." *Social Psychiatry* 2 (1967): 158–167.

Editorial Note

Jerome D. Frank's chapter offers an excellent illustration of the relationship between types of therapy and the sociocultural events that are thought to be important in the development of psychiatric disorder. In keeping with our integration-disintegration frame of reference, this chapter provides a view of therapy as a set of social and psychological skills which maximize social adaptation. More precisely, Frank points out that the need for psychotherapy is usually the consequence of some form of social breakdown.

Therapy attempts are old and varied in technique. Frank's concerns are with psychotherapy based on current naturalistic concepts of human nature and the proliferation of different types of therapists far in excess of traditional psychiatric manpower. But we are also reminded that religio-magical healing attempts are ancient; the questions of basic identity and elementary fear are among the very first ones posed in the Bibical view of the human situation.

It is also important to note that Frank's view of prevention involves provision of integrative social supportive opportunities. How can these best be supplied and evaluated?

The kinds of therapies that we have, or have had, are reflections of our society as well as of our theories about disease and health. Therefore, we may ask how therapy alternatives can best be fitted to sociocultural contexts.

Frank sees all psychotherapies as aimed to combat "demoralization" (i.e., helplessness, isolation, sense of failure, powerlessness). Should program efforts be directed toward a better epidemiological picture of this demoralization?

B. H. K.

CHAPTER 7

New Therapeutic Roles

JEROME D. FRANK

THE CURRENT psychotherapeutic scene displays a bewildering profusion of individual and group activities proffered by various nonprofessionals as well as professionals to a wide variety of people in many diverse settings. A recent text requires some 300 pages simply to summarize the psychotherapies now extant.[55] This proliferation is in response to a burgeoning demand for psychotherapeutic services. Since professionals could not meet this demand by themselves, they have undertaken to train nonprofessionals to organize and administer agencies providing mental health services on a community-wide basis. This extension of the target of psychotherapy from the individual to the community arises from the recognition that the kinds of distress and disability for which psychotherapy is offered are related to breakdown of the person's adaptation to his environment, leading to expansion of the therapeutic goal to include prevention by efforts to ameliorate environmental stresses. As a result, mental health professionals find themselves today in the roles of educators, consultants to agencies concerned with various aspects of social welfare, and even community organizers.

In view of this situation, any attempt at a definitive presentation of new therapeutic roles would be premature and will not be attempted. Instead, this chapter offers a brief historical review as the best means of gaining a perspective on the current scene, followed by consideration of encounter groups and community mental health centers. As the two most innovative therapeutic activities at opposite ends of the spectrum, they highlight the major issues involved. A

111

third section attempts to reduce the apparent confusion of the current scene by the hypothesis that the primary target of all forms of psychotherapy is demoralization, which takes protean forms, and that the effectiveness of all psychotherapies lies primarily in certain shared features that combat this state of mind. Finally, a few very tentative predictions as to future developments are offered.

The Current Scene in Historical Perspective

Religio-magical healing.   Since this chapter confines itself to forms of psychotherapy based on naturalistic concepts of human nature, it may be well to start with a reminder that these exclude a large class of healing methods and theories which probably attract more sufferers than those we shall discuss. From time immemorial humans have turned to supernatural forces to combat their sense of meaninglessness and confusion and to gain power over themselves, other persons, and natural events.

For several reasons, religio-magical healing was for centuries the treatment of choice for forms of suffering now classed as mental illness. The sufferer saw himself as in the grip of phenomena that lay outside his normal experience or that of his fellows. They likewise must have been puzzled by his report of experiences that seemed to have no natural causes, such as hallucinations, or by behavior that seemed motivated by forces that they could not understand. Moreover, these conditions often included feelings of guilt or other emotions inseparably linked to questions of ethics and the meaning of existence. Thus religio-magical healers and healing sects have never ceased to flourish throughout the world, even in those societies in which the scientific world-view dominates, as evidenced by the popularity of Christian Science and healing evangelists in the United States. Today we are witnessing an invasion of mystical sects from the Orient, such as Sufi, Hare Krishna, and transcendental meditation, which offer spiritual peace and bodily health. (A strong selling point of the last is that the bodily changes it produces are demonstrable by scientific methods.) A disquieting phenomenon is the upsurge of interest in less benign cults such as witchcraft and Satanism, which gain their appeal, I believe, because they promise their adherents control over the menacing phenomena of modern life, including those emanating from fellow humans. The popularity of astrology may have the same source, especially because of its claim to prophesy coming events.

The emergence and proliferation of naturalistic psychotherapies.   Turning our backs, with some reluctance, on this fascinating area, we may note that naturalistic psychotherapy first appeared on the Western stage in the late eighteenth century under the somewhat disreputable sponsorship of Franz Anton Mesmer, who, as a physician whose theories contained a large admixture of the occult, represented a fusion of the religio-magical and scientific traditions. Mesmerism had many features of therapies popular today. Patients were treated in groups by a charismatic therapist whose methods included thinly veiled sexual stimulation and the creation of emotional states in the participants sufficiently powerful to send many of them into prolonged convulsions.

Mesmer's theories, which ran counter to the intellectual climate of the Enlightenment, coupled with his flamboyant, contentious personality, led to his being branded a charlatan and driven from France. Mesmerism, however, continued to arouse lively interest and evolved into the more respectable hypnotism, which has continued to flourish until this day. The creator of psychotherapy as a distinct discipline with an organized body of knowledge and theory linked to a special procedure, Sigmund Freud, came to psychoanalysis via hypnotism.

Until mid-twentieth century, psychoanalysis and its modifications dominated psychotherapy, and its practitioners were almost exclusively psychiatrists. While only a small minority are psychoanalysts, psychiatrists still have the highest prestige in the field in the eyes of the general public. Social workers, initially handmaidens of physicians who dealt with the environmental problems of patients, became involved relatively early in psychotherapy, especially with children, under the rubric of casework. Like their psychiatrist teachers, they practiced forms of interview therapy aimed at fostering the patient's self-understanding.

In addition to psychiatrists and psychiatric social workers, members of a variety of nonmedical helping professions conducted activities resembling psychotherapy, although not labeled as such, for help seekers who were not seen as patients. The largest group among these help givers were the clergy, to whom about half of persons with personal problems went first for help,[29] followed by parole officers, school counselors, and the like.

The range of persons for whom psychotherapy was considered appropriate was small. They were mainly middle- and upper-class, educated city dwellers suffering from forms of distress that Freud and his followers had identified as psychoneuroses and who had heard of psychoanalysis as a means of getting help—a group which has been termed "the friends and supporters of psychotherapy." [30] Persons with problems of child-rearing and married life also came to psychotherapists.

Developments since World War II—New training programs. The psychotherapeutic explosion, in which we are still living, seems to have been initiated by World War II which, by making psychotherapy available to military personnel and their families, created an awareness of its existence and potential helpfulness among large segments of the population who had been hitherto ignorant of it. The immediate response of the military to the resulting increased demand was to use psychologists in addition to psychiatrists as psychotherapists, and to start treating soldiers in groups rather than individually, two innovations which have become firmly established.

Since the war, extensive programs of mental health education, conducted by private and public agencies, have led more and more people in all walks of life to define their troubles as treatable by psychotherapy. One gains the impression that we have become a psychotherapy-intoxicated culture, demanding of psychotherapy that it perform many of the functions previously carried out by helpful family members and friends, as well as expecting it to supply meaning and significance to life, hitherto the province of traditional religions.

This cultural attitude soon found tangible expression in the provision of federal funds for the expansion of training programs, especially for psychiatrists and psychologists, and the extension of psychotherapeutic services. A landmark was the Mental Health Act of 1946, providing for expansion of existing mental health programs and creation of new ones for rehabilitation and prevention of mental illness on a community-wide scale. In 1963 came the further step of the creation of community mental health centers, with a wide range of therapeutic and preventive services. By purporting to make these services available to large new segments of the population, notably in the slums of the cities, community mental health services have further contributed to the demand for psychotherapy.

The first response to the increased demand was the expansion of training programs for professionals. A recent survey indicated that there were about 20,000 psychiatrists, 23,000 social workers, and 23,000 clinical psychologists.[23] One would think that this small army would be sufficient, but it is not. As the realization has dawned that a high level of expertise is not necessary to be able to help many recipients of psychotherapy, and that the effectiveness of professionals could be multiplied if they devoted more time to training others and less to doing therapy themselves, emphasis is shifting from the training of mental health professionals to programs which use them to train para- and nonprofessionals to perform many of their functions.[43]

Within mental hospitals, psychiatric nurses and aides have for years been trained to do simple psychotherapy and, especially, to conduct groups of patients on the wards.

Since the vast majority of persons considered suitable for psychotherapy are not hospitalized, the great bulk of new training programs are directed toward members of the community. A recent count revealed some 150, covering the entire educational spectrum.[56] Some programs are offered to members of other professions, such as general physicians, ministers, lawyers, public health nurses, and teachers, as well as welfare workers, probation officers, and vocational counselors. The programs endeavor to teach them three categories of mental health skills—evaluation, intervention by means of individual interviews and group discussions, and referral.[37]

A much larger pool of potential psychotherapists consists of laymen with a college degree,[22] especially those with the kind of life experience that has familiarized them with developmental and adjustment problems, notably housewives who have raised or are raising a family. A pioneer program for this group, which is being widely emulated, consists of two years of intensive training with main emphasis on supervision. Graduates receive an M.A. degree and are termed "mental health counselors." [10] They work primarily in professional settings and carry out all therapeutic activities of psychiatrists except the prescription of medications. They also are capable of assuming considerable administrative responsibilities.

An example of an intermediate level program is one offering an Associate in Arts (A.A.) degree after two years to new high school graduates, women with grown children, and existing subprofessional workers who wanted to upgrade their skills, salary, and prestige. It includes specialized courses and field experience in mental retardation, emotional disturbances, community programs, and social welfare. The program also includes extensive participation in small groups conceptualized as laboratories in human relations training. Graduates are termed "mental health generalists." [19] A similar program terms its graduates "mental health technicians"; their training qualifies them to carry out primary patient care, crisis intervention, and triage.[12]

At the lowest educational level, community mental health centers offer brief programs for members of the communities they serve, as will be considered more fully below.

The programs outlined so far have been created and are conducted by mental health professionals. To complete the survey of new therapeutic roles, two additional groups must be mentioned. One of these is so amorphous and variegated that its members cannot be categorized. It consists of the leaders of the vast panorama of activities included under the rubric of encounter groups or personal growth centers.[2] The leaders range from highly skilled professionals,[42,47] through persons who have worked with these professionals, to persons who, having attended one or two such groups, proceed to conduct groups of their own. These fade into the final category, that of sufferers from various forms of distress or disability who have banded together to help themselves and, in so doing, train themselves to help others. Notable examples of these peer self-help psychotherapy groups [27,45] are Alcoholics Anonymous, Recovery Incorporated,[52] and self-help programs for drug addicts, of which Synanon is the pioneer.[50]

Personal Motivations of Psychotherapists. The motivations of many persons who seek careers in psychotherapy are the same as those for any career: the opportunity to earn more money and gain enhanced status and self-esteem by performing a socially valued function. These operate especially in housewives with grown children who are searching for a new role, in members of the lower echelons of health services, in young people who have not completed their educations, and in slum dwellers who view these careers as opportunities to escape the underclass and become integrated into the larger society. However, motives specific to this particular career may also be involved. It has been suggested that psychotherapy is a form of therapy for the therapist as well as the patient.[53] Many leaders of encounter groups do not hesitate to ask the group's help for their own problems, and these groups provide ready gratification of the leader's desires for power, attention, and intimacy.

It has been noted that in the larger cities mental health professionals are drawn preponderantly from marginal, upwardly mobile subcultures, and would therefore be expected to be sensitized to the personal impact of social oppression.[25] Many have personal backgrounds that fostered a sense of isolation and heightened awareness of inner events. For them, "the psychic gains of intimacy are made in the office and not in the home" (p. 53).[24] Along the same lines, a study of psychiatric residents concluded that most are emotionally conflicted and achieve personal integration through their professional and therapeutic role.[13] By virtue of having problems of their own, psychotherapists are able to empathize more readily with the similar problems of their clientele.

Personal Growth Centers and Community Mental Health Centers

To bring the new psychotherapeutic roles into clearer focus, it may be helpful to look more closely at the two most actively innovative areas: the personal growth centers and community mental health centers. These two very different responses to social demands, tailored to two ends of the social and economic spectrum, offer sharp contrasts in almost all respects. At the same time, they have raised profound questions as to the nature and goals of psychotherapy and, concomitantly, the role definition of the psychotherapist—questions which at this writing remain largely unanswered.

Personal growth centers. Reasons for the phenomenal growth of personal growth centers and encounter groups have been discussed elsewhere.[2,14,16,28] In any case, their growth has been spontaneous, unplanned, and uncontrolled. They represent a response to the demands of a particular segment of the population—well-educated, relatively affluent, mobile, and suffering from malaises they attribute to such features of American life as careerism, bureaucratization, and impersonality. Many have had, or are in, psychotherapy. Bored, restless, feeling isolated, satiated with mechanical, impersonal stimuli such as television, and having doubts as to the meaning of existence, they seek experiences to overcome these demoralizing states of mind. Participants are self-selected, unscreened, and usually have to expend considerable money and effort in order to participate.

Encounter groups foster open, nondefensive, intimate interactions with others and fuller communication with one's own feelings. They strive to expand the consciousness of their participants, and sometimes to help them find a new meaning in life through transcendental experiences.

Although most of the leaders of these groups initially had some professional training in the mental health field, as mentioned earlier, many leaders have no particular training other than participation in an encounter group themselves.

The settings for encounter groups are equally diverse, ranging from hotel rooms and private homes to public meeting halls or personal growth centers such as Esalen. Their only common feature is that they are separated from the participant's usual environment. The experiences they provide last several hours at a minimum, and may last for a week or so.

The procedures of these groups are so diverse as to defy classification, and their leaders seem to be engaged in a frantic competition for innovativeness and novelty. Most stress emotional arousal, usually fostered by some sort of bodily interaction, and freedom of verbal expression. [26,47] The goal is to provide rewarding personal experiences for the participants, even if the behavior necessary to achieve them would be considered outrageous outside the group. There is no concern with the relationship of the participants to others in the community. As a result, many participants have a "reentry problem" as they try to carry over behaviors learned in the group to their customary settings.

Community Mental Health Centers. At the other end of the psychotherapeutic spectrum are the community mental health centers. These are manifestations of a humanitarian effort by members of the dominant culture to mitigate the subjective distress and disruptive behavior of members of the lower classes. They seem to be a response on the one hand to increasingly insistent and intrusive demands from the disadvantaged for mitigation of the hardships of their lives, and on the other to what may be termed "mental health imperialism"—the redefinition of social and ethical dilemmas and problems as "mental illnesses" requiring "treatment" (Chap. 3).[49] This conceptualization is epitomized by the title of a brochure of a community mental health center: "Mental Health Affects Everyone." It has been strengthened by surveys showing a large amount of "significant psychopathology" among stratified samples of citizens.[48]

Thus the impetus toward the creation of community mental health centers comes not from consumers but from providers of mental health care. These centers were created by legislation drawn up by health professionals and supported by public funds.

The mission of community mental health centers was conceived as basically twofold: treatment and prevention. In contrast to the personal growth centers, which seek to enrich experience, the goal of treatment was conceived as helping the patient to improve his behavior. The assumption was that his distress was primarily caused by maladaptive ways of behaving, and that if he could learn to cope more effectively with the stresses of his environment, he would feel better. This usually implies changing his behavior to make it more acceptable to the community. In addition to direct services, these centers were to provide consultative and educational services to other agencies concerned with community and personal problems. These activities were somewhere between treatment and prevention.

The concept of prevention grew out of the recognition that: *"There is an intimate relationship between the social organization of the community and the individual psychological organization of its residents"* (p. 60, italics in original).[39] Prevention, therefore, meant improvement of the quality of life of the community, especially through the efforts of the citizens themselves. Citizen involvement was seen by some as sociotherapy, "a professionally guided treatment modality for the supposed apathy and lack of motivation of the poor," (p. 174)[3] which involved two aspects: participation by personnel of the center in community development, and participation of community members not only in community betterment but also in determination of the policies and programs of the centers.

In contrast to the encounter groups, mental health centers are expected to take full responsibility for the effectiveness of their services, and this responsibility is squarely located in the professional staff. Because it was recognized that there would not be nearly enough of these to go around, however, and also in pursuance of the aim of fostering community participation, all mental health centers train members of the community to serve in various ways. Training programs for these "indigenous nonprofessionals" [21] of "new careerists," [54] to give two typical appellations, are usually brief and stress observation and learning by doing under close supervision. They may include participation in training groups and role playing.[39,46] Some see a covert goal of these training programs as offering a kind of therapy for the trainees: "Under the umbrella of training we may be able to . . . encourage effective coping behavior rather than decompensation in the face of insoluble personal and reality problems" (p. 1183).[40]

In sharp contrast to encounter groups, the clientele of community mental health centers is defined by the location of the center, typically in slum areas, and therefore typically consists of lower-class members of disadvantaged groups. Since these centers had to create a demand for their services, the clientele needed to be informed that such services were available and could be helpful. Some, of course, get the services whether they want them or not. As has already been implied, the target is not primarily the individual, but the individual in relation to his community.

The treatment programs of these centers are essentially conventional. They include much simple guidance and counseling. Most make heavy use of group and family approaches and psychodramatic methods, all of which have been found to be especially helpful with lower-class patients.

With respect to the organization and functioning of these centers, except for the fact that professionals make final decisions, roles are loosely defined. Professionals not only conduct conventional therapy but also run programs of education and become involved in community organization. The roles of the nonprofessionals are equally varied. In one program, the "mental health aide" is described as a " 'friend in need,' a potential counselor, a model and a sustainer of hope. . . . He relies most heavily on techniques of giving information, advice and counsel, persuasion and environmental manipulation. He also participates in community action, community education and social planning . . ." (p. 769).[21] In another program, organized in terms of therapeutic teams, each team contains some nonprofessionals, and on each team one member is designated the "primary contact person," who is ideally the intake interviewer. This person may be any member of the team. "Everyone, regardless of discipline, is a primary therapist" (p. 9).[44] In another program the nonprofessionals participate in and eventually act as co-therapists in various patient groups and carry their own caseloads.[7]

Psychotherapy As a Social Institution

The activities of both encounter groups and community mental health centers can be viewed as psychotherapeutic in the sense that both aim to relieve psychologically induced distress. As such, both highlight certain culturally interrelated problems with respect to the place of psychotherapy as a social institution with reference to the larger society, the appropriate targets and goals of psychotherapy, the training and role of the psychotherapist, and psychotherapeutic procedures themselves.

Most of these problems are highlighted better by the community mental health centers than by personal growth centers because the policies of the former are explicit and the procedures are organized. Therefore, what follows will focus mainly on them.

In general, they have thus far fallen short of their professed aims for a variety of reasons.[8] Being innovative in many respects, they were not adequately conceptualized or funded for some of the functions they were expected to perform. The expectations of the granting agency were not always effectively communicated to the staffs, nor were the community expectations clear. The staff members had not received training for the new roles, and these themselves were unclear.[11,34]

Within the centers, these unclarities inevitably created power struggles among the professionals and tensions in their relations with the nonprofessionals, to whom their attitudes often fluctuated between patronizing overacceptance and covert or overt rejection. The nonprofessionals often found failure to live up to the promises of advancement implied by the program, with resulting resentment.[4]

The aim of preventing mental illness through promotion of the mental health of the community, which implies shifting the primary focus from the distressed individual to the living conditions which stress him, has opened a Pandora's box for all involved. Professional staffs found themselves expected to function as mental health educators, consultants to teachers, police, welfare workers, and members of other agencies in direct contact with the populace, and even to work for better schools and housing. Not having been trained for these activities, many fell back on trying to be therapists—by, for example, trying to give their clients "insight"—with unfortunate results.[38]

The statutory requirement of community participation has led to embroilments between the centers and the communities they serve. This participation has usually been nominal, with control of the programs remaining firmly in professional hands, which becomes a source of community resentment. When genuine community participation has been achieved, it typically has degenerated into a struggle for control of the agency's policies and programs, with the community pressing for more social action than the professionals find comfortable.[3] This has activated conflicts latent in the center's dual mission of providing clinical and preventive services, creating confusion within the agency as well as struggles between it and the community. Caught squarely in the middle are the new careerists who, as members of the community, are torn between offering therapy and leading marches on City Hall to seek redress of community grievances.[4]

From a broader perspective, this uncertainty as to mission raises questions as to how far a publicly supported agency dare go in attacking the institutions on which it depends for support.[51]

In any case, as the experiences of community mental health centers make clear, psychotherapy can be a significant social force. This is explicit with the encounter groups, which see themselves as exemplifying a counterculture standing for values and behavior patterns superior to those of the larger community, but at present rejected by it. Community mental health centers could function as both conservative and radicalizing forces. As the former, they are supported by the community and therefore can be viewed as agents for maintaining the status quo. One writer even used the term "fire insurance" to describe them, seeming to imply that by ameliorating stresses or, more fundamentally, by teaching the clientele to conform to the dominant values, they could reduce the revolutionary pressures of the slums.[3] This aspect is also revealed in the fact that certain attitudes and forms of behavior which would be regarded by slum dwellers as appropriate to their condition, notably suspiciousness and resentment, are easily regarded by mental health professionals as signs of psychopathology. Perception of the community mental health center as an institution created by the power structure to pacify malcontents and dissidents is well expressed by some black paraprofessionals: "We must not allow the establishment to use us to pacify the community. We must . . . not become flunkeys doing the dirty work of our agency to 'cool out' the poor, especially blacks" (p. 600).[4,41]

On the other hand, anyone who takes the goal of prevention seriously is bound to recognize that it involves social reform.[17,20] As an eminent psychologist put it:

> We go on trying to fix up damaged adults in one-to-one relationships when a more proper professional function would be to spend a considerable portion of our energies trying to fix up a society in ways that will increase the strength and stability of the family, thereby affecting positively the mental health of generations to come . . . for prevention people like ourselves would be needed as teachers, researchers and, especially, as radical social activists, proselytizing for changes in our society to make it more supportive, less dehumanized (p. 875).[1]

In the light of such statements, it is easy to see how members of the extreme right could view the mental health movement as a threat to traditional customs and values. In their code this makes it a Communist conspiracy to undermine the American way of life.

With respect to the target of therapy, uncertainty as to the relative importance of the individual and the community has just been considered. As to individual recipients of therapy, many participants in encounter groups and clients of community mental health centers do not define themselves as candidates for psychotherapy. Yet many of both groups have symptoms or behave in ways which are considered appropriate targets for psychotherapy. In either case the distinction between therapist and patient is blurred. Thus some encounter group leaders make no distinction between themselves and other group members and feel free to ask the group to help them at times with their own emotions. The concept that training programs for nonprofessionals represent therapy for the nonprofessionals indicates a similar blurring of the distinction in the community mental health centers.

Both encounter groups and the mental health centers raise questions as to how much and what sort of professional training is necessary for the successful conduct of their activities. Encounter groups have simply avoided this issue because they have no standards, but it seems clear that leaders who have had no training other than participation in such groups themselves can be helpful to others. The matter has received more systematic attention in community mental health centers. Although some nonprofessionals, having found a career line, may develop scorn for their less fortunate clientele, nonprofessionals tend to be in closer touch with their patients than are professionals. Because they have not acquired the habit of categorizing behavior as symptomatic of a particular psychiatric disorder, they can more readily be empathic, and this is further facilitated by shared background and life experiences. Moreover, if they have overcome their clients' problem, they can serve as hope-inspiring models. Thus ex-drug addicts are particularly effective with addicts,[5] and ex-alcoholics do very well with alcoholics. The minimum amount of training, therefore, would seem to be enough to enable the therapist to become familiar with some sort of simple therapeutic rationale and procedure. Professional sanction is useful to give legitimacy to their activities, and may also be important from the standpoint of the assumption of responsibility for what transpires.

The Demoralization Hypothesis

This glance at the extreme limits of the settings to which patients with problems considered suitable for psychotherapy gravitate makes clear that we are dealing with a widespread social phenomenon that has no clear boundaries and which is in a state of flux approaching chaos. In general, it appears as if practically any kind of joint activity is helpful to some people, provided they and the therapist believe that it will help. In all probability this situation will persist for some time before clarity emerges. In the meanwhile, a few generalizations concerning consumers and methods of "psychotherapy" may be ventured as the beginnings of a framework for bringing some order into the field.

The consumers have certain similarities beneath their variegated appearances. First, all are suffering and many cause persons close to them to suffer. Second, these manifestations involve the total person, especially his communications with himself and others. Third, whether or not the suffering has bodily components, the main disturbance is at the symbolic level—very few persons come to psychotherapy only because they have physically attacked someone or have an organic disease.

Perhaps one can go further and suggest a common cause behind these phenomena which, as a first approximation, can be termed "demoralization." [15,16] The demoralized person feels, to varying degrees, hopeless, helpless, and isolated. He cannot cope with some aspect of his life and blames himself for his failure. He feels alienated from others, uncertain of the future, discouraged, and, especially in our generation, may have rejected traditional values without finding acceptable substitutes. Acute demoralization has been termed "crisis response"; [6] a more chronic form is called the "social breakdown syndrome." [18]

How a person shows demoralization depends on his sociocultural milieu, his personality, and his specific vulnerabilities. As a result, demoralization has innumerable manifestations, including drug or alcohol addiction, chronic bitterness at those he sees as the sources of his difficulties, social withdrawal, anxiety, depression, and the whole gamut of neurotic and psychotic symptoms. While many of these are not caused exclusively by demoralization, they interact with it. Symptoms like hallucinations and specific fears wax and wane with the person's general state of demoralization and, by reducing his coping capacities, aggravate it, creating a vicious circle.

Not all demoralized persons receive formal psychotherapy. In all probability, for most the stress is temporary, and many get sufficient informal help from family and friends. Some distrust psychotherapy, as indicated earlier, and some are so hopeless that they despair of seeking help from anyone.

The morale of an individual is powerfully affected by the morale of his group. This has been defined as "the capacity of a group of people to pull together consistently and persistently in pursuit of a common purpose" (p. 781),[31] and it depends on faith of the members in this purpose, in the leadership, and in each other. A group with high morale maintains the morale of its members by giving them a sense of purpose, power, and close linkages to each other—the antithesis of demoralization. The view advanced here that psychopathological symptoms reflect demoralization is consistent with the finding that their incidence goes down when group goals are strong and the society cohesive, as in wartime, and with the general finding that incidence of psychopathology is a function of the level of disorganization of the society.[33]

It needs no social scientist to observe that society in the United States is in a demoralized state, with citizens lacking a common purpose and evincing massive distrust of their fellows, leaders, and institutions. Demoralized persons, feeling powerless to help themselves, look for help from others. In stable periods this help is provided by traditional institutions such as the family and organized religions. In times of very rapid changes, such as today's, these institutions, having been formed under radically different conditions of life, fail to provide adequate psychological security, values, and guides for behavior.

The mushrooming of psychotherapies, which typically occurs in periods of social transition,[36] can be seen as society's effort at filling the gap until new institutions and value systems appropriate to the conditions of modern life emerge. This hypothesis is consistent with the massive demand for psychotherapy, its institutional support, and its social impact both as a reinforcer of old values and a promulgator of new ones.

In view of the enormous range of psychotherapeutic theories and procedures, the reader must be wondering by now what the justification could be for referring to psychotherapy as an entity. The reason is my belief that, since the common purpose of all psychotherapies is to combat demoralization, the features they share which have this effect are much more important than their differences. These features, which have been elaborated elsewhere,[14,15,32] combat hopelessness, helplessness, and isolation.

All psychotherapies involve a help giver who enters into an emotionally charged, confiding relationship with a help seeker, to whom he offers a conceptualization and a procedure in which both participants have faith. In conjunction, these make sense of the person's difficulties and suggest new ways of coping with them. The conceptual scheme may bolster the patient's current value system or offer a new, more viable one for guiding his conduct and giving meaning to life. The relationship, conceptualization, and procedure restore the patient's links to his fellows and instill new hope, courage, and confidence that he can master his problems. These therapeutic components can be discerned in the activities of all therapists, from the new careerist who guides the discouraged slum dweller through the maze of welfare bureaucracy to the encounter group leader who helps the group member to undergo a peak experience, although, of course, their relative salience may vary considerably, depending on the patient's problem and the therapist's approach.

Implications for the Future

If the hypothesis that the essential function of all forms of psychotherapy is to combat demoralization is valid, then one must wonder how long the widespread enthusiasm and public support for it will last. At present it has usurped functions usually performed by religion, education, and politics. Perhaps in time these traditional institutions of social adaptation will change so as to be able again to perform their proper functions, society will become better integrated, demoralization and its manifestations as psychopathological symptoms will be less prevalent, and the role of psychotherapy will become more limited.

For the present and near future, however, mental health professionals will continue to perform three roles: diagnosis and therapy, in which the target is a suffering individual; prevention, in which the target is the community; and training, the task of which is to train others to carry out the first two roles.

With respect to diagnosis and therapy, certain functions will probably remain the province of psychiatrists by virtue of their medical training. These include the evaluation of possible organic factors in mental illness and their management by medications. Along the same lines, unless the legal system is changed, psychiatrists will continue to bear the prime responsibility for care of persons whose behavior leads society to demand that they be removed from circulation as "patients" rather than "criminals." On both counts, psychiatrists will probably continue to look after persons with major psychoses.

For persons for whom psychotherapy is the treatment of choice, although diagnosis will probably remain a prerogative of professionals, in the absence of any evidence that current diagnostic categories bear any relationship to the relative effectiveness of different psychotherapies, it is impossible to predict what the proper diagnostic categories will be. Perhaps they will primarily concern evaluation of the patient's expectations, based on aspects of his background and personality, regarding the type of therapist and therapeutic approach that he would find most congenial.

As to therapy itself, we must face the fact that successful therapy, for the great majority of persons who come to psychotherapy, does not require that the therapist have any kind of elaborate training or an academic degree. In fact, for many patients nonprofessionals or fellow patients can serve as more persuasive models or be better able to empathize than professionals, by virtue of similar life experiences. However, it seems probable that professionals will maintain their preeminence with respect to some aspects of therapy.

Many persons will continue to insist on being treated by those who have an advanced degree and have mastered a particular approach because this is necessary for them to have faith in the therapist's competence. Because they embody the healing tradition, psychiatrists may continue to have a special advantage in this regard.

Among professionals there may well develop a division of labor, determined by patients' expectations as revealed by whom they seek out and the mode of communication by which they indicate their distress. It may be, for example, that psychiatrists will focus on patients who express their demoralization primarily through disturbances of bodily functioning; psychologists will work mainly with those who offer specific subjective or behavioral symptoms; clergy, with those who couch their demoralization in ethical or spiritual terms; and social workers, with persons who place major responsibility for their difficulties on environmental stresses.

Since demoralization results from an imbalance between personal coping capacity and environmental stress, the mental health professional cannot avoid attention to the amelioration of social evils. This brings him face-to-face with the problem of prevention. To what extent is it his responsibility to bring about beneficial changes in child-rearing practices and family structure, combat oppression, and foster community integration, and how should he go about it? The first point to bear in mind is that all hypotheses as to environmental causes of mental illness are tentative. It does not require professional insight to know that broken homes, malnutrition, and poor housing are demoralizing and injurious to both physical and mental health, but the most effective way to combat gross evils such as these is through the political process. If the mental health professional believes that socioeconomic reform should be his major concern, his most effective action would be to get elected to public office.

When it comes to subtler influences on mental health, such as blurring of family roles, certain forms of parental discipline, and so on, it is well to preserve a becoming humility. As has happened in the recent past, overenthuiastic claims and actions have produced only disillusionment, followed by a reduction in health professionals' effectiveness.

Moreover, the most effective point in the community structure at which to intervene to foster desirable changes is far from clear. When should it be the courts, when the schools, when the public housing authority? Nor can the effects of an intervention be predicted with any assurance, and sometimes they turn out to be the opposite of what was intended. [9]

While recognizing the importance of treading carefully and being ever mindful that hell is paved with good intentions, many mental health professionals will undoubtedly continue to participate in programs of prevention, like all clinicians doing the best they can in the light of imperfect knowledge and understanding.

It is obvious that, in the present state of ignorance, no preventive program should be contemplated that does not include provision for evaluation. However, this admonition, uttered countless times, will probably continue to be largely disregarded, mainly because evaluation is so difficult and doing something is more fun than evaluating what you have done.

Current programs for training the mental health professional have two features which should prove useful for all preventive activities. They confer status, which enables the professional to gain a respectful hearing, and they sensitize him to problems of communication and how to overcome them. However, it is clear that traditional programs do not fit mental health professionals for the roles of educator, consultant to community agencies, administrator of community mental health centers, or community organizer. Therefore, training in these roles will probably find an increasingly extensive place in these programs.

By and large, professionals possess better articulated conceptual schemes and methods, and many probably have greater verbal skill and higher intelligence, than most nonprofessionals. By virtue of these qualities, as well as their status, professionals will continue to conduct training programs and supervise the therapy of nonprofessionals. For the same reason, they will probably continue to play a leading part in planning, organizing, and running institutions supplying mental health services. However, it seems probable that much of training, supervision, and administration will gradually be taken over by nonprofessionals whom the professionals have trained. How far this process will go cannot be predicted, but a complete takeover by the nonprofessionals seems unlikely. More probable is that some point of relatively stable equilibrium will be reached.

REFERENCES

1. Albee, G. W. "Emerging Concepts of Mental Illness and Models of Treatment: The Psychological Point of View." *American Journal of Psychiatry* 125(1969):870–876.

2. Back, K. W. *Beyond Words: The Story of Sensitivity Training and the Encounter Movement.* New York: Russell Sage Foundation, 1972.

3. Bolman, W. M. "Community Control of the Community Mental Health Center: I. Introduction." *American Journal of Psychiatry* 129(1972):173–180.

4. Boyette, R.; Blount, W.; Petaway, K.; Jones, E.; and Hill, S. "The Plight of the New Careerist: A Bright Horizon Overshadowed by a Dark Cloud." *American Journal of Orthopsychiatry* 42(1972):596–602.

5. Borenstein, D. "The Relative Value of the Medical Staff versus Addicts in the Rehabilitation of the Drug Users in a Drug Abuse Program." *Johns Hopkins Medical Journal* 129(1971):290–297.

6. Caplan, G. "Emotional Crises." In *The Encyclopedia of Mental Health*, edited by A. Deutsch and H. Fishman, vol. 2, pp. 521–532. New York: Franklin Watts, 1963.

7. Christmas, J. J. "Group Methods in Training and Practice: Nonprofessional Mental Health Personnel in a Deprived Community." *American Journal of Orthopsychiatry* 36(1966): 410–419.

8. Chu, F. D., and Trotter, S. *Community Mental Health Centers.* Washington, D.C.: Center for the Study of Responsive Law, 1972.

9. Dunham, H. W. "Community Psychiatry: The Newest Therapeutic Bandwagon." *Archives of General Psychiatry* 12(1965):303–313.

10. Elkes, C.; Godenne, G. D.: and Stone, A. R. "The Making of Mental Health Counsellors." *HSMHA Health Reports* 86 (1971):307–313.

11. Enelow, A. J., and Weston, W. D., Jr. "Cooperation or Chaos: The Mental Health Administrator's Dilemma." *American Journal of Orthopsychiatry* 42(1972):603–609.

12. Fink, P. J., and Zeroff, H. "Mental Health Technology: An Approach to the Manpower Problem." *American Journal of Psychiatry* 127(1971):1082–1085.

13. Ford, E. S. C. "Being and Becoming a Psychotherapist: The Search for Identity." *American Journal of Psychotherapy* 17(1963):472–482.

14. Frank, J. D. 1971. "Therapeutic Factors in Psychotherapy." *American Journal of Psychotherapy* 25(1971):350–361.

15. ———. "Psychotherapy: The Restoration of Morale." *American Journal of Psychiatry* 131(1974):271–274.

16. ———. "An Overview of Psychotherapy." *Overview of the Psychotherapies*. Edited by Gene Urdin, pp. 3–24. New York: Brunner/Mazel.

17. Glidewell, J. "Priorities for Psychologists in Community Mental Health." In *Issues in Community Psychology and Preventive Mental Health*, edited by G. Rosenblum, pp. 141–153. New York: Behavioral Publications, 1971.

18. Gruenberg, E. M. "The Social Breakdown Syndrome—Some Origins." *American Journal of Psychiatry* 123(1967):1481–1489.

19. Hadley, J. M.; True, J. E.; and Kepes, S. Y. "An Experiment in the Education of the Preprofessional Mental Health Worker: The Purdue Program." *Community Mental Health Journal* 6(1970):40–50.

20. Halleck, S. L. *The Politics of Therapy*. New York: Science House, 1971.

21. Hallowitz, E., and Reissman, F. "The Role of the Indigenous Nonprofessional in a Community Mental Health Neighborhood Program." *American Journal of Orthopsychiatry* 37(1967):766–770.

22. Hansell, N.; Wodarczyk, M.; and Visotsky, H. M. "The Mental Health Expediter: A Review After Two Years of the Project and One Year of the Expediter in Action." *Archives of General Psychiatry* 18(1968):392–399.

23. *Health Resources Statistics*. Rockville, Md.: U.S. National Center for Health Statistics, 1969.

24. Henry, W. E. "Some Observations on the Lives of Healers." *Human Development* 9(1966):47–56.

25. ———; Sims, J. H.: and Spray, S. L. *The Fifth Profession*. San Francisco: Jossey-Bass, 1971.

26. Howard, J. *Please Touch: A Guided Tour of the Human Potential Movement*. New York: McGraw-Hill, 1970.

27. Hurvitz, N. "Peer Self-Help Psychotherapy Groups: Psychotherapy Without Psychotherapists." In *The Sociology of Psychotherapy*, edited by P. M. Roman and H. M. Trice, pp. 84–138. New York: Jason Aronson, 1974.

28. Jacobs, R. H. "Emotive and Control Groups as Mutated New American Utopian Communities." *Journal of Applied Behavioral Science* 7(1971):234–251.

29. Joint Commission on Mental Illness and Health. *Action for Mental Health: Final Report of the Joint Commission on Mental Illness and Health*. New York: Basic Books, 1961.

30. Kadushin, C. *Why People Go to Psychiatrists*. New York: Atherton, 1969.

31. Leighton, A. H. *Human Relations in a Changing World*. New York: E. P. Dutton, 1949.

32. ———. "Contribution to the Therapeutic Process in Cross-Cultural Perspective—A Symposium." *American Journal of Psychiatry* 124(1968);1176–1178.

33. Leighton, D. C.; Harding, J. S.; Macklin, D. B.; Macmillan, A. M.; and Leighton, A. H. *The Character of Danger*. New York: Basic Books, 1963.

34. Leopold, R. L. "Urban Problems and the Community Mental Health Center: Multiple Mandates, Difficult Choices." *American Journal of Orthopsychiatry* 41(1971):144–149.

35. Lieberman, M. A.; Yalom, I. D.; and Miles, M. B. *Encounter Groups: First Facts*. New York: Basic Books, 1973.

36. May, R. "Contribution to the Therapeutic Process in Cross-Cultural Perspective—A Symposium." *American Journal of Psychiatry* 124(1968):1179–1183.

37. Modlin, H. C., and Taylor, J. B. "Professional Role Deveopment for Mental Health Tasks." *Archives of General Psychiatry* 20(1969):524–527.

38. Papanek, G. O. "Dynamics of Community Consultation." *Archives of General Psychiatry* 19(1968):189–196.

39. Peck, H. B.; Kaplan, S. R.; and Roman, M. "Prevention, Treatment and Social Action: A Strategy of Intervention in a Disadvantaged Urban Area." *American Journal of Orthopsychiatry* 36(1966):57–69.

40. Peck, H. B.; Levin, T.; and Roman, M. "The Health Careers Institute: A Mental Health Strategy for an Urban Community." *American Journal of Psychiatry* 125(1969):1180–1186.

41. Pinderhughes, C. A. "Urban Mental Health Issues." *American Journal of Psychiatry* 125(1969):1721–1722.

42. Rogers, C. R. "The Process of the Basic Encounter Group." In *The Proper Study of Man: Perspectives on the Social Sciences*, edited by J. Fadiman, pp. 211–227. New York: Macmillan, 1971.

43. Roman, P. M., and Trice, H. M., eds. *The Sociology of Psychotherapy*. New York: Jason Aronson, 1974.

44. Rusk, T. N. "Evaluation of a Rapid Access Crisis-Oriented Mental Health Service." Unpublished paper, presented at Fifth World Congress of Psychiatry, 1971, Mexico City.

45. Scheff, T. J. "Reevaluation Counseling: Social Implications." *Journal of Humanistic Psychology* 12(1972):58–71.

46. Scherl, D. J., and English, J. T. "Community Mental Health and Comprehensive Health Service Programs for the Poor." *American Journal of Psychiatry* 125(1971):1666–1674.

47. Schutz, W. C. *Joy: Expanding Human Awareness*. New York: Grove Press, 1967.

48. Srole, L.; Langner, T. S.; Michael, S. T.; Opler, M. K.; and Rennie, T. A. C. *Mental Health in the Metropolis*. New York: McGraw-Hill, 1962.

49. Szasz, T. *Ideology and Insanity*. New York: Doubleday Anchor, 1970.

50. Volkman, R., and Cressey, D. R. "Differential Association and the Rehabilitation of Drug Addicts." *American Journal of Sociology* 69(1963–1964):129–142.

51. Wachspress, M. "Goals and Functions of the Community Mental Health Center." *American Journal of Psychiatry* 129(1972):187–190.

52. Wechsler, H. "The Self-Help Organization in the Mental Health Field: Recovery, Incorporated, A Case Study." *Journal of Nervous and Mental Diseases* 130(1960): 297–314.

53. Whitaker, C. A., and Malone, T. P. *The Roots of Psychotherapy*. New York: Blakiston, 1953.

54. Wilcox, A. F. "The New Professionals." *Mental Hygiene* 54 (1970):347–355.

55. Wolberg, L. R. *The Technique of Psychotherapy*. New York: Grune & Stratton, 1967.

56. Young, C. E.; True, J. E.; and Packard, M. E. "A National Survey of Associate Degree Mental Health Programs." *Community Mental Health Journal* (1974):466–474.

Editorial Note

Kiev's discussion of psychiatric problems and the outlook for their resolution in the world's developing nations is an appropriate bridge between the focus of Part II on patient care and that of Part III on interventions in the social environment. The author is concerned both with treatment of vulnerable populations and with the effort to restructure disjunctive elements in a changing social system. At heart Kiev, like Mertens in Chapter 14, addresses the issues of social change and the psychiatrist's role in helping exposed populations live healthily with change by overcoming their resistance to it. But if organizational change in the advanced industrial societies presents difficulties (as Mertens suggests), how much more wrenching and psychologically challenging is the massive thrust of change in a society's move from a traditional agricultural to a "modern" industrial model?

This chapter points to the need for a general understanding of the economics of the process of modernization as a context for the psychological health of the participants and for the activities of helping agents. It is especially cogent in tracing out the relations among such gross features of economic development as industrialization, urbanization, capital investment requirements, and agricultural needs, and the psychosocial hazards these features pose for individuals caught up in them. Kiev illustrates such relations by noting health problems that pile up in groups at highest risk: the woman cut off from supporting kin ties and religious involvement; the urban migrant unequipped for industrial employment; the unattended child roaming city streets.

While he does not do so in any detail, the author might well have speculated about the peculiar demands posed for personality functioning by the exigencies of modernization. He does mention the demands for "factory discipline" in terms of the precise, compulsive orientation toward clock time. We might also inquire into other aspects, such as the link between savings/capital formation and the inclination toward "deferred gratification" of individual needs; or the strains implicit in grafting the "need for achievement" (seemingly so central to the technocratic enterprise) upon persons nurtured in a traditional static culture.

One of the unusual themes of this account is the emphasis on the intertwining of physical and mental well-being. The large impoverished sector of the developing countries' populations is at high risk of infectious disease, malnutrition, and unrepaired chronic disability. These conditions may link up directly with psychological health (as in the influence of malnutrition upon cognitive development), or more indirectly and insidiously (as in the implications of chronic ill health for diminished self-esteem and mental depression). Further, the capricious undertone of prolonged exposure to infectious attacks may contribute importantly to the attitude of fatalism, which Kiev rightly identifies as an obstacle to occupational striving and to vigorous health maintenance measures.

In the developing societies, even more than in the United States, it is apparent that the clinical treatment model alone is an inadequate response to the magnitude of mental health problems. Hence this chapter underlines the pressing requirement for many of the "extended" strategies discussed in Part III. Kiev argues persuasively for the employment of indigenous institutions, such as schools, and indigenous agents, such as teachers and folk healers, in meeting social psychiatric challenges.

We are reminded, finally, of the great dependence of mental health efforts upon shared public values and upon the political sphere of national life. Just as the contemporary fate of community mental health centers in America hinges on these factors, so do they emerge in exaggerated form in the poor societies. The making of choices, the setting of priorities, is the kernel of politics. In their straitened circumstances, the developing nations find it exceedingly hard to allocate monies for, e.g., primary prevention, when that goal must compete with building a steel mill or fertilizer factory. Yet, as the author insists, successful modernization may rest as heavily upon the cultivation of superior human resources as it does on sheer economic investment.

R. N. W.

CHAPTER 8

Psychiatry Programs for the Developing Countries

ARI KIEV

IN EARLIER REPORTS and in a recently produced series of documentary films,* I have outlined some of the programs most feasible for developing countries, placing emphasis on utilization of the therapeutic potential of indigenous healers and on the introduction of short-term psychiatric facilities emphasizing the use of psychopharmaceuticals for reaching the largest number of people possible with the limited resources available.[2,12,13,14] This chapter examines the relevance of psychiatric theories and strategies to the broader issues of development.

While existing psychiatric institutions need upgrading, more personnel, and a higher funding priority in governmental programs, and general practitioners must be educated regarding the use of psychopharmaceuticals and methods of community psychiatry, psychiatrists must also address themselves to the subtle problems of motivation and initiative which prevent people from becoming fully committed to the development process. Psychiatry can indeed be of great help to developing countries by helping to introduce programs designed to develop more useful strategies for daily living which will better tap the human resources of the population, assisting them to function better and ultimately to

* A 16 mm documentary film series covering several aspects of Transcultural Psychiatry in Nigeria, The Sudan, Mexico, and Jamaica can be obtained from the Social Psychiatry Research Institute, 150 East 69th Street, New York, N.Y.

seek more participation in the modernization process. I am not suggesting that psychiatrists should impose their values on others, but rather that psychiatrists, as behavioral strategists, can help people to accomplish their objectives by overcoming internalized obstacles to progress and activity. Psychiatry can help people to overcome culture-specific obstacles to individual self-actualization. It can also help to find ways to introduce alternative patterns of behavior within existing institutions by minimizing the obstacles to action inherent in all organizations.

The Economics of Development

The "Third World" or "developing" countries, in Asia, Africa, the Caribbean, and Latin America, have developed since World War II. Differing historically, they have all been characterized by increasing use of technology, industrialization, and large-scale migrations from rural into urban areas.

Barbara Ward, the noted economist, has pointed out that the underdeveloped countries have not benefited from "an intellectual revolution of materialism and this-worldliness, the political revolution of equality, and above all the scientific and technological revolution which comes from the application of technology and the sciences to the whole business of daily life." [21] Emphasis on influencing nature through technology and science rather than through magic and prayer was lacking until recently due in part to the emphasis on tradition and maintenance of the status quo in these societies. This rigid, stratified world stifled opportunity and motivation for self-improvement, preventing the development of a middle class.

Slowly, however, Western colonialism has brought new impetus to the developing world. It has made people aware of the disparities between rich and poor, stimulated interest in modern techniques, and brought improved health to these areas. The local people saw how scientific, industrial, and technological society enjoyed "almost irresistible power." Through training of local personnel and the introduction of transportation and communication systems, an industrial base was developed in many countries. Today the forces of tradition and modernization struggle in the developing societies. The rivalry between the Western nations and the Communist world, both of which offer different methods for harnessing the revolutions of population, science and equality, complicates the turmoil.

The revolution of materialism has created many sources of discontent. Many feel that there is an inadequate distribution of consuming power and not a sufficiently large independent class to make for an adequate development of the economy. Because of the continued increase of power and wealth of a few families, there continues to be much social unrest and discomfort, despite the increasing industrialization of the developing world.

The motivation for equality and popular government increases the resistance of the wealthier classes to relinquishing power and influence to the developing middle classes increasingly anxious to participate in their own political fate. Communism opposes both the old landlords and the new entrepreneurs, while advocating an approach to rapid patterns of development and rapid capital accumulation which will benefit the majority of the masses.

Population increase strains the economy and food production, preventing savings or capital accumulation for expansion of the economy. An expanding population should provide more workers for new industries and more consumers, but this cannot happen until the traditional society becomes a modern industrial one, and production increases. The increasing population eats up the means of living, producing starvation, disease, and high death rates. Concentration of the population in the young age groups creates problems. The young are nonproductive and do not contribute much to the work force. To improve things birth rates must decline and life expectancy must improve so that the age composition of the population is altered, producing a larger working-age segment.

According to Ward, the means of ending the disproportion between people and resources is to apply capital massively to the resources. The difficulty is to secure this massive saving when rising population forces up the levels of consumption. If the rate of increase is 2 percent a year, as it is in India, or even 3 percent as it is in parts of Latin America, can people save on anything like an adequate scale? According to Ward, to keep pace with the 3 percent increase in population (since you have to invest three times as much capital to secure one unit of income), a nation has to increase 9 percent of its national income each year. This is well beyond the 4 or 5 percent of traditional society. In order to get ahead of the high birth rates, it may even be desirable to get 12 to 15 percent of the national income devoted to productive capital in order to achieve breakthrough to a period of sustained growth. This is difficult when population increase exceeds productivity.

Crucial to economic development are savings, which lead to surplus, which permits a diversion of energies and equipment to other tasks and changes in the techniques of productivity. One way of achieving this economic breakthrough is to force savings, as was done in Russia and in China. Another way of increasing savings is to decrease the population growth. Still another approach is to get money from elsewhere. This last technique has, until recently, been consonant with the strategy of the Free World, which has provided considerable economic aid to poor nations.

Once sustained economic growth occurs, the rates of expansion of the population can diminish, as people realize the economic value of small families. Export industries can secure foreign exchange through sales abroad, as was done by Sweden, the United States, and more recently Japan and Israel. Unfortunately, there are few things to export, and political insecurity makes people reluctant to invest in their country and/or to bring in foreign capital.

The obstacles to industrialization in a handicraft and primitive agrarian economy include primitive agricultural technology and migration of excess farm labor to the city. Not only services and trade but manufacturing must develop in the city, with capital derived from saving or foreign investment. While this last source is the most plentiful, it is often difficult to obtain because of the risk of takeover, lower returns on investment, and potential ideological conflicts. Programs to improve education, health, and hygiene are also crucial at this stage.

New sources of power growing at a rate at least equal to the growth of industries using power, an adequate supply of trained labor, and an adequate supply of trained managers, engineers, and skilled workers must be developed.

Lack of capital has prevented industrial "takeoff." The monopolistic nature of the economic system and heavy government control have also hindered the growth of free markets crucial for a balance of trade. There is at present very little overall planning for the developing world as a whole, which might, according to some economists, resolve some of this problem. Common markets or broad markets for industrial expansion must serve as sources of support upon which nations with poor resources can rely. In the past, declines in world market prices reduced trade in exports such as coffee and sugar. Such declines reduce available money for importing raw material needed for industrial expansion. Difficulty in importing also results from reductions of foreign exchange reserves. Industrial expansion reduces reliance on the export of goods or the importation of foreign exchange in the form of loans or gifts.

Traditions tend to perpetuate the separation of society into the rich and the poor, creating much resentment, social unrest, and discord. There are inadequate funds for schools, roads, and health services. Large landowners have no real incentive to save the land by using cover crops, and thus much erosion develops. Many of the landlords invest their profits abroad or use them for lavish living, and do not reinvest their earned profits in machinery and improved techniques. Large areas of land go uncultivated, particularly in periods when the prices of export crops are low. This creates underemployment of agricultural labor and prevents the use of land for much-needed food.

Thus, there is a pattern to progress and expansion. In the preinvestment phase the country lacks the essentials for investment, especially the infrastructure of power, transport, harbors, and housing. In this preliminary planning stage investments must be made in education and training, in the establishment of the infrastructure, and in a survey of resources.

In the next stage investments begin to show. The ground has been laid and rapid growth in the economy and industry can be obtained. At this point, large-scale capital aid from abroad can offset local poverty and lack of capital, and may prevent the government from using totalitarian methods to compel people to save. Each country must develop its own strategy in terms of its own capacity, its resources, the scale of its internal markets, and its export prospects. Investment and education are crucial. Some studies suggest that between 50 and 60 percent of the gains in productivity made in the West in the first part of the twentieth century came from better-trained minds, more research, and a more systematic use of intelligent and educated people. Most of the economies of the developing world are in need of this advance in education.

The third area of expansion is industry. Each country must plan in terms of its particular need and resources. According to Ward, "A developing government should aim its policies at insuring the quickest rate of capital accumulation. Profits should be strongly encouraged in public as in private enterprise and tax systems arranged so that all the incentives are towards their reinvesting. . . . Profits are one of the chief means by which resources can be put at the disposal of the investors in society." [21]

A Mental Health Orientation to Development

Most people who have discussed the "developing" countries have focused, like Barbara Ward, on the basic problem of reaching a point of sustained economic growth by forced saving or foreign aid. The focus has been developing industry, so that these countries can take advantage of the scientific and technological progress of the past thirty years. In general, health, education, and welfare programs have been deemphasized without adequate recognition of the critical need to develop the human resources of the developing nations. What programs have developed have, in general, concentrated on infectious diseases and malnutrition, with mental health programs being relegated to the lowest priority. Failure to recognize the significance of human resource programs could prove disastrous.

Given the fact of rapidly expanding populations and declining infant mortality rates, with the advent of modern medical care, personnel and resources for medical and educational programs will be less adequate than at present to meet the needs of these countries in the future. The United Nations estimates that by the year 2000 there will be more than 7 billion people in the world, the bulk of whom will be in these developing countries. It is doubtful, for example, that a country such as Liberia, with 1.5 million people and one psychiatrist now, is going to have sufficient numbers of psychiatrists in twenty years. There probably will not be sufficient numbers of paramedical personnel either.

Therefore, innovative programs must be planned to meet specific human needs, if any kind of viable and self-sustaining modern society is to develop in the developing countries.

SOCIAL CHANGE

Social change constitutes the most fundamental and characteristic stress of developing countries. The shift from rural to urban areas, the increase in industrialization, and the breakup of traditional patterns of stability associated with the family and traditional religion have led to much turmoil, resistance to progress, and the appearance of many vulnerable groups of people. Acculturation stress, loss of traditional ways, discrimination, and difficulty in adjusting to a more complex, technologically oriented urban situation have proved stressful for almost all groups, especially minority groups who have long met with injustice.

A variety of social changes ranging from industrialization and urbanization to changes in agricultural, health, and sanitation techniques, plus changes in the political and economic spheres, have contributed to much social unrest and personal uneasiness throughout the developing world. The developing areas of the world are characterized by poor standards of health, education, and technological development, and an excessive rate of population growth due to high birth rates and increasing longevity.

Excessive population growth has resulted from improved public health measures such as insect control, sewage disposal, and improved water supplies, leading to a combination of increased birth rates, reduced child mortality rates, and increased survival rates. Still, the economy cannot adequately feed, clothe, and educate the populations. In many places the urban population exceeds in size and rapidity of growth the rural population. Urban industry and employment opportunities are generally not at a level commensurate with population increase.

With increasing industrialization, one can expect an increased life expectancy and a reduced mortality followed by reduction in fertility, as happened following the Industrial Revolution in Europe. As more women work outside the home and seek better educations for their youngsters, they will probably be positively motivated to decrease the birth rate. The maldistribution of people on unstable land and in overcrowded urban areas presents additional problems of crowding and inadequate food production to nourish the population adequately. Because of the relatively young age of the population, the government and the family must assume large burdens for the care of children. Educational programs must prepare sufficient numbers of technically trained people to meet the needs of modernization. A good portion of the young people cannot enter into the labor market for some time. Because a great number of children reach school age each year, there are always a lot of young people looking for jobs and a lot of families seeking homes. To keep pace with these increasing population pressures, the number of places in schools, jobs, and dwelling units must rise more than 3 percent each year. Population growth interferes with economic advancement by creating a surplus of labor on the farms, which holds back the mechanization of agriculture and also decreases the income which might otherwise be utilized for long-term investment in education, equipment, and capital needs. Much of the income must be spent to support the consumption needs of the growing population.

Food production has not kept up with the population increase. To maintain economic growth in the face of increasing population, it is necessary for industrialization and agriculture to expand considerably. Most of the jobs have to come in industry, and this implies a continuing large-scale movement of population from the agricultural rural areas to the urban areas. It also implies a need for heavy investments to provide sources of employment, and also an increased need for urban housing and services. In many places the urban population is increasing faster than housing and services can be provided.

A large lower population stratum can be found in most of the developing countries. This group has not benefited from economic progress up to the present and suffers multiple deficiencies: lack of employment at tolerable living wages; lack of education; lack of skills and working habits; inadequate housing, sanitation, and diet, which reduce working capacity; unstable family life contributing to and fostered by the other deficiencies. With rapid population growth and continuing reallocation of population from rural to urban areas, it is likely that this group will continue to grow even in the face of industrialization, improved standards of living, and improved conditions for the remainder of the people.

URBANIZATION

The major change in the developing world entails a shift from a rural agrarian world to an urban industrial one, with attendant problems of overcrowding, poor hygiene, poor sanitation, and migration. Where regional planning does exist, there is as yet no device for coordinating physical planning with economic change, partly because academic training in planning is provided almost entirely by schools of architecture.

CHANGES IN INSTITUTIONS

Urbanization has disrupted the family, another vulnerable group. Socioeconomic changes have altered the status of women, enabling them to vote, to divorce, and to own property. Increasingly, the state has assumed family functions (as in public education and social insurance), which further alters the traditional role of the family. Some countries have begun to develop urban centers without having first established sufficient industrial growth to absorb the increased city population. This has resulted in crowded urban slums, which have devastating psychological effects for traditional people who leave the intact rural cultures where family and community ties protect the psychological integrity of individuals.

The lower classes suffer from malnutrition, endemic tuberculosis, high death rates, and infant mortality rates which slow economic development. The growing number of poor, illiterate, untrained, and unemployed people in the crowded slums present a major problem in terms of unstable families, illegitimacy, illness, crime, and violence; these individuals drain the economy while they slowly seek to adjust to new values, customs, and institutions. Few of their children complete school.

A more advanced stage of urbanization is characterized by an increasing proportion of the population living in cities of 100,000, industrialization, a middle class, and nationalism. In a few traditional agricultural societies, the emphasis is on industrial rather than urban growth, leading to an imbalance between urban and economic growth. The imbalance is seen in inadequate housing, minimal living standards, chronic unemployment, and urban discontent. Problems in these countries are most notably related to industrialization and urbanization. Social tensions are increasingly acute relative to gaps in improvement among various sectors of the society. Social unrest and competition across class lines also occurs in the more advanced of the developing societies. New middle groups in cities include entrepreneurs, small shopkeepers, and public and private white-collar workers. They value higher-status education for their children, have incomes above the subsistence level, and are conscientious about participating in national, political, and cultural life.

Industrial workers, many of whom have unionized in some countries, increasingly seek to improve their status and attain a better life. The material aspirations of the middle class often rise faster than their incomes, which do not benefit from the national per capita income gain. Changes in interpersonal relationships and in the roles of women and adolescents have further contributed to instability and dissatisfaction.

MANPOWER PROBLEMS

Urbanization and industrialization have also created significant manpower problems. Migration to urban areas has reduced the rural work force (which, with an expanding dependent population, needs to be larger), while not proportionately increasing the urban labor force. Because of lack of training and paucity of jobs, newcomers to the cities are underemployed or unemployed. There are not enough trained people for certain jobs and too many for others. The universities and technical institutes have not produced adequate numbers of skilled people for the new industries.

To make up for shortages, people with inadequate qualifications are often hired. The skilled workers may go unemployed or move into less skilled but technical jobs. This occurs because the shortage of workers at intermediate levels is more serious than that of highly skilled workers. One remedy for this unbalanced employment market has been in government planning and programs to absorb the unskilled labor surpluses and to assure the upgrading of employed workers through correspondence and on-the-job training, or multipurpose training to facilitate transfers from one occupation to another.

Industrialization is thus not absorbing enough of the urban labor force, and surplus labor continues to filter into service occupations of low productivity. These people cannot afford to live anywhere but in the ever-expanding shantytowns. While low-cost housing projects have in some areas alleviated overcrowding among the lower middle classes and the better-paid workers, they have done very little for the populations of the shantytowns whose housing is extraordinarily substandard.

Some attempts have been made at urban and regional planning to correct for unemployment, illiteracy, and poor housing. Attempts to develop agriculture, establish industries, villages, land reforms, rural electrification, and community development, as in Yugoslavia, have been rare. A balanced redistribution of the population, as in Israel, has not been tried either, nor have there been efforts to decentralize new industries and establish industrial estates, as in India and Italy. To check the flow of rural migrants to the crowded cities, there have been attempts to decentralize economic administrative activities by developing areas and towns such as Ciudad Bolívar in Venezuela and Brasilia in Brazil. There has been very little city planning on a regional scale, partly because, as noted earlier, academic training is provided almost entirely by schools of architecture. Where regional planning does exist, there is as yet no device for coordinating physical planning with economic change.

Social Change and Mental Illness

The complexity of studying the frequency and distribution of psychiatric disorder in underdeveloped and developing societies is underlined by the diversity of conclusions reached by various investigators, ranging from reports of no psychoses found to reports of an increased incidence of paranoid disorders attendant upon social changes such as detribalization, urbanization, and industrialization, which have been wrought by Westernization.

Although most studies have drawn attention to a number of important epidemiological questions, they have in the main been inconclusive because of various methodological inadequacies. Without knowing hospital usage patterns, the number of untreated cases, and the kinds of alternative treatment facilities available, hospital studies have been unable to draw definitive conclusions about the actual number of cases at a given time (prevalence) or the rate of inception of new cases in a given time period (incidence) solely on the basis of admission data. Comparability of most studies has been limited by the use of different criteria and differing methods of investigation. Thus while one cannot conclusively state that the incidence and prevalence rates for mental illness are universally rising in the development situation, one can look more closely at the psychodynamic factors involved in the phenomenon of social change by way of elucidating probable relationships between social processes and psychological events.

Social change upsets institutions which support emotional stability and provide care for disturbed individuals. Highly complex urban societies, as well as the transitional slums in developing societies, may foster anomie and social isolation which may render certain individuals more vulnerable to psychological disturbance than others from the same group.

While the milieu per se does not cause certain behavioral patterns, it plays a critical role in certain individuals predisposed both by personal experience and cultural labeling. New towns may predispose to mental illness because of the absence of social supports. Recent studies suggest that many psychotic symptoms traditionally associated with chronic schizophrenia may derive from specific cultural or situational factors rather than from the underlying disorder. Certain environments both foster certain conflicts, and facilitate the expression of certain symptoms. Industrialization, urbanization, and social change have led to increased rates of mental illness, drug addiction, alcoholism, crime, prostitution, and delinquency in a number of developing countries, albeit the rates do not reach the magnitude found in the more developed countries. Evidence of social breakdown appears to derive mainly from crowded urban areas and shantytowns of Asia, Africa, and Latin America, where there has been a weakening of primary institutions, increased isolation, and large-scale shifts of the population with concomitant breakdown of family ties, all of which has predisposed to increased anxiety and emotional disturbance.

EPIDEMIOLOGICAL STUDIES

The information obtainable about morbidity varies from country to country. With numerous dialects, languages, and kinship groups, the developing nations have been hard pressed to accomplish a census of the population, let alone establish a medical register. In many instances superstitions and stigma discourage reporting. The absence of comparable reporting systems makes valid international comparisons of statistical data almost impossible. Nevertheless, statistical data within countries may suggest trends and relationships which can be compared and may point to groups which are more vulnerable.

VULNERABLE GROUPS

In some societies stress is greatest for those most closely involved in social change, for whom opportunities open up new avenues for achievement, new expectations, higher goals, and simultaneously the opportunity for greater failure, frustration, shame and guilt, and isolation. The data suggest that social change may take many forms—from a change in relationships to a shift in residence to a shift in the degree of Westernization and urbanization.

VIOLENCE AND SELF-DESTRUCTIVE BEHAVIOR

In some cultures the decline of social controls leads to violence and crime as well as higher suicide rates. This observation is supported by a world-wide panel of psychiatrists contributing to a symposium on transcultural studies of suicide and attempted suicide.[13] In rural Senegal, according to Collomb, violence is associated with ritualized acts of vengeance.[5] Elsewhere, alcoholism predisposes to violent crimes. L. Bryce Boyer reports that the crime rate among the Mescalero Apache in the United States is ten times the national average and is correlated with a high rate of alcoholism.[3] Violence in Latin America occurs in the context of the machismo tradition, which makes a virtue of excessive alcoholic intake.[6] Violence also serves as an index of social anomie and discord. Evidence of high rates of violence are likely to be accompanied by a high incidence of suicide.

In India the daughter-in-law is a particularly high suicidal risk because of the nature of the planned or arranged marriages and the social pressure and tremendous social expectations which require that she do the bidding of the mother-in-law.[17] In Africa deculturalization or detribalization is the most significant pressure among the young.[10] The highest suicide rates occur among those in the twenty-five to forty age group, with the educated and professionals the most affected.

The highest rate among the White Mountain Apache occurs among women who are no longer protected by kin or the subcultural belief.[9] This contrasts with the high suicide rates among married men who can't fit into the matrilineal system of the Mescalero Apache.[3]

STATUS CHANGE

Social change, acculturation, and immigration lead to shifts in status which can be stressful. The loss of the social control and support provided by traditional tribal beliefs and practices reduces the capacity of rural African migrants to cope in urban areas.

In Rhodesia the Shona improve their status by losing their identity in the Clan Brotherhood.[10] But this increases their vulnerability when they enter the urban area and have few habits of self-reliance. The same holds for those whose marriages are arranged in India.[17] Violation of status expectancy brings dishonor in Japan, leading to hara-kiri, a culturally prescribed method of dealing with shame or loss of face.[7]

Marginality sometimes makes for greater vulnerability, particularly in acculturation situations. Sometimes tradition or other obstacles to acculturation serve to protect the individual from other more noxious stresses, as in the case of the blacks in New Orleans who have very little sense of failure to achieve.[4] A sudden improvement in standard of living may prove stressful, as happened in Scandinavia,[1,8,19] or may have no effect, as in Australia,[20] where industrialization did not lead to any particular increase in suicide rates.

Among the White Mountain Apache, the acculturated have a greater fear of suicide than those who have adhered to tradition.[9] Acculturation correlates with high rates of suicide, alcoholism, crime, drug abuse, and violence in Africa [10] and in other parts of the world, and yet in some instances, as for example Australia,[20] the most acculturated experienced the lowest rates.

Death of a spouse may also cause a change in social status. Widowers, widows, and the divorced have high rates of suicide compared with those not exposed to a change in relationship, which may be further compounded by isolation.

In India, poverty and unemployment may lead to the suicide of an entire family.[17] Failure to secure adequate income in Japan is correlated with failure to achieve a sense of social responsibility, and thus in turn leads to suicide.[7] Indeed, such economic pressures relate to the increase of suicide rates.

In India, impotence is a commonly reported cause of suicide among men.[17] Suicide rates in Africa are higher among women, and are generally associated with an increase in education and the absence of strong group supports in urban settings. In East Africa suicide is highest among the educated groups, while in Rhodesia a greater proportion of African than European men die from suicide.[10] This relates to the increased vulnerability caused by social change and acculturation. At times, though, individuals are insulated from acculturation pressure by traditional supports.

A Strategy for Developing Countries

Shortages of personnel, lack of basic statistical information, lack of government planning agencies, and powerful political groups which favor the status quo all contribute to lack of progress. The ministries of health and the governments must establish national goals for health. They must modify fragmented programs by improving communication among various competing bureaucratized agencies dealing with the overlapping health, education, and welfare needs of the same population groups.

It makes sense to take an overview of the entire society, and to work out ways for establishing contact between the government and the population. Like the general practitioner of old, one health worker might very well screen all problems at the family level, referring people to the appropriate agencies which provide comprehensive services. The work of individuals skilled at contact work would not have to be duplicated. Similarly, other tasks ought not to be duplicated. Recognition of the interrelatedness of health and sustained economic growth must be clarified for all. Psychiatry must address itself to the various population groups made vulnerable to psychological disorder and malfunctioning by virtue of exposure to specific social stresses. To the extent that the urban slums are pockets of revolution, resentment, nonproductivity, and crime, attention must be focused on helping people in these areas enter comfortably into the modern world as productive people. Physical health programs must be supplemented by mental health programs, many of which can be introduced in school situations.

The rural migrant to the urban area must contend with considerable anxiety in adjusting to a new environment in the absence of traditional sources of support. He must find ways of gaining greater personal strength within himself, and must be helped to get on a track which utilizes his talents and which enables him to set personal goals and pursue them toward a more fulfilling personal life.

The urban slum dweller lacks a sense of social identity in part because he lacks goals. The typical slum dweller lacks a sense of purpose, is confused over incompatible goals, and experiences conflicts over the incompatibility of values between rural and urban areas. The urban setting emphasizes personal responsibility rather than group responsibility. The individual may have great difficulty in developing a new attitude toward time, personal responsibility, and autonomy. Lacking such experience, he may have difficulty in adjusting or adapting to a stressful urban setting.

The absence of kin and the anomic environment of the city make it difficult to establish meaningful relationships. Families are less stable and the role of the woman is undermined. While she may have been able to involve herself in domestic chores in the rural area, she may have to work outside the home in the city and may have to support her family. She has fewer supports as a result of the decline of the extended family and the weakening of the church, and at times must contend with her husband's resentment of her economic independence.

Ignorant, superstitious, and failing to understand the workings of the urban area, the individual has great difficulty in setting meaningful goals. He may not be able to find opportunity to express traditional religious goals. He may lack links to others and may feel cut off from the source of his goals and traditional customs which gave his life meaning.

HEALTH PROBLEMS

The health of an area is related not only to the state of public health measures but to social and economic conditions as well. Environmental factors further increase the risk of poor health. Adding to the existence of agents of disease associated with inadequate sanitation, the crowded city provides breeding grounds for certain psychological disorders such as delinquency, crime, and suicide.

Cultural and dietetic customs, as well as inadequate food, contribute to nutritional disease, as, for example, in the classical A vitaminoses and protein deficiencies such as kwashiorkor which reduce resistance to stress. Lack of educational training and public health facilities adds to the health burden. Many customs must be overcome before people will conscientiously utilize the resources of the modern facilities which do exist. The number of doctors is inadequate and there is a great need for public health programs related to the eradication of a variety of infectious, parasitic, and nutritional diseases. The psychiatric dimension of these conditions and the related psychological spinoff of these problems cannot be minimized. Psychiatrists working together with other members of the mental health team, which ought to include psychiatric social workers, psychologists, drug abuse specialists, and so on, have an opportunity to introduce programs relating to education and the development of new life styles. That is, psychiatry may act as a catalytic agent facilitating modernization.

A case in point is diarrheal diseases, which still account for the death each year of a quarter of a million children under one year of age in certain developing countries, a figure 98 percent greater than that for the United States. These diseases are preventable with available and proven techniques. What is lacking in much of Latin America is their application on a national basis, although some progress has been made since 1930, when the mortality rate in seven countries of the Americas ranged from 65 to 234 per thousand live births. Thus, in 1960, the same countries showed rates ranging from 26 to 132. This mortality and morbidity problem of children relates to a variety of factors having to do with customs, beliefs, ignorance, agriculture, nutrition, and water supply.

Clearly, psychiatry has a part to play in illuminating the role of these factors when dealing with a situation of inertia. The psychiatrist studies such problems as motivating the population to adopt a program, or getting the medical establishment to modify its views of native healers. How can one assess the signs and symptoms of resistance? How can the psychiatrist help in the development of the introduction of sensible programs? These are the key issues. Since we are dealing here with modification of behavior and attitude, it becomes crucial to understand the investment people have in existing patterns of behavior and institutions, and the extent to which they feel dissatisfied. To what extent are they feeling unfulfilled? What are their dreams? What are their resources? Can you motivate an entire community? Or must you seek out the natural leaders and encourage them to take the lead? Who are the innovators? How do you find them? How do you mobilize an anachronistic institution to focus more attention on the needs of the impoverished? How do you elicit the involvement of the elite classes? To what extent are psychodynamic formulations of value in assessing these individuals? What about the problem of women?

There is need to develop a variety of national health programs for infectious diseases and nutritional conditions. Nutritional and food supplementation programs can be introduced into communities by educational health teams, which can simultaneously introduce concepts of mental health.

The problem is basically one of educating and motivating the population as regards modern concepts of physical and mental health. Poor countries may have to utilize some of the resources of the large industrial organizations that have their activities in these countries. One way, for example, would be to have health representatives entering into the community to promote a particular style of life which ensured that the maximum benefits possible were being introduced to the population, and to see that people understood the harmfulness of certain practices and the benefits of others.

Emphasis should be on the positive features of new programs rather than on downgrading the traditions. One cannot ignore the fact that the traditional practices persisted because they allayed anxiety and reinforced the group's values. When new programs prove to fill these needs, they will be accepted as well.

Vulnerable groups most in need of preventive and/or treatment programs must be identified. Knowledge about attitudes toward illness can be significant in understanding the persistence of poor hygienic practices in the face of modern facilities. Denial of reality, investment in myth, and reluctance to change because of a culturally acceptable fatalism relate to psychiatric as well as medical problems. These attitudes reinforce an inertia and fear of innovation and perpetuate the status quo. Fatalism perhaps more than ignorance underlies much of the reason for the nonacceptance of modern medicine and modern psychiatry.

Government planners, eager to monumentalize their term in office and to deal in tangible and measurable products, tend to focus on high-visibility projects such as building programs, to the neglect of more important long-range education or preventive programs. While foreign aid, direct capital investment, direct loans, and gifts receive emphasis, insufficient attention is directed toward teaching people to assume responsibility for their own destinies. Blinded by poverty and oppressed lives, the local and imported experts are often too willing to take over solution of the problem, failing to recognize that the solution is only temporary unless they help the people to develop their own solutions. And so, both developing country and foreign government involve themselves in a folie à deux, both believing that material progress alone may suffice to get a country moving toward sustained economic growth.

Psychiatrists and social scientists can play an important advisory role by providing the governments of developing countries with an understanding of the broader issues involved in the implementation of foreign aid programs, which may create problems in the wake of modernization and industrialization.

Mental health professionals can assist as well in other areas of activity relating to such issues as leadership selection and training, community organization and education, principles of innovation and creativity, and in the development of self-reliance and such technical skills as bargaining and negotiating.

If mental health services are to be introduced to the developing countries, an accurate appraisal of the patient groups likely to be in most need of such services must be determined. The types of programs and personnel required must be designed to fit the particular needs of these groups. A case in point are the children of the developing world.

Large-scale population movement from rural to urban areas depletes the rural areas, and creates overcrowded slums in the city with massive problems secondary to the breakdown of the extended tribal family. Barefooted, malnourished young children wander the streets of the urban ghettos of the world, begging and stealing and creating a large source of potential delinquents. They must be a high priority in any kind of mental health program.

Provision must be made for housing, clothing, and educating these children, who very often suffer from deprivation syndromes or behavioral disorders secondary to malnutrition and relative neglect. Programs must be developed to provide for their education and welfare needs; efforts must also be made to integrate the urban migrant into the mainstream of society. Such programs have as a major objective prevention of a delinquent subculture whose members can enter the larger social situation only with difficulty. Such programs ideally might be developed in school situations where children would be given experience in making their own decisions, participating in decision-making processes of the class, and functioning in a setting with a minimum of external restraints. Emphasis should be placed on personal responsibility and autonomy.

Modern mental health programs also focus on the persistence of numerous tribal customs which impede the development of antonomy and psychological independence among the young. Slavery, various mutilations (which are customs), and other repressive measures must be eliminated because of their deleterious effect on mental health at the most crucial periods of time in the lives of young people. This is a difficult task because of the obvious difficulty in changing social patterns and taking an imperialistic or Western stance regarding these customs. However, to the extent that modernization is introduced, one must recognize the effect of these customs and seek ways to modify them. A sensible strategy is to develop alternative activities to such an extent early on that there is little time or motivation to become involved in the culture-specific customs; e.g., if children are in special schools, it will be very difficult for them to engage in tribal customs.

School becomes the mainstay of any program. It also provides a ready group of paraprofessionals who, through their work as teachers, can significantly influence the motivation and ultimately the mental health of young people. Teachers should be trained in mental health concepts and techniques so as to be able to utilize the fact that the young are to some extent a captive population in this particular institutional setting.

EDUCATION

Education is perhaps the best defense against adversity and has always been one of the main avenues for social progress. Education, particularly at the college level, has been the prerogative of the elite and the upper classes in the developing nations. Thousands of students, especially poorer ones, drop out each year and derive minimal advantage from their incomplete courses. This is particularly true in rural areas. Indian children in some Latin American countries attend school without ever being able to speak the official language. This prevents their essential identification with and assimilation to the larger society. For others, education leads to overtraining and hence unemployability. Many from rural and peasant backgrounds, having obtained an education, have been unwilling to work with their hands, and have sought white-collar jobs. Thus in many instances educated people form part of the unemployed population, since there are insufficient jobs for those with so-called good educations. A large number of dropouts occur in the lower middle classes, where children are given little incentive to remain in school. In the 1950s, according to the *Report On The World Social Situation*, "the process of democratization was at work by which secondary education was coming to be regarded as right (in some cases a compulsory duty) for all children; the idea of secondary education as a prerogative of a chosen few (with discrimination in favor of the elite or in favor of boys) was declining more rapidly in some countries than others." [18]

The proportion of its young people enrolled in secondary schools can be used as a good indicator of a country's wealth and human resources. Generally, educational development correlates with economic prosperity.

THE NEEDS OF CHILDREN

Efforts must be made to understand the origins and development of such social psychiatric problems as malnutrition in the midst of sufficient food, high incidence of accidents among children in urban areas, vagrancy, exploited child labor, child prostitution, and child drug addiction. The roots of psychological and behavioral problems inextricably interact with some of the same environmental factors that relate to infectious and nutritional diseases.

Rural areas suffer special problems, since in general the fathers migrate to the urban areas, leaving behind a strenuous situation for mothers and children.

The high rural death rate would be lowered by mother and child health services, sanitary education, nutrition education, mobile units for medical care and immunization, and communicable disease control programs. Illiteracy, illegitimacy, and abandoned children also constitute serious social problems. The mental health specialist can contribute some understanding to the overall management of individuals in different age groups. Given manpower shortages, it might make sense to incorporate psychiatric principles into general medical and nutritional programs.

RURAL DEVELOPMENT

Rural development programs are among the crucial steps necessary for improving general conditions. It has become clear that for stability of a growing industrial-based economy, such programs are necessary to reduce inflationary pressures and reduce the balance of payment crises by increasing the rate of agricultural production, particularly food for domestic consumption, and by developing the standard of living in the rural areas so as to increase the number of consumers. Furthermore, improvement of the rural situation will reduce the pressure to migrate to the city slums. In some areas the peasants are becoming more politically conscious of their relatively poor status. Elsewhere, land reforms have led to a considerable change in the life of some rural people.

Other countries have laws and plans for redistributing public lands and in some places for expropriating unused private lands. Most programs have difficulty in implementing their plans to resettle large portions of the population. Because the people are scattered, it is difficult to introduce health or educational programs or to provide market outlets. Migrant squatter groups lack social organizations and have numerous problems of their own.

This urban group will also require special programs to assist them in adapting to new circumstances. Programs in acculturation, language, and development of basic skills will have to be introduced. Here is a terrific opportunity for social psychiatric programs to be introduced, particularly in helping people who are adjusting to totally new cultural and socioeconomic conditions.* In particular, the development of tribal associations in African urban areas seems to be a

---

* Along these lines, I have had considerable success in assisting inner city youth to develop self-reliance and a sense of autonomy with an audio-cassette series on "Strategies For Daily Living." Relying on the spoken rather than written word, these cassettes lend themselves to repetitive reinforcement and familiarization with common sense principles which increase personal choices. Further information about these tapes can be obtained from The Psychodynamic Research Corporation, Englewood Cliffs, New Jersey 07632.

reasonable way to develop an institutionally viable structure which can have preventive significance for the bulk of African migrants.

In Latin America, where Indians have difficulty integrating into the Latin culture, other types of programs may be needed. Special programs must also be developed to meet the needs of the migrant group. Not only housing, but also training programs in basic hygiene and nutrition must be provided. A general reorientation regarding time and the type of work available in factories must be transmitted to individuals.

CONCLUSIONS

Using a team approach in alliance with professionals from allied mental health fields, as well as paraprofessionals, educators, and other relevant personnel, psychiatry can do much to introduce preventive programs by considering the particular needs of people in transition from rural to industrial economies, e.g., learning how to work in terms of time schedules in factories, accepting the authority of the foreman, adapting to periods of isolation, and learning how to interact with people from different backgrounds.

Psychiatry, Folk Medicine, and the Development Process

The psychiatrist can provide a perspective to help individuals and organizations develop better ways of coping with existing stresses, and improve the utilization of resources, by identifying areas where talent is underutilized and by establishing goals and strategies to tap such resources. A case in point is the area of indigenous healing practices, which have much to offer developing countries with limited medical resources. Additionally, the competition between modern medical programs and folk healing systems has special significance because it raises crucial issues relevant to all modernization schemes, affording an opportunity to clarify the question of imposing Western values on the countries of the developing world. Should we recognize the validity of folk healers? Should we compete with them?

Should we co-opt them into our systems? What harm results from interfering with them? How disruptive to a society can abolition of folk healing systems be? How helpful can folk healers be to the introduction of modern medical practice?

Do folk healers reach the same groups? Do they serve similar or different needs? Do they function in the same way? How do they differ in their functions? If we work with them, what must we know?

Folk medicine represents a major focus of belief systems and social action patterns in all societies. Folk healers and healing institutions provide tremendous psychological support and social integration, especially in periods of social change, as evidenced by an increase of such activities as a reaction to colonialism.

Any effort to change or eliminate folk healing has a major impact on the economy, family stability, and other institutions, and must be approached cautiously. We must develop standards for consulting and appraising the value of folk medicine as well as other traditional beliefs and practices. Where does it work? For what conditions? How can we educate folk healers in order to reach the people themselves? What is the politics of such consultation? This is, of course, part of the larger question of how to contend with inherent obstacles to introducing change, such as tribal conflict, revolution, political instability, and the competing ideologies of the advanced nations. This is particularly true today, with the increased popular demand for folk medicine and other nativistic practices for dealing with the increasing anxiety associated with urbanization, mass migration, and social change. The population explosion floods the scarce modern resources and facilities, thus also perpetuating the demand for folk medicines.

There are dangers in imposing one's values on developing societies, particularly if one disrupts folk belief institutions and does not guarantee sustained support. To prohibit folk medical practices without recognizing their value may create a situation in which efforts to educate the populace and the healers about modern preventive concepts may fail. In the least developed or undeveloped countries folk healers are often among the leadership group and are key representatives of the major value systems. It is often impossible to implement mass innoculation or other modern programs without their help.

In the next stage of development, or *underdevelopment*, it may be possible to incorporate folk healers into treatment centers as religious leaders, or even as interviewers in epidemiological surveys, as Lambo has done in Nigeria. In most developed societies folk healers may be organized into guilds, or trained as bilingual health workers, as has been done among the Navajo.[15,11]

In most advanced societies the folk healer may serve the needs of the disenfranchised and disadvantaged. The Mexican-American curandero is a case in point.

We must recognize the dialectic process in development so as to be able to anticipate the development of conflicts and resistances to development. Development is not a unilinear, uniform process, but a succession of adjustments and accommodations to new patterns and life styles. Excessive planning is not good.

Eradication of folk healing systems fails to recognize that they may be meeting social and cultural needs over and above medical needs, and that modern medicine alone may not serve these multifaceted needs. Developers must be patient and recognize that once social change processes get underway they develop an antonomy and a momentum of their own. If not pressed too hard, naturally occurring patterns will eventually evolve with cultural coloring and adaptation which meet significant needs. So the developer must not try to control the processes too tightly or the program will not develop in the way most appropriate for the culture. Technical advisors must learn restraint when dealing with social systems which are unprepared for adopting their recommendations as speedily as they would like. Preparation of such advisors should pay attention to the different time and progress perspectives they will meet in developing countries. They must be alert to their own susceptibility to look for shortcuts which can lead them to undesirable involvements in intracultural power struggles between elitist and populist approaches.

We must approach general development questions with the same attitudes as we approach folk medicine. We cannot push too fast and ignore the relevance of folk beliefs and practices to the developing society. We must regularly examine our own views and approaches, searching for a mutuality of objectives. The folk healer can be a key pivot in providing leverage to those introducing change, and his cooperation can help. Study of his role behavior may also assist in clarifying crucial values which he supports and needs he fulfills, to learn what gives him his leverage so as to be able to recognize crucial attitudes. These efforts are important not only to facilitate development but also to avoid those impositions which may disrupt the societal equilibrium.

REFERENCES

1. Achte, K. "Finland." In *Transcultural Studies of Suicidal Behavior*, edited by A. Kiev.

2. Argandona, M., and Kiev, A. *Mental Health in the Developing World: A Case Study in Latin America*. New York: Free Press, 1972.

3. Boyer, L. B. "Mescalero Apache." In *Transcultural Studies of Suicidal Behavior*, edited by A. Kiev.

4. Breed, W., and Swanson, W. C. "New Orleans Blacks." In *Transcultural Studies of Suicidal Behavior*, edited by A. Kiev.

5. Collumb, H. "Senegal." In *Transcultural Studies of Suicidal Behavior*, edited by A. Kiev.

6. de Paiva, L. M. "São Paulo, Brazil." In *Transcultural Studies of Suicidal Behavior*, edited by A. Kiev.

7. DeVos, G. "Japan." In *Transcultural Studies of Suicidal Behavior*, edited by A. Kiev.

8. Ettlinger, R. "Sweden." In *Transcultural Studies of Suicidal Behavior*, edited by A. Kiev.

9. Everett, M. W. "White Mountain Apache." In *Transcultural Studies of Suicidal Behavior*, edited by A. Kiev.

10. Gelfand, M. "Salisbury, Rhodesia." In *Transcultural Studies of Suicidal Behavior*, edited by A. Kiev.

11. Kaplan, B. and Johnson, D. "The Social Meaning of Navaho Psychopathology and Psychotherapy." In *Magic, Faith, and Healing: Studies in Primitive Psychiatry Today*, edited by A. Kiev.

12. Kiev, A., ed. *Magic, Faith, and Healing: Studies in Primitive Psychiatry Today*. New York: Free Press, 1964.

13. ―――. *Curanderismo, Mexican American Folk Psychiatry*. New York: Free Press, 1968.

14. ―――. *Transcultural Psychiatry*. New York: Free Press, 1972.

15. ――― ed. *Transcultural Studies of Suicidal Behavior*. Unpublished symposium.

16. Lambo, T. A. "Patterns of Psychiatric Care in Developing African Countries." In *Magic, Faith, and Healing: Studies in Primitive Psychiatry Today*, edited by A. Kiev.

17. Rao, A. V. "India." In *Transcultural Studies of Suicidal Behavior*, edited by A. Kiev.

18. *Report on the World Social Situation*, United Nations, N.Y., 1967, 1970.

19. Retterstol, N. "Norway." In *Transcultural Studies of Suicidal Behavior*, edited by A. Kiev.

20. Stoller, A. "Australia." In *Transcultural Studies of Suicidal Behavior*, edited by A. Kiev.

21. Ward, B. *The Rich Nations and the Poor Nations*. New York: W. W. Norton, 1962.

Part III

Habilitation and Environmental Enrichment

IN THIS SECTION there are three chapters on competence, three chapters on social interventions to create more competent life styles, and a case illustration of drugs as a substitute for competence. All these chapters deal with fundamental questions: Can the social system be strengthened to maximize individual health? How? Can children be better provided with competence and/or mastery skills as they grow up? Can life styles be changed to provide the necessary coping opportunities and skills? Can organizations be made responsive to noxious aspects of their functioning? Can noxious social environments be changed?

Is shared psychosocial health attainable? Can social systems function more humanely, be more protective of self-esteem and other crucial needs? Are positive sexual identity, private and public self-esteem, social support and coping skills among the basic behavioral predictors of mental health?

It is also important to classify cultural systems as to the ease or difficulty posed in meeting basic human needs such as affiliation, love, dependence, etc. Other basic processes such as aggression vs. peacefulness, the level of anomie vs. structural regularity, ease of social change vs. social inflexibility, sexual satisfaction vs. sexual inhibition also need to be classified, perhaps as a continuum of health to destructive behavior. The parallel intended is that of high blood pressure, high cholesterol, and heavy smoking as a set of important predictors of heart disease.

Editorial Note

It is a truism that for generations the attention of psychiatry and psychology has been fixed on illness behaviors. Only in the recent past have we seriously approached the study of individual effectiveness and successful coping. Although Hamburg, Adams, and Brodie do not assert a claim in the following chapter to have developed a model of mental health, their analysis of the ways in which people maintain a going concern in the face of stress is surely a contribution to such a model. Their discussion of "tasks" and "strategies" adopted under the pressure of adversity might usefully be compared to the descriptions of efforts to measure healthiness in Chapters 10 and 16. The authors' tone, particularly when they examine responses to severe burns and leukemia, is reminiscent of Albert Camus's wise reflection that the goal is not to be cured, but to live with one's ailments.

The thrust toward competence and health exemplifies Leighton's basic propositions on social processes and mental health in that positive inner and outer features might be said to conspire to arrest and even reverse the propensity to become psychiatrically ill.[22] Temporary disturbance of the essential psychical condition is weathered and the individual moves forward to fresh tasks. One of the most striking features of the authors' rehearsal of strategies for coping is the nice articulation of inner resources and social supports that seem to be required for a viable strategy. That is, a sufficient basis for healthiness under duress is found in a combination of individual resources (previous coping experience, ego-strength, cognitive mastery, and other assets) and environmental resources (interpersonal guidance, confirmation, shared experience).

An encouraging note in this chapter is especially evident in the concluding sections discussing peer counseling and "anticipatory guidance" as preparatory techniques in coping. Here we glimpse the promise that efficacious behavior may not only be scientifically understood, but may be explicitly taught and learned. These techniques are relevant to Frank's description (Chapter 7) of new therapeutic roles and to Hollister's analysis (Chapter 13) of primary prevention. Indeed, the peer counselor could be described as a front-line therapist, simultaneously giving and receiving help in a fashion that may forestall any later need for more obtrusive treatment measures.

In conclusion, it should be remarked that Hamburg and his colleagues consistently regard the human being as capable of mastering self and circumstance. In contrast to so many writers on psychological health and dis-ease, they abjure the image of the individual as passively subject to inner turmoil and environmental whim. He is seen, under varying magnitudes of genuine stress, as the mover as well as that which is moved. This is a salutary reminder of Henry A. Murray's dictum that man's behavior is characterized by "pro-action," not merely by helpless reaction.[25] It is also akin to Leighton's identification of the exercise of positive force or volition as one of the central human strivings.

R. N. W.

CHAPTER 9

Coping Behavior in Stressful Circumstances: Some Implications for Social Psychiatry

DAVID A. HAMBURG
JOHN E. ADAMS
H. KEITH H. BRODIE

Coping Behavior Under Stressful Conditions: A Perspective

RESEARCH on coping behavior brings into focus the means by which individuals or groups are effective in meeting the requirements or utilizing the opportunities of the specific environments they encounter. It highlights possibilities for enhancing the competence of individuals through developmental attainments, including ways of learning from exceptionally difficult circumstances. Despite the fact that everyone is exposed to a variety of stressful events throughout the life cycle, only a small proportion of those exposed are shattered by such experiences. The literature of psychiatry and closely related fields has provided abundant documentation of the ways in which such common life events can be traumatic. Some of these experiences are inherent components of the life cycle; others represent acute and unpredictable crisis situations; and still others reflect major features of urbanized, technologically complex societies. Examples of common stressful experiences which have been emphasized in recent research and clinical discussions include: (1) separation from parents in childhood; (2) displacement by siblings; (3) childhood experiences of rejection; (4) illness and injuries of childhood; (5) the initial transition from home to school; (6) puberty; (7) later school transitions, e.g., from grade school to junior high school, and from high school to college; (8) competitive graduate education; (9) first full-time employment; (10) marriage; (11) pregnancy; (12) severe illnesses and injuries of the adult years; (13) illness and death of parents; (14) menopause; (15) periodic moves to a new environment; (16) adult unemployment; (17) rapid technological and social change; (18) wars and threats of wars; (19) experiences of prejudice and social depreciation; and (20) forced migration.

Despite the omnipresence of such threatening experiences, the human species displays remarkable resilience in adaptation. This has been significantly neglected until recent years in both clinical observation and systematic research. What do we typically do in the face of distressing experience? In the past quarter century, much clinical attention has been directed to ways in which people avoid such experiences, even if this process requires extensive self-deception. The classical mechanisms of defense such as repression, denial, reaction formation, isolation, and rationalization are centrally involved with this avoidance by minimizing recognition of, or otherwise distorting, potentially distressing aspects of personal experience. Such mechanisms, however, represent only one important class of responses to threatening elements of experience. There is a wide range of individual differences in response to such situations. Appraisal of threatening elements rests heavily on their personal meaning—which in turn is strongly influenced by a succession of past environments, especially in the family, and dispositions that have become internalized. The salience of a given element to motives or values of the person, and conflict among these motives, is crucial to the individual's threat appraisal. When the appraisal indicates to the person that trouble lies ahead, *many* responses are possible, including some that reach far beyond avoidance of threat. Although such considerations have been a part of psychiatric literature for some time, behavioral scientists have lately been making significant progress in the understanding of these responses. They have been variously described as coping, problem solving, and adaptive behavior. This interest is strongly reflected in several published sources.*

* See, for example, references 2, 3, 4, 5, 7, 12, 14, 15, 20, 21, 23, 27, 28, 30, and 31.

Information developed from these research efforts is beginning to suggest ways in which such stressful circumstances may be modified to diminish human suffering. The findings and implications of these studies are already becoming useful in psychotherapy, counseling, rehabilitation, preventive intervention, and in the practice of physicians, nurses, social workers, and teachers. Additional information about coping patterns under specified conditions could help individuals acquire coping skills and assist in anticipating typical or recurring coping exigencies. While stressful circumstances, especially major transitions of the life cycle, occur in a fairly predictable way, so far only a few of these have been the subject of multiple studies that provide reasonably dependable information in some depth. For most stressful situations we must do the best we can with fragments of information about the tasks embedded in the situation and about the ways in which these tasks can be met effectively. Future research should make it possible to elucidate a roster of stressful situations; the tasks embedded in each of these situations; the range of strategies employed in the general population in meeting these tasks; the distribution of these strategies by age, sex, and ethnic group—and the risks, costs, opportunities, and benefits associated with each strategy in each situation, taking into account cultural and subcultural settings. Increasing availability of such information should be useful in the social psychiatry of the future.

In the present chapter our aim is to summarize some information on coping behavior under stress, derived largely from studies in which we have participated, and to illustrate the application of such information in social psychiatric intervention efforts. The series of collaborative studies to be described explored the variety of ways in which individuals drawn from a broad range of the population cope with difficult circumstances. These studies deal with a major psychosocial transition (going away to college) and with situations of life-threatening illness and injury (severe burns, severe poliomyelitis, and childhood leukemia). Our review will be largely in terms of *tasks* and *strategies*. By tasks we mean requirements for effective adaptation; by strategies we mean the variety of ways in which these requirements may be met. Coping functions are considered to involve not only containing distress within tolerable limits but also maintaining self-esteem and interpersonal relationships, and meeting environmental conditions. Behavior is considered to serve a coping function when it increases the likelihood that a task will be accomplished according to standards tolerable both to the individual and to the group in which he lives.

Coping Strategies in an Adolescent Transition

Using these criteria, a series of coping studies was carried out at the National Institute of Mental Health in Washington, D.C., on groups of adolescents who were experiencing the transition from high school to the freshman year in college.[9,26] The effort was to delineate the tasks and strategies of this important educational transition. These groups were chosen from the senior class in an urban middle-class high school on the basis of interpersonal and academic effectiveness during the high school years. One group was studied prior to admission to college; the other was followed through the first year of college.

The transition experienced by these young people involves several prominent stresses whose resolution has substantial bearing on the individual's future. These stressful elements of the situation constitute tasks of this transition, tasks that also reflect more general characteristics of adolescent experience. These tasks may be seen broadly to include: (1) separation from parents, siblings, and close friends; (2) greater autonomy in regard to making important decisions, assuming responsibility for oneself, and regulating one's behavior; (3) establishing new friendships; (4) pressures (internal and external) toward greater intimacy and adult sexuality; and (5) dealing with new intellectual challenges.

Although some adolescents respond to this situation with increasing anxiety and disorganization, most of those in the competent high school groups studied were not overwhelmed by the anticipation of change. In general, they met these tasks effectively. We will summarize some of the principal strategies through which these tasks of adolescent development were met.

1. *Reaching out for new experience.* The majority of students were positively oriented toward new experiences. This characteristic had been apparent for at least a few years prior to the high school–college transition.

2. *Seeking activity.* They were active in facing the tasks of the transition. This characteristic reflected itself in the purposeful, autonomous way in which they assumed responsibilities for making preparations for college.

3. *Referring to analogous past experiences.* The students often identified elements in the new situation with some experience in their own past which they felt was analogous. By reference to their ability to handle this analogous experience, they could reassure themselves about their ability to handle this situation and other similar ones in the future.

4. *Referring to continuity with the present self-image.* The students expressed in various ways the feeling that the step to college represented a modest increment in a continuous process of maturation. They tended to see a narrowing gap between themselves and their image of college students. Long in advance of the actual departure for college, a pattern of anticipatory detachment from

parents supported the students' self-images as people ready for change. This preparatory behavior may have also served the function of warding off feelings of depression associated with loss.

5. *Learning about the new situation in advance.* Another part of matching the self-image with the requirements of the new situation is to find out more in advance about what will be required in the new situation. Confidence tends to grow as the ambiguity of the new situation is reduced. These students used a variety of channels for getting advance information about the new situation: correspondence with the college, catalogues, talks with college friends, counselors, teachers, and parents, visiting college campuses, and reading books about college.

6. *Role rehearsal.* Most students prepared themselves for college by rehearsing forms of behavior which they associated with college students. This process is related to the pattern of anticipatory socialization described by Merton and Kitt: "For the individual who adopts the values of a group to which he aspires but does not belong, this orientation may serve the twin functions of aiding his rise into that group and of easing his adjustment after he has become part of it." [24]

7. *Group Identification.* Another mechanism for the students' self-assurance that they would do well at college was to identify themselves as part of a group which shares a reputation for being adequately prepared for college.

8. *Modifying the level of aspiration.* Some students, previously characterized by very high aspirations, lowered their sights in terms of what they were going to expect of themselves in college. It was as if they were redefining an acceptable self-image that would permit them to maintain a feeling of satisfaction in their performance if it were at a lower level than in high school. Nevertheless, a floor was also placed under performance, thus delineating a range of acceptable performance.

9. *Selectively perceiving encouraging elements in the new situation.* The students tended to perceive college as a potentially friendly environment. The encouraging elements, especially interpersonal, could offset difficult aspects of college life.

10. *Supportive function of shared experience.* Almost all of the students expressed the view that the anxiety they were experiencing was not unusual. Thus, being aware of anxiety did not make the student feel uncomfortably different from others.

11. *Usefulness of worry.* The work of worrying in preparation for dealing adequately with a stressful reality situation has been pointed out by Janis [20] in his studies of surgical patients. These students were similarly concerned about the situation ahead; however, these concerns did not lead to a circular ruminative preoccupation. Their concerns tended to focus on specific matters about which something concrete could be done.

12. *Present activity in anticipating future concerns.* Some of the students' behavior seemed important, not only in dealing with elements in the present situation, but also in dealing with an anticipated future concern. For example, one student had some concern about whether his widowed mother could handle certain household chores in his absence. He tried to get everything done around the house before he left for college. Such behavior provided a reference point for handling anticipated guilt he might experience about leaving his mother.

13. *Rehearsal of future behavior in fantasy.* This was another way of dealing with some future contingency by imagining what kind of behavior could deal with it.

14. *Clarifying new self-definitions and career possibilities.* Students were able to experiment with new alternatives in regard to choices of major subject and career plans by rehearsing these possibilities with others in informal discussions. New friendships provided the freshman with opportunities: (a) to free himself of the need to reciprocate with stereotypical expectations on the part of others; and (b) to experiment with new patterns of behavior in different kinds of relationships and new career plans.

15. *Intellectual stimulation through informal discussion groups.* Such sessions provided opportunities for discussing class assignments, books they were reading, new subject matter, "wild" ideas, and in general expanding their intellectual horizons.

16. *Learning through pooling of information and coping skills.* Informal discussions help in building up a predictable environment; resources are identified and expectations are delineated, e.g., regarding prevalent values.

17. *Learning through role complementarity.* A common experience during college life is a subtle process by which friends exchange coping skills, helping each other in their respective areas of strength, whether or not they are aware of doing so. For example, one student may help another by providing a model for the development of effective study habits and personal organization, and perhaps receive in return a model of effectiveness in the sphere of sex and dating behavior.

18. *Support in time of crisis.* The uses of friendship are extremely varied and ubiquitous in dealing with academic and interpersonal disappointments.

19. *Sounding board for other points of view.* By meeting peers of different cultural and subcultural backgrounds, a student could recognize the impact of his behavior on others and become aware of values other than his own.

Other coping mechanisms employed by the college freshmen to maintain their self-esteem and manage anxiety in social and academic situations include: (1) projecting a clear self-image as an effective doer; (2) mobilizing new combinations of skills; (3) regulating acceptable risk in different areas of commitment; (4)

using assets to test new images of growth potential; (5) selecting upperclassmen as resource persons; and (6) learning through part-identifications with faculty.

Coping Strategies of Patients with Serious Physical Impairment

Although socioacademic stress may be traumatic in many ways, it is perhaps reasonable to expect that normal, competent adolescents should be able to cope with expected transition. On the other hand, severe physical disability, coming on quite suddenly, is an extreme test of coping resources. Indeed, a plausible case can be made for expecting uniformly devastating results. One might suppose that the vast majority of severely damaged patients would be psychologically overwhelmed and left with lasting disturbances.

Yet clinical experience indicates that the outcome is sometimes surprisingly favorable. A few systematic studies on outcome indicate that a substantial proportion of severely injured patients make impressive psychosocial recovery. Existence of such favorable outcomes, even if they were rare, would be significant in the analysis of human coping behavior. What types of coping behavior contribute to favorable outcomes?

In studies of patients with serious illness, we have primarily directed attention to those aspects of behavior which related to one or more of the following broad tasks: keeping distress within manageable limits; maintaining a sense of personal worth; maintaining or restoring relations with significant other people; enhancing prospects for recovery of bodily functions; and increasing the likelihood of working out a personally valued and socially acceptable situation after maximum physical recovery has been attained. This is what we mean by coping behavior in the context of severe long-term illness.

In studies of burn patients [18,19] and acute polio patients,[29] we were concerned with the psychological responses which enabled these patients to deal with their predicament. We attempted to clarify the following questions: What are the most difficult and disturbing aspects of the adaptive problem faced by severely ill or burned patients—i.e., the specific tasks of this situation? What psychological strategies do such patients predominantly utilize in attempting to cope with these problems?

When a severely injured or acutely ill patient is admitted to the hospital, he may not only be in a state of severe physical pain, but is also undergoing serious emotional disturbances. Many of these patients are difficult to manage because of their inability to adjust to their physical status and their surroundings. Some are noisy, loud, and demanding; others are markedly depressed; some are sullen and uncooperative in treatment. Although the adaptive problems in such patients have important elements in common, they also differ considerably, not only in different patients, but in the same patient at different times.

The primary adaptive tasks are associated with the injury or illness itself. They are: a distinct threat to survival; fear of permanent physical damage and disfigurement; considerable pain and prolonged physical discomfort; the possibility of frequent surgical or other unpleasant medical procedures; and a long, tedious convalescence.

These problems directly associated with the injury or illness are complicated by other problems that appear, in varying combinations, in many patients. Prominent examples of these complicating problems are:

1. *Sense of responsibility for damage.*   When the patient believes that the burn or illness was caused by his own negligence or through the fault of a person he trusted, intense distress may ensue. Patients who have strong feelings of guilt may interpret the injury as punishment. Repetitive anxiety dreams and compulsive rumination often occur under these conditions.

2. *Separation from family and friends.*   Separation from family and friends, which is frequently inevitable in obtaining the specialized care required, deprives the patient of his main sources of emotional gratification at a time when he needs them most. An overwhelming feeling of loneliness and homesickness often leads to depression and self-pity.

3. *Effect of disability on future plans.*   The effect of disability on future plans is one of the commonest sources of concern. For example, the patient whose livelihood depends on manual dexterity is likely to be especially disturbed by burns of the hands. The possibility of intereference with a nonvocational activity that means a great deal to the patient may be equally disturbing, with burns of the lower extremities or the prospect of permanent paralysis being particularly threatening to young men who had obtained their greatest satisfaction from physical activity.

4. *Feelings of inadequacy.*   Feelings of inadequacy in comparison with other people are likely to become exaggerated by physical helplessness. Some patients are disturbed by the enforced extreme dependence on others. This occurs chiefly in those who have had serious doubts about their ability to cope with adult responsibility before their illness or injury. If these doubts have been counteracted by a facade of great independence, the disability is especially menacing in its implications.

5. *Sexual problems.*   Burns of the genitalia and perineum are not uncommon in military or industrial populations. Their management generally is relatively simple, but minor burns of the genitalia are more distressing to many patients than serious burns elsewhere. Women are likely to be concerned over their

fertility, particularly if the menses are interrupted as a result of the physical stress. Concern over expected sexual problems associated with residual paralysis was frequent in the polio group.

6. *Personal rejection.* Many patients interpret their disability as a threat to their capacity to be loved by others. These patients are often hypersensitive to the slightest indication of personal rejection and are in constant need of attention.

7. *Hostility.* A considerable amount of hostility toward others may be aroused by circumstances connected with the injury or illness or by difficulties in subsequent care. The difficulties of patients who have had serious concern in the past over the handling of hostile feelings may be intensified. This may lead to sullenness, depressive reaction, or resentful outbursts.

The many grave psychologic threats of a nearly fatal injury or severe prolonged illness place the patient in danger of being overwhelmed by emotionally painful stimuli. Most patients were found initially to attempt to keep unpleasant thoughts and feelings out of awareness either consciously (suppression) or unconsciously (repression), and to minimize painful stimuli that do enter consciousness by tight control of all emotions (constriction). The patient's attitude is, in effect, "I will not think about any of these unpleasant things, but, if I cannot avoid them, I will not allow myself to have any feelings about them." A few patients go so far as to avoid any recognition of injury itself (denial). Patients in whom this type of response is very prominent generally have used similar adaptive mechanisms to a lesser extent before injury.

This form of adaptation was illustrated in the case of a burn patient who died two weeks after injury. Although she preferred not to think about the circumstances and nature of her injury and avoided the subject whenever possible, she remembered it clearly. Within a few days, however, she developed the attitude that she was not seriously ill at all, but practically well. She then recalled having been afraid of dying immediately after the injury, particularly when she first went to the operating room, but she said that when she had survived this ordeal she knew that she would be all right; she felt there was no doubt that she was now practically well, that she would require little further care and would soon be back to a normal family life. She said that she was not helpless, but to a considerable extent could care for herself. She talked rather lightly and comfortably for the most part. She felt that she would be sufficiently improved in a few days to be able to go home and take care of her children. This patient made such statements calmly and deliberately while she lay helpless on a frame in grave condition.

In the polio group, over half of the patients either did not recognize that they had polio or were quite skeptical of the diagnosis. A less serious illness such as flu was substituted. This defense appears to serve a useful function in preventing the patient's being overwhelmed, thus permitting him to make a more gradual transition to the exceedingly difficult tasks that lie ahead. In the early phase following serious injury there are many ways in which the threatening impact can be controlled, regulated, even minimized. But in the long run, other processes come into play that have the effect of facing threatening implications in dealing with them.

Most of the patients in these studies sooner or later came to face the actual conditions of their illness, sought information about the factors relevant to their recovery, and assessed the probable long-term limitations. The time of transition from denial or other protective strategy to acceptance varied greatly from patient to patient, sometimes occurring within a few weeks after onset, and in other cases requiring a much longer period of adjustment. A variety of coping strategies, employed at every level of awareness, were used by the patients in making this transition.

Interaction with other patients was usually beneficial. Severely disabled patients were placed next to patients less disabled or making significant recovery. This situation favored the development of a sense of security in the more helpless patient and a sense of competence for the other. An "open ward" arrangement, as opposed to private rooms, served to increase interpersonal contacts and the availability of nursing care. Sometimes fellow patients served to orient a newcomer to ward procedures and treatment techniques when staff instruction had only induced resistance.

The importance of close relationships in providing emotional support for the patient during this transition was manifested in various and sometimes paradoxical ways. One of these was a pattern observed in several women in their thirties who were mothers. These women were quite eager to be at home, where they felt a strong sense of being important and needed emotionally. Even though severely handicapped physically, they felt a sense of power in being able to exert control over their families' lives and a sense of pride in being able to use their experience to guide the actions of others. A few of the polio patients found some retrospective satisfaction in their own illness, in the sense that they would prefer to have the illness themselves than to have their children suffer from it. One young husband, who explained that he was almost happy he got polio instead of his wife or children, said he had much experience of active life, while his children had their whole lives to look forward to. He thought his wife was vulnerable and could not withstand such an illness. He, meanwhile, could take illness and disappointment and it would be less of a problem to him to bear. By viewing the situation in this way, he was able to enhance self-esteem and sustain hope. Similarly, wives who had polio expressed relief for economic reasons that they were stricken rather than their wage-earning husbands.

A role of importance in the community was also supportive to these patients. One patient, an adolescent girl, reported with considerable pride her experience upon returning home in which the ambulance driver had turned on the siren and thus attracted considerable attention and greetings from many people. Sometimes a patient became a community symbol for strength and endurance in the face of adversity: newspaper articles, radio programs, and community projects centered about them. A patient who had become somewhat depressed and disillusioned because her family lived 150 miles away from the hospital and could not visit was mentioned in the column of a popular Chicago columnist. She received almost 400 letters, some containing money or gifts, and became much more hopeful. For the first time she was willing to accept adaptive appliances in order to answer her "fan mail."

The effectiveness of coping behavior is strongly related to the feeling that one's presence is not only valued by significant other people but is virtually indispensable to them. Psychological recovery also hinges to a substantial extent on physical conditions. Physical progress can provide a powerful stimulus for the patient's emotional growth. When the polio patient sees clear evidence, for example, that he is regaining the use of his hands, he is likely to feel great encouragement to make new efforts for continued progress.

In the effort to achieve a long-term physical goal, the patients studied showed a strong tendency to set intermediate goals.[11] These goals appeared to be quite useful as vehicles of effort and transition. Such intermediate goals have certain common characteristics that probably contribute to their usefulness: (1) the time unit is relatively short-term (measurable in weeks, sometimes one to two months); (2) the goal is readily visible, bearing a recognizable relation to the patient's capabilities at the time that goal is set; (3) the goal is probably attainable. Attainment of such goals tends to be intrinsically rewarding. In these circumstances, such attainments provide repeated reinforcement for effort, and stimulus for further effort.[11] They strengthen a self-concept encompassing capability of change. As limits of recovery are gradually reached, further aspirations are also lowered in a stepwise progression.

Almost all these patients had to settle for considerably less in the way of physical recovery than they had hoped for. In most cases severe limitations or disfigurement remained even after several years of treatment, effort, and suffering. How was it possible for them to bear such disappointment? Most patients experienced a series of successive approximations through which they eventually faced and accepted the physical limitations they would so much have preferred to avoid. These approximations amounted to a series of small steps leading to ultimate recognition of a painful reality. With this recognition came a progressively increasing tendency to adapt to the new situation, to make use of whatever potentialities it offered for dependable gratifications, self-respect, and reliable relationships with significant other people.

Had these patients been faced at the outset with the certain prospect of their ultimate disability, it might well have been overwhelming for many of them. At the least, it would have been highly discouraging and probably disorganizing for many patients; quite likely, such reactions would often have impaired cooperation in treatment and the many organized, sustained efforts so important in utilizing whatever potentials that remain. It appeared that these patients did not suddenly, abruptly face the likelihood of their ultimate disability. Rather, this occurred gradually, in small steps, in slow transition from a self-concept of physical vigor to one of physical limitation. It seems that the stepwise nature of this transition makes the whole process more bearable. The loss of cherished capabilities thus occurs in small increments, with some personality reorganization taking place in each intermediate phase.

A major component of this final step in successful adaptation to permanent disability has to do with the individual's environmentally sanctioned image of himself as "different." The important distinction is between being "sick" and being "different." As long as the disabled individual sees himself and is seen by the environment as *sick*, he continues to demonstrate appropriate illness behavior and to have appropriate expectations of getting well. Basic to adequate coping with permanent disability is the awareness and acceptance by the individual and his environment that he is no longer sick, but different. If this transition is successfully made, he may then function in some sense as a different kind of human being, with distinctive needs, problems, and ways of adapting.[1]

Parents of Leukemic Children

Study of parents of leukemic patients [13] revealed that they experienced reactions similar to those of polio and burn patients, with slight variations in effect and interpretation. Without exception, the parents recalled a feeling of "shock" or of being "stunned" when hearing the definitive diagnosis. Only an occasional parent reported a concomitant feeling of disbelief, though in retrospect most parents feel that it took at least some days before the meaning of the diagnosis "sank in." Thus, the majority of parents appeared to accept the diagnosis intellectually, rather than to manifest the degree of disbelief and marked denial found in some burn and polio patients. There was an active seeking for hope-sustaining beliefs. Perhaps the diagnosis was in error, the disease not truly fatal. There was a tendency for the parents to be overwhelmingly impressed by the hospital after their child had been admitted. This reaction was associated with revived hope, expressed by statements such as: "If any place can save my child, it will be here." Remissions in the course of the prolonged illness also tended to revive hope. As the full implications of the illness began to be accepted, patterns of adaptive responses were again observed in many of the parents.

As we have indicated, resolution of the problem of responsibility is in general an important task for people in life-threatening situations. Once the diagnosis of leukemia was made, the parents would, almost without exception, initially blame themselves for not having paid more attention to the early nonspecific manifestations of the disease. They wondered whether the child would not have had a better chance of responding to therapy if the diagnosis had been made sooner. Although such reactions of guilt were extremely common, most parents in this study readily accepted assurance from the physicians that they had not neglected their child. Particularly reassuring to the parents was the information that the long-term prognosis in most cases of childhood leukemia is esentially the same no matter when the diagnosis is made.

A search for some meaning in the tragedy of the illness often seemed necessary. Most parents found it intolerable to think of their child's leukemia as a chance or meaningless event. Therefore, they tried to construct an explanation for it, displaying a certain amount of urgency until one appropriate to their particular frame of reference could be accepted. A few parents were content with a deferred explanation. They were satisfied with the knowledge that it would be some years before a scientifically accurate answer becomes available to explain why their child had developed leukemia. Parents in this category were all relatively well-educated and had some orientation to the nature of scientific work. A greater number of parents appeared to need a more immediate answer. They would eagerly accept one of the more recent theories concerning the etiology of leukemia, with some additional explanation which was a composite of scientific facts, elements from the parent's past experiences, and fantasies. Though in the majority of cases their concept of etiology served partially to resolve any feelings of being responsible for the child's illness, the synthesis sometimes appeared to reflect parental self-blame. In these instances, the guilt appeared to be less anxiety provoking than the total lack of a suitable explanation for the leukemia. Such observations highlight the significance of the search for meaning of life-threatening events.[6]

Most parents found religious beliefs comforting, as had many of the burn and polio patients. They frequently made such comments as: "It helps us be more accepting," "At least we know he will be in Heaven and not suffering." Only a few individuals thought about their child's illness primarily in a religious context, believing that "This is the Lord's way of protecting him from an even worse fate." Such parents were inclined to accept the illness as an expression of God's will. In the course of several years' work with parents of leukemic children, it was common for them to report a return to religion and to express sympathy for parents who did not have sufficient religious faith to help them in this crisis.

Hope, viewed as a favorable alteration of the expected sequence of events, was universally emphasized by the parents. Feeling hopeful tended to support active responses in meeting the situation. Persistence of hope for a more favorable outcome did not require that the child's prognosis be seriously distorted.

As the disease progressed, hope diminished. Early in the course of the illness, many parents hoped for the development of a curative drug. As the child became increasingly ill, they hoped only for one further remission. They no longer made long-range plans but lived on a day-to-day basis. They would, for instance, focus on whether their child would be well enough to attend a movie, rather than think about his ultimate fate. This gradual narrowing of hope appeared inversely related to the emergence of anticipatory grief.[23]

The amount of grieving in anticipation of the forthcoming loss varied greatly among the individual parents. In most, grief was apparent by the fourth month of the child's illness, frequently being precipitated by the first episode in the child's disease. Grieving then gradually evolved as the child's condition worsened. The death of another child on the ward had an exacerbating effect on the sense of loss in other parents.

The process of resigning oneself to the inevitable outcome was frequently accompanied by statements of wishing it was all over. The narrowing of hope and the completion of much of the grief work was described by one mother: "I still love my boy, want to take care of him and be with him as much as possible . . . but still feel sort of detached from him." She continued, however, to be very effective in caring for and comforting her child. This anticipatory mourning appears to be useful in preparing for the eventual loss; the few parents in our study who did not display such behavior experienced more severe distress after the child's death than did parents who had largely worked through the loss in advance.

Applications of the Stress-Coping Perspective in Social Psychiatry

We have given examples of coping strategies useful to persons of various ages, both sexes, and different socioeconomic backgrounds in facing a variety of tasks in several stressful situations: serious illness and injury, as well as adolescents in a major transition. Certain common themes recur. All these studies suggest that, under stressful conditions, people seek broadly for information about the following questions: (1) How can the distress be relieved? (2) How can a sense of personal worth be maintained? (3) How can a rewarding continuity of interpersonal relationships be maintained? (4) How can the requirements of the stressful task be met, or the opportunities utilized? Psychological preparation, which amounts to the development of effective coping behavior, requires time to obtain answers to these questions prior to a threatening event. If the threatening event occurs without warning (as in the burn and polio situations), time for "preparation" is likely to be bought by temporary self-deception, in such a way as to make recognition of threatening elements gradual and manageable. A time scale of weeks or a few months for preparation, as in the leukemia sitution, appears to have considerable utility. Where a time scale of many months or even a few years is involved, as in the transitions of youth, very gradual, thorough, preparation is likely to occur.

Coping strategies are developed in many ways and from many sources: directly and indirectly, overtly and covertly, in fantasy and in action. Strategies for obtaining and utilizing information are formed at all levels of awareness and may be employed over long periods of time. Strategies that are established in a person's psychological repertoire, and that have served similar functions in earlier stressful experiences, are likely to be employed first. But distress of high intensity or long duration is a powerful impetus to the formation of new strategies, integrating internalized orientations and current opportunities. Such new strategies, if effective, are likely to become available for use in future crises, and indeed may broaden the individual's adaptive capability.

This approach leads itself to application in predictable stressful circumstances. It should be feasible to utilize knowledge of tasks and strategies in a situation of major transition in such ways as to heighten the effectiveness of most individuals in coping with difficult aspects of the experience.

Many people can benefit from specific information regarding tasks and strategies relevant to their current circumstances. When a new pattern of action is undertaken that holds reasonable promise of effectiveness, emotional responses tend to change concomitantly. The more effective the action, the less the distress. A gain in confidence and reduction in anxiety tend to follow effective performance of an act that had previously been subject to considerable misgiving. This approach implies that we must learn what strategies are useful in which situations, and which of these are closest to the individual's available repertoire. Behavioral science could help many individuals cope with their predicaments if investigations could build a substantial inventory of: (1) common problem situations; (2) feasible strategies; and (3) probability of preparation for each strategy in various human populations. Such information is most likely to be widely useful if developed within a broadly bio-psycho-social framework.[8]

Several attempts have been made to apply the coping concepts described in preventive contexts, and we shall now briefly describe two of these. One of the most interesting such applications has been in the preparation of volunteers for service in the Peace Corps.[10] This program involved a carefully formulated attempt to convey, to a group of volunteers going to a given country to do a given job, some reasonably vivid and accurate account of what it would be like to be in that place, at that time, and doing that kind of job. Efforts were made to anticipate and describe both problems likely to occur (tasks) and possibly useful solutions (strategies). Thus, if one was to be a teacher in rural Ghana, one would need to learn something about Ghana in general, something about the ways of the countryside, and something about schools. In addition, one should anticipate the features of likely encounters with students, African teachers, and officials in that particular setting. The volunteers were brought into extensive contact with people who had prior experience in the culture to which they were going, and given ample opportunity for discussion and rehearsal. In later years, returned Peace Corps volunteers who had been through that very experience were used as "teachers." This proved particularly salient for the new volunteers. Nationals of the country in question were also increasingly drawn into the training experience. Finally, fairly explicit basic information on human relations was included as part of the preparation for overseas assignment. This entire approach has been called "anticipatory guidance" and has striven for a kind of emotional inoculation for stressful experience.

A second preventive application of coping models is in a recently developed peer-counseling program for early adolescents.[16] Early adolescence is an important and neglected phase of human development which lends itself to analysis in terms of developmental tasks and coping strategies. The coming of age in modern societies is an increasingly long and complex process. Since the Industrial Revolution there has been a secular trend toward earlier onset of biological puberty, whereas full social maturity is acheived later and later. The former presumably rests upon nutritional and hygienic changes; the latter has to do with increasingly complex educational rquirements for a highly technological society. There is thus about a decade in which, by most criteria, the individual is neither child nor adult. Contemporary evidence of manifest distress in this age group suggests that we need clarification of the tasks and strategies of this difficult period, not only by sex and by age level, but also by social class and ethnic group. There are preliminary indications of significant differences in tasks and strategies among these various subsets of adolescents, even though there is overlap as well.

As an example of the complex interaction of biological and social factors in coping, the earlier onset of puberty means that, on the average, it tends to coincide in American society with the transition from elementary school to junior high school. There are marked differences in the junior high school and the elementary school as social environment, and thus a drastic change in environmental conditions occurs both internally and externally at about the same time. This is a heavy load upon the organism and a sharp discontinuity with past experience. A great many adolescents are inadequately prepared to cope with this conjunction of stressful events.

As an approach to this problem, a peer-counseling program was developed for junior and senior high schools which rests upon an analysis of developmental tasks and coping strategies. Utilizing the credibility of peers in adolescence, the program trains students to help other students. It does so largely by clarifying the tasks and potential strategies for this phase of the life cycle in a particular social setting, by providing information on the complex processes of interpersonal relationship, and by providing continuing supervision of the student counselors. Preliminary findings suggest that the program is useful for both counselees *and* counselors. The long-range objective of this project is to develop a self-sustaining peer-counseling program which can function effectively within a school system, with a minimum necessity for involvement of mental health professionals. A detailed curriculum for the training of peer counselors has been evolved, and a training program for teachers and professional counselors has been developed to aid them in selecting, training, and supervising students as peer counselors. Criteria and rating measures for estimating the effectiveness of the student in his performance as a peer counselor have been worked out. Social indicators such as level of school achievement in relation to potential, truancy, dropout rates, disciplinary school actions, incidence of drug abuse, incidence of violence or vandalism in the schools, and teacher turnover rates are utilized to estimate the overall impact of the program.

These examples of anticipatory guidance in the Peace Corps and a peer counselor program in the high schools are suggestive of ways in which a stress-coping framework may be employed in future social psychiatric efforts. Such work is still at an early stage of development. But enough experience has accumulated to encourage responsible innovation with systematic assessment in this field. In our judgment, growing knowledge of coping behavior in various stressful situations will permit much relief of human suffering and an enhancement of effectiveness in dealing with inevitable life transitions.

REFERENCES

1. Adams, J., and Lindemann, E. "Coping with Long-term Disability." In *Coping and Adaptation*, pp. 127–128, edited by G. Coelho, D. Hamburg, and J. Adams. New York: Basic Books, 1974.

2. Benedek, T. "The Psychosomatic Implications of the Primary Unit Mother-Child." *American Journal of Orthopsychiatry* 19(1949):642.

3. ———. "Climacterium: A Developmental Phase." *Psychoanalytic Quarterly* 19(1950):1.

4. Bibring, G.; Dwyer, T.; Huntington, D.; and Valenstein, A. "A Study of the Psychological Processes in Pregnancy and of the Earliest Mother-Child Relationship: I. Some Propositions and Comments." *Psychoanalytic Study of the Child* 16(1961):9–24.

5. ———. "A Study of the Psychological Processes in Pregnancy and of the Earliest Mother-Child Relationship: II. Methodological Considerations." *Psychoanalytic Study of the Child* 16(1961):25–72.

6. Chodoff, P. "Adjustment to Disability: Some Observations of Patients with Multiple Sclerosis." *Journal of Chronic Diseases* 9(1959):653.

7. Cobb, S., and Lindemann, E. "Coconut Grove Burns: Neuropsychiatric Observations." *Annals of Surgery* 117(1943):814–824.

8. Coelho, G.; Hamburg, D.; and Adams, J.; eds. *Coping and Adaptation.* New York: Basic Books, 1974.

9. Coelho, G.; Hamburg, D.; and Murphy, E. "Coping Strategies in a New Learning Environment." *Archives of General Psychiatry* 9(1963):433–443.

10. D'Andrea, V. "Mental Health Training for Overseas Volunteer Service." *International Journal of Social Psychiatry* 12(1966):192–198.

11. Davis, F. "Definitions of Time and Recovery in Paralytic Polio Convalescence." *American Journal of Sociology* 61(1956):582–587.

12. Erikson, E. "Identity and the Life Cycle." *Psychological Issues* 1(no. 1), 1959.

13. Friedman, S.; Chodoff, P.; Mason, J.; and Hamburg, D. "Behavioral Observations on Parents Anticipating the Death of a Child." *Pediatrics* 32(1963):610–625.

14. Grinker, R. R., and Speigel, J. *Men Under Stress.* New York: McGraw-Hill, 1945.

15. Grinker, R. R., Sr.; Grinker, R. R., Jr.; and Timberlake, J. "Mentally Healthy Young Males (Homoclites)." *Archives of General Psychiatry* 6(1962):405–453.

16. Hamburg, B., and Varenhorst, B. "Peer Counseling in the Secondary Schools." *American Journal of Orthopsychiatry* 42(1972):566–581.

17. Hamburg, D., and Adams, J. "A Perspective on Coping Behavior: Seeking and Utilizing Information in Major Transitions." *Archives of General Psychiatry* 17(1967):277–284.

18. Hamburg, D.; Hamburg, G.; and DeGoza, S. "Adaptive Problems and Mechanisms in Severely Burned Patients." *Psychiatry* 16(1953):1–20.

19. Hamburg, D.; Artz, G.; Reiss, E.; Anspacher, W.; and Chambers, R. "Clinical Importance of Emotional Problems in the Care of Patients with Burns." *New England Journal of Medicine* 248(1953):355–359.

20. Janis, I. *Psychological Stress.* New York: Wiley, 1958.

21. ———. "Psychological Effects of Warnings." In *Man and Society in Disaster*, pp. 55–92, edited by G. Baker and D. Chapman. Basic Books, 1962.

22. Leighton, A. H. *My Name is Legion.* New York: Basic Books, 1959, p. 142.

23. Lindemann, E. "Symptomatology and Management of Acute Grief." *American Journal of Psychiatry* 101(1944):141.

24. Merton, R., and Kitt, A. "Contributions to the Theory of Reference Group Behavior." In *Continuities in Social Research*, edited by R. Merton and P. Lazarsfeld. Chicago: Free Press, 1950.

25. Murray, H. A. *Explorations in Personality.* New York: Oxford University Press, 1938.

26. Silber, E.; Hamburg, D.; Coelho, G.; Murphey, E.; Rosenberg, M.; and Pearlin, L. "Adaptive Behavior in Competent Adolescents." *Archives of General Psychiatry* 5(1961):354–365.

27. Smith, M. "Research Strategies Toward a Conception of Positive Mental Health." *American Journal of Psychology* 15(1960):673–681.

28. ———. "Explorations in Competence: A Study of Peace Corps Teachers in Ghana." *American Journal of Psychology* 21(1966):555–566.

29. Visotsky, H.; Hamburg, D.; Goss, M.; and Lebovits, B. "Coping Behavior Under Extreme Stress." *Archives of General Psychiatry* 5(1961):423–448.

30. White, R. "Ego and Reality in Psychoanalytic Theory." *Psychological Issues* 3 (no. 3), 1963.

31. ———. *Lives in Progress.* New York: Holt, Rinehart, 1966.

Editorial Note

In the mid-1950s the editors identified the study of concepts of normality and abnormality as the first key issue for a social psychiatry. The issue is still with us, but the present chapter, together with Chapter 16 (on health measurement), affords evidence of a considerable advance in both conceptualization and empirical inquiry. There appears to be a substantial accumulation of evidence and convergence of thinking about what constitutes healthy psychological processes. The core of agreement is that the mentally well-functioning individual must be characterized by both "internal" criteria (such as life satisfaction and self-esteem) and "external" criteria (such as effective participation in a network of social roles). A sophisticated conception of healthiness is central to each of the selections in Part III; they all describe efforts to elevate in some way the health of populations. And as Hollister points out, the advocates of primary prevention in community psychiatry are recurrently challenged to state the goal of their efforts, the sought condition of "mental health."

Beiser and Leighton offer the exceedingly interesting suggestion, borne out by other researchers as well, that health and illness may be composed of two distinct ranges of phenomena, rather than being simply the opposite poles of a single continuum. This necessarily complicates our view of behavior, but is at the same time probably a more accurate rending of social and psychological reality. In particular, it allows us to think of the individual as a mixed, complex entity, an organization of both positive and negative processes. Perhaps we can seldom make the extreme, blanket judgment that a given person is healthy or unhealthy; instead, we are impelled to look closely at his array of strengths and weaknesses, the balance of forces enabling him to maintain a going concern—or not to do so. As Beiser and Leighton (and others like Robert W. White) emphasize, the study of "normal" lives in "natural" settings tends to convince us that most people combine elements of effective coping with other, less salutary responses. The problem for social psychiatry is not, then, some impossible agenda of producing uniform superpsychological healthiness, but a shrewd and modest program designed to capitalize on individual assets and mitigate the force of the inevitable deficits. The authors wisely remark, for example, that "chronic anxiety can more often be neutralized and brought under control than eliminated. Sometimes, indeed, it can be converted into an asset that helps the individual to be productive and attain his goals."

Despite our recognition of the potential yield from investigating healthy behavior, we suffer from a paucity of ideas and observations concerning what Halbert Dunn termed "high-level wellness." [14] Thus the authors of this chapter insist that "a need still exists for ways in which to conceptualize and measure well-being and excellent, in addition to adequate, role performance." One might almost argue that we applaud and reward extraordinary competence but do not learn from it. There is a palpable but largely unexplored relationship between psychological health and such yea-saying qualities as creativity, executive capacity, empathic interpersonal talents *(for instance, those exhibited in effective helping or healing or teaching), and* leadership *(exemplary activity). Clearly, not all the incumbents of social roles that manifest these properties are paragons of mental health; that outstanding individuals are often flawed in manifold ways is a truism. Our proper study, however, should not be of the alcoholism of novelists or the anxieties of statesmen; it should be of the intra- and interpersonal strategies that coalesce in importantly contributory social psychological conduct. There is an ancient Chinese imprecation: "May you live in interesting times." In our very interesting and very troubled times, there is some urgency in pursuing models of heightened human capacities.*

R. N. W.

CHAPTER 10

Personality Assets and Mental Health*

Morton Beiser
Alexander H. Leighton

The Concept of Health

THE TOPIC of positive mental health brings us directly into the realm of values, a realm which has until recently been generally avoided by those in the field of medicine. It has seemed more practical, as well as more appropriate to the task of treating the sick, to accept absence of disease as the best measure of health. It has also been considered more objective and scientific.

Yet, numbers of people have been troubled by the fact that absence of pathology and good functioning are not simply two sides of the same coin. For example, there can be restoration of function without the disappearance of pathology. This may occur as a result of natural compensation, as can be seen in certain cases of damage to the cerebral cortex. It can also be brought about by "therapeutic" intervention, as with insulin in diabetes, or digitalis in cardiac disorders.

* This work, conducted as part of the Harvard Program in Social Psychiatry, was supported by Public Health Service Grant MH-12892 from the National Institute of Mental Health.

There are analogues in the field of mental health. Chronic anxiety can more often be neutralized and brought under control than eliminated. Sometimes, indeed, it can be converted into an asset that helps the individual to be productive and attain his goals.

In spite of these and similar observations, symptoms have, until fairly recently, continued to be the overriding concern of the mental health professions.

A review of the psychiatric literature suggests that in the last twenty years a change in emphasis can be discerned. Increasing interest in positive mental health has been paralleled by a shift from armchair speculation to actual studies, and these have in turn stimulated new ways of looking at the problem. Three major currents seem to run through the recent literature:

1. Conceptualization of health as a process (functioning) rather than as some unspecified territory at an opposite pole to illness.
2. The view that health (like individual growth and development) has to be considered in a societal context.
3. The appearance of empirical studies reporting on the behavior of people living "normal" lives in "natural" settings. (This is in contrast to the more common studies of groups identified in terms of medical criteria together with what are, as a rule, rather inadequately defined controls.)

Health As an Adaptive Process

"Health as process" constitutes a general theory, and the identification and measurement of the process requires an approach using multiple criteria. Pioneering work in this field comes primarily from those interested in mental health. Thus Jahoda [21] emphasizes the need for multiple criteria in assessing health in her review of the literature up to 1957. Gurin, Veroff, and Field [18] employed multiple criteria in designing their nation-wide study. They interviewed a sample of adults about various aspects of their own well-being and feelings of distress. Analysis of the responses showed that statements of happiness and statements of difficulty and worry were not related in any simple, reciprocal fashion. Eighty-nine percent of the sample said they were "very happy" or "pretty happy," while 25 percent said they worried a lot, or all the time. In other words, at least 14 percent were both worried and happy. Furthermore, younger people were more apt to describe themselves as happy, but also as worrying a great deal, whereas older people worried less but were also less happy.

Gurin and associates mentioned the implications which their findings could have for assessment procedures. If a single criterion, such as absence of worries, was taken as the sole indicator of mental health, older people might look healthier than the young. If the indicator chosen was reports of happiness, the conclusions could be exactly opposite.

Norman Bradburn and coauthors in a later study [6,7] have developed this argument further. Also using a survey method, they asked about overall happiness and then in addition posed a battery of questions concerned with "positive effect." These were:

During the past few weeks, have you felt:
a. Excited or interested in something?
b. Proud because someone complimented you?
c. Pleased about having accomplished something?
d. On top of the world?
e. That things were going your way?

There were also a set of "negative affect" items.

During the past few weeks, have you felt:
a. So restless that you couldn't sit long in a chair?
b. Very lonely or remote from other people?
c. Bored?
d. Depressed or very unhappy?
e. Upset because someone criticized you?

As expected, there was a high degree of interrelationship among items in the positive set and among items in the negative set. But a predicted negative association between items in the two sets did not obtain. Furthermore, the relationship of both to statements about overall happiness was complex. Bradburn says:

A person's sense of well-being can be understood best as a function of the relative strengths of the positive and negative feelings he has experienced in the recent past. The data show clearly that these two distinct and independent dimensions are associated with different aspects of a person's life. Forces contributing toward increased negative feelings, such as anxiety, marital tension and job dissatisfaction, do not produce any concomitant decreases in positive feelings, and those forces which contribute toward the development of positive feelings, such as social interaction and active participation in the environment, do not in any way lessen negative feelings. Thus, it is possible for a person who has many negative feelings to be happy, if he also has compensatory positive feelings. Only by knowing the relative balance of feelings can one make predictions about people's happiness (pp. 56–57).[7]

Health in Societal Context

In a general way it has long been recognized in medicine that both health and illness are concepts which have meaning only in terms of context. Winton and Baylis,[35] for example, make the statement that "Health and disease are primarily sociological concepts."

As in the case of the concept of "health," so also in the matter of social relativity, medicine has tended to shy away from explicit investigation. It has been, rather, in sociology and cultural anthropology that both systematic work and speculation have been undertaken regarding relationships between sociocultural and illness patterns. The investigators have tended to phrase their definitions of health in terms relative to the social context in which behavior occurs. A. F. C. Wallace[34] defines (mental) health as a "state in which the person is performing to his own and others' satisfaction the roles appropriate to his situation in society." The use of terms like "appropriate" again raises the question of values. What if it is the society that is wrong rather than the individual?

Many people feel that the concept of health is so value-laden and socially relative as to be outside the possibility of scientific investigation. We believe that there are two points to be made in this connection. The first is that, as Winton and Baylis suggest, "illness" is a concept no less value-laden than "health." People have a strong negative value with regard to the state called "illness," but this does not interfere with conducting scientific investigation regarding the phenomena brought to attention by the value. The difference that marks the concept of "illness" from "health" is not so much the absence of value judgment as such, but rather that the value is widely shared and fairly uniform. This uniformity of view and feeling creates the impression of dealing with something factual. With "health," on the other hand, there are numerous differing values, and this makes them more obvious as such.

The second point is to suggest that, with both "health" and "illness" concepts, the important thing is for one to be explicit regarding the valuative component and to make this part of the phenomena under scrutiny. In this way it will not operate as a covert assumption on the part of the observer, and exert unperceived effects on the results.

Talcott Parsons,[25,26] in developing theory centered about health in social context, uses the term "system" as a conceptual bridge to refer both to functioning at the individual level and at the level of society:

> In a relative sense, the functioning of systems must be evaluated: they are more or less well adapted to their situations, more or less well integrated, and so forth. A conceptual scheme which makes values a

central category cannot evade this consequence, and should not attempt to.

He further suggests that individuals as systems must be assessed in particular situations according to the norms (values) governing that particular situation. This indicates a research strategy, and is quite different from becoming tangled in posing questions and counterquestions about the relativity of value judgments in terms of a broad ethical perspective.

The research strategy is that groups be identified that are distinct from each other by the intragroup values they hold, values that are relevant to illness and health. The desirability of this is most obvious where there are marked cultural contrasts, as between an African and a North American community. The orientation can, however, be applied to other groupings, such as ethnic minorities within North American society, socioeconomic classes, urban versus rural groups, members of particular occupations that tend to have certain strongly shared values (e.g., the medical profession), and so on. The frame of reference may also be applied to groupings derived from a somewhat different point of view, namely according to sex or according to age, where again the values may differ sufficiently to require a different basis for rating health.

Empirical Studies of Normal People in Natural Settings

In spite of their difficulty, studies of health in nonclinical populations have begun to accumulate and to contribute important insights into the process of adaptation and the nature of health. These studies have dealt, by and large, with accessible populations, such as children and adolescents in schools,[11,24,28,29] college students,* and workers in industry [8] or other special-interest groups.[15,32] Some have also been general community surveys.†

Many of these studies have been devoted to elucidating factors related to functioning, rather than to making a statement as to what the criteria of health might be. The strategy has been to study the adaptive patterns of "average" (and in that sense "normal") people in particular life situations.‡

Still other studies have specified indicators of health and then studied factors, including personal capacities which might be related to these health dimen-

* See references 1, 5, 12, 17, 19, 20, 30, and 31.
† See references 2, 3, 4, 6, 7, 16, 18, and 23.
‡ See references 10, 17, 19, 24, and 28.

sions. Indicators which have found fairly wide acceptance and which have been used in survey research are:

1. A relative absence of structured psychiatric symptoms. [18,22,33]
2. A sense of well-being.*
3. Effective performance in major social roles. [5,8,15,32]

Too often, however, the criteria adopted have suffered from being either unidimensional and/or minimal, rather than optimal measures. They are often apt to be criteria rooted in man's deficits rather than his excellences.

A need still exists for conceptualizing and developing measures of optimal functioning. Once this has been done, these could be combined with measures of psychic distress (which are, by and large, more highly developed) to form meaningful systems for classifying people.

The Stirling County Research in Positive Mental Health

In our own field studies in rural and urban areas, we began many years ago by defining mental health as the absence of illness. In time an intensive longitudinal study of a small group (123) of symptomatic and asymptomatic people living in a rural area in Nova Scotia led to refinement of some of our concepts and methods.

A team of psychiatrists came to live in Stirling County for a period of one to two months each year for five consecutive years. During this time in the field they conducted interviews with the respondents, collected structured material as well as ancillary medical and psychological data from family doctors and other key informants, and held weekly clinical conferences. Field workers engaged in other aspects of the research frequently attended these clinical sessions and contributed to the psychiatrists' understanding of the social and cultural context in which the respondents lived.

In addition to a relative lack of symptoms, two features were used time and again in describing the people judged to be the most healthy on clinical and intuitive grounds: a subjective sense of well-being and evidence of participation as a contributing member in community or social groups.

These observations in turn led to a search for methods of measuring well-being and community contribution. In this chapter we shall report on some of the studies related to well-being.

* See references 2, 3, 4, 6, 7, 16, 18, 23, and 27.

WHAT IS AN ADEQUATE MEASURE OF WELL-BEING?

During one field period the psychiatrists administered a twenty-six-item questionnaire containing, among other items, a modified version of the ten developed by Bradburn and his associates. With the use of factor analysis, we were able to identify three separable dimensions which could be treated as mental health scales.

We have called these Negative Affect, Sense of Pleasurable Involvement, and Long-Term Satisfaction. The three scales are described in Table 10.1. They are also described in more detail in previous reports.[2,3]

Factors I and II are obviously very similar to Bradburn's negative and positive affect scales.

One item on Bradburn's positive affect scale showed no consistent pattern of covariation with the four defining variables in our Pleasurable Involvement factor. Further analysis of the qualitative responses to this item, "During the past few months have you felt on top of the world?" confirmed the impression that it

TABLE 10.1
Positive Health Scales

FACTOR	ITEMS
I. Negative Affect	During the past few months have you felt: a. bored? b. very unhappy? c. very lonely or remote from other people? d. upset because someone criticized you? e. so restless that you couldn't sit long in a chair?
II. Pleasurable Involvement	During the past few months have you felt: a. pleased about having accomplished something? b. that things were going your way? c. proud because someone complimented you for something you had done? d. particularly excited or interested in something?
III. Long-Term Satisfaction	a. Considering the way your life is going at the moment, would you: 1. like it to continue in much the same sort of way? 2. like to change some parts of it? 3. like to change many parts of it? b. How successful have you been at planning your life, in your work, and with your family? Would you say: 1. very? 2. somewhat? 3. undecided? 4. a little unsuccessful? 5. very unsuccessful? c. Do you feel you have accomplished most of the things you would have liked to, up to this point in your life? Answer yes or no.

is a meaningless idiom in this particular setting. We eliminated it, therefore, from further consideration.

The emergence of factor III is somewhat surprising, in view of the similarity of some items which load here as compared with those which load in factor II. Notice in particular item a. of the Pleasurable Involvement scale and item c. of Long-Term Satisfaction. Both refer to accomplishments, and one might have expected some degree of halo effect. Yet the first one, tied to the past few months, and the second, requiring a more philosophical view of one's whole life, showed no covariation.

Among the studies we previously cited for their focus on well-being, most have utilized, in one way or another, a question which has come to be known as the global happiness item: "Taking all things together, how would you say things are these days—would you say you are very happy, pretty happy, not too happy?"

In view of the extensive use of this item, and its appealing face validity, it seemed worthwhile to study its relationship to the three affective dimensions—Negative Affect, Pleasurable Involvement, and Long-Term Satisfaction.

All three proved to be highly correlated with global happiness, and partial correlations revealed that these relationships are independent of the interaction among the three affects themselves. A multiple regression analysis demonstrated that an index composed of the three "predicts" scores on global happiness far better than any one dimension in isolation.[2]

The suggestion that feelings of "global happiness" may be a result of several simultaneously interacting affects has some importance. It suggests that useful inquiry might be directed at the more microscopic rather than global levels. It may also help to resolve some of the discrepancies in the literature on which at least one author has commented extensively.[13] Some of these discrepancies result from the use of global measures or from treating well-being as synonymous with absence of psychic distress.

ASSETS IN THE CONTEXT OF STIRLING COUNTY

Besides trying to conceptualize and develop measures of mental health, the Stirling County work has involved a search for assets, both personal and situational, which promote the emergence of positive patterns.

The influence on well-being of age, sex, educational level, physical health, and socioeconomic status was considered. We were also interested in personal capacities enabling an individual to achieve his own brand of happiness. Two of these are considered in this report: interpersonal reactivity and role-related planning abilities.

It is probably safe to assert that it requires personal capacities in order to utilize opportunities presented by the environment. On the other hand, an extremely impoverished environment will tax even the most richly endowed personality. Thus, we have called the final group of variables to be considered *interactive*, in that they depend on an interaction between personality readiness and resource availability. They include participation in formal community activities, community satisfaction, and household satisfaction.

The 123 respondents were chosen after a larger community survey to constitute a panel with equal numbers of men and women falling into three different age groups—young adults, middle-aged, and elderly. They live in twelve different communities presenting a range of socioenvironmental circumstances. They are also extremely heterogeneous from a mental health viewpoint, ranging from people with few or no psychiatric symptoms and therefore "healthy," according to one definition, to people who would be considered frank "cases" by any clinical psychiatrist.

Roughly one-third of the panel are of Acadian-French extraction, are Catholic, and speak French at home, although most are also bilingual. Most of the others are of English-Protestant stock and speak only English. A small percentage of the respondents are blacks.

Although there have been some instances of intermarriage among the three groups, and although relationships are at least overtly cordial, they have maintained, for the most part, remarkably segregated communities.

One feature which characterizes both the French and English socioculturally integrated communities is a shared sentiment of intragroup superiority. The basis for these feelings differs; the English-Protestant group, for instance, considers its way of life superior, whereas the French-Catholic group, who are a minority in the province, feel that they are superior to others in spiritual things, although perhaps weaker in economic and political matters. An individual sense of pride is an important feature of positive functioning, and life in integrated communities probably fosters this attribute by means of the prominent and supportive web of sentiments. We studied this proposition by asking our respondents: "On the whole, are you satisfied with the community you live in, yes or no?"

The family is another source of pride. Family status and an extended web of kinship determine a great deal of social interaction in the county. It is difficult to formulate unobtrusive questions about family life, but one which was helpful was simply phrased as: "Are you satisfied with the household you live in, yes or no?"

About a third of our respondents have a grade ten education; about 20 percent have had only three or four years of formal education. These are, by and large, the older people, who grew up when the laws pertaining to education were more lax than they are now. Only about 10 percent have completed high school, and a handful have had some college training.

In general, the occupational profile reflects the relatively low educational level. As in most small town and rural areas of North America, however, there are also real limitations with regard to occupational opportunity in this region. We have been amazed at the skill and ingenuity some of the respondents display in overcoming personal and environmental limitations. The ability to plan for the future, taking into account realistic personal and environmental limitations, as well as seeing real possibilities where they exist and capitalizing upon them, is a skill which we came to view as related to positive mental health.

The work role is, of course, extremely important, but people simultaneously occupy many others. In the integrated communities there is considerable emphasis on maintaining balance. For instance, in the French-Catholic communities, the picture of a "good man" is one who works hard and enjoys his job, is a fervent Catholic and fulfills religious duties, and participates in community activities. The prominent sentiments in the Protestant integrated communities are similar, although perhaps not so explicitly articulated. In these instances, it is clear that people are called upon to fulfill many different roles simultaneously. The potential for conflict between roles has received some attention, primarily in the sociological literature. In contrast to the model of role incompatibility and clashes, we have been struck by the ability of some of our respondents to maintain a balance, a role harmony. There is, after all, an element of freedom of choice in assuming and performing various roles. We have begun to think that people who are able to allocate time and resources appropriately and economically among the roles they occupy, and even to deal with some of the normative incompatibilities which may exist among roles, are displaying a personality attribute which has mental health implications. Basing their judgments on the wealth of accumulated clinical data, the psychiatrists rated each respondent on a dimension called "role-related planning abilities."

To a great extent men and women lead separate lives, both at work and at play. Some of the men are avid sport fishermen and hunters, and this area is particularly advantageous for them. Golf, curling, and hockey are other local sports. Stock car racing is a local "craze" and some of our respondents take part in competitions and enjoy tinkering with their cars in spare time. There is also a certain amount of visiting and "hanging around" at the local service station or at the canteen, which the men in particular seem to enjoy.

For women, even more than for men, life is with people. Women visit each other in their homes, hold card parties, and attend various church-sponsored activities together. The company of relatives and friends compensates in large measure for the lack of many physical conveniences, the relative isolation from shopping and cultural activities they might enjoy in a city, and the hardships wrought by long and often harsh winters. Interpersonal reactivity, the ability to meet people and to interact comfortably with them, and the ability to secure emotional support from appropriate sources, such as family and friends, become exceedingly important attributes under such conditions.

There are also many formal organizations—religious, civic, fraternal, and sororal—to which men and women in the county belong. We constructed an index of the intensity of a respondent's participation by asking questions about the number of organizations to which he or she belonged, the amount of time devoted to the organization, and whether participation was as a member or as the incumbent of an office.

SELECTED FINDINGS

Some selected findings are summarized in Table 10.2.

TABLE 10.2
Correlates of Affective States

	NEGATIVE AFFECT	PLEASURABLE INVOLVEMENT	LONG-TERM SATISFACTION
A. Social and "control" variables			
Age	0	0	0
Sex	0	0	0
Education	0	0	0
Socioeconomic status	(−)	0	0
Number of physical conditions *	(+ +)	0	(−)
B. Personal variables			
Role-related planning abilities	0	(+ +)	0
Interpersonal reactivity	(−)	(+)	(+)
C. Interactive			
Participation in community activities	0	(+ +)	0
Household satisfaction	0	0	(+ +)
Community satisfaction	(− −)	0	(+ +)

0 = No significant association
(−) = Significant negative association, less than 0.3
(− −) = Significant negative association, more than 0.3
(+) = Significant positive association, less than 0.3
(+ +) = Significant positive association, more than 0.3

* The number of physical and psychophysiologic conditions which the respondent had, as judged by the psychiatrists.

Numerical values have been omitted in this table, in the hope of simplifying a fairly complex presentation. For the interested reader, most of the statistics have been presented elsewhere.[2,3]

The most striking overall finding is that the pattern of associations for each of the affective variables is different. Negative Affect has been found elsewhere [2,6,7] to relate to measures of frank psychiatric disorder, and here it behaves most like other measures of psychic distress in relating to socioeconomic status and number of physical conditions. Negative Affect is also related to Interpersonal Reactivity and Community Satisfaction.

Pleasurable Involvement, as its name implies, is related more to those variables which reflect an intense involvement in work and community roles and in dealings with other people. Neither Negative Affect nor Pleasurable Involvement are related to the variables of age, sex, and education.

Long-Term Satisfaction is also not related to these control variables. Like Negative Affect, it is related to physical health, and like both other affect scales, it is related to interpersonal reactivity. However, the strongest relationships are with those variables connoting satisfaction with situations and activities which are perhaps less ephemeral than membership in organizations. For Long-Term Satisfaction, the associations are with positive feelings emanating from one's family and household, and one's general community.

CONCLUSIONS AND DISCUSSION

The value of our data is primarily heuristic. We cannot make claims about causality, such as that belonging to a number of formal organizations promotes feelings of Pleasurable Involvement, since the reverse is equally tenable. We do feel, however, that the value of approaching mental health as a multidimensional construct, rather than as a unitary phenomenon, is compellingly illustrated.

If one were to study "general happiness," for example, rather than attempting to break it down into its component parts, it might be possible to demonstrate a relationship between happiness and socioeconomic status. This would lend support to the old adage that money can buy happiness. However, on the basis of our data, we might be more inclined to propose that it makes its contribution to alleviating negative feelings, but it does not ensure that a person with money will necessarily feel any sense of short-term or long-term pleasure.

The potential impact of physical illness on psychological well-being has been largely neglected in the research literature. One exception is a study by Norman Maitlin [23] involving 1,417 respondents selected from a random sample of families in Puerto Rico. Using number of illnesses reported as the independent variable, and Bradburn's negative and positive affect scales (what we have called Negative Affect and Pleasurable Involvement) as the dependent variable, Maitlin found that people who are more ill also report more negative feelings. On the other hand, number of illnesses is not related to reports of positive feeling, a finding strikingly parallel to our own.

It would seem that alleviation of physical ailments may contribute to overall happiness by reducing negative feeling states, and this is obviously of direct relevance for health care programs. It is also plausible to think that the *way in which medical services are delivered may directly affect positive feeling states*. For instance, Rosenberg has demonstrated a relationship between self-esteem and positive feeling states.[28] One might conjecture that service models which enhance rather than diminish self-esteem levels of the clients will have an important bearing on health.

Age, sex, and educational level bear no relationship to any of the affects in this sample. This is somewhat at variance with other studies, in which a positive relationship between education and Pleasurable Involvement, for example, has been demonstrated.[6,7]

There are two possible explanations, one methodological and one substantive. From the methodological point of view, it may be that the range of educational levels which our panel represents is narrower than that found in the kinds of population in which a relationship between years of schooling and positive affect has been demonstrated. Only 10 percent of our sample have completed high school, and a handful have had some college education. With this restriction in variance, the chances of finding statistical associations are diminished.

Another possible explanation is more substantive, and brings us back to a consideration of the question of the context, in this case the rural area known as Stirling County. Even though it is not related to affect scores, educational level is related to socioeconomic status, role-related planning abilities, and participation in formal community activities. When we did a multivariate analysis, in which all the latter variables were controlled, a relationship between education and Pleasurable Involvement emerged—but it was negative, rather than positive. The suggestion from all this is that education may indeed foster some of the capacities and activities which relate to contentment in Stirling County. However, well-educated people who are not integrated into the life of their community are not likely to be very happy. Poorly educated people may lack some of the tools required for successful participation, and their attempts at involvement in community activities may backfire.

This finding is reminiscent of one reported by Brenner in his study of some 5,000 high school students in New York State.[9] Brenner also used Bradburn's positive affect scale as a dependent variable, and found that participation in extracurricular activities, which increases with social class, was an advantage for middle- and upper-class students but a disadvantage for lower-class students. On the other hand, time spent out of work for pay, a factor which decreases with social class, had a favorable set of associations with well-being among lower-class students.

Earlier we mentioned that men and women live in somewhat different worlds in Stirling County. This in turn suggests that the sources of happiness for each may vary. When we did separate analyses by sex, we did indeed find differences. Our data indicate that Pleasurable Involvement for men is closely related to job satisfaction and role-related planning abilities, i.e., to the performance of instrumental activities related to their role as workers and providers in this setting. For women, interpersonal relatedness and participation in formal community activities, activities suggesting a dimension of interrelatedness with other people, seems more important.

To sum up, it seems that the study of human happiness can be a legitimate topic for scientific scrutiny as well as an ethical problem. It would be advantageous, however, to think of happiness as a complex construct, rather than as a global dimension.

In studying the factors related to achieving and maintaining happiness, the socioenvironmental context must be taken into account. If this is done, it will aid in the selection of relevant factors for study. It will also militate against simplistic thinking on the order of "It's good for people to join clubs because it makes them happy."

Achievement of personal happiness depends upon a complex interaction between personal capacities and the opportunities presented by the environment. The patterning of interactions between person and environment which lead to success are probably dependent upon situational features such as education, available sex roles, and socioeconomic status. The study of these patternings in different settings and at different times promises rich rewards for future research.

REFERENCES

1. Barron, F. *Personal Soundness in University Graduate Students*. Publications of Personal Assessment Research, monog. M.1. Berkeley: University of California Press, 1954.

2. Beiser, M. "Components and Correlates of Mental Well-Being." *Journal of Health and Social Behavior* 15(1974):4.

3. Beiser, M.; Feldman, J. J.; and Egelhoff, C. J. "Assets and Affects: A Study of Positive Mental Health." *Archives of General Psychiatry* 27(1972):545–549.

4. Berkman, P. L. "Measurement of Mental Health in a General Population Survey." *American Journal of Epidemiology* 94(1971):105–111.

5. Bond, E. D. "The Student Council Study: An Approach to the Normal," *American Journal of Psychiatry* 109(1952):11–16.

6. Bradburn, N. M. *The Structure of Psychological Well-Being*. Chicago: Aldine, 1969.

7. ———, and Caplovitz, D. *Reports on Happiness*. Chicago: Aldine, 1965.

8. Bray, D. W., and Grant, D. L. "The Assessment Center in the Measurement of Potential for Business Management." *Psychological Monographs* 8(1966):625.

9. Brenner, B. "Social Factors in Mental Well-Being at Adolescence." Ph.D. dissertation, University of Michigan, 1970. Microfilmed.

10. Coelho, G., et al. "Coping Strategies in a New Learning Environment." *Archives of General Psychiatry* 9(1963):433–443.

11. Coopersmith, S. *The Antecedents of Self-Esteem*. San Francisco: W. H. Freeman, 1967.

12. Cox, R. D. "The Normal Personality: An Analysis of Rorschach and Thematic Appercep-tion Test Responses of a Group of College Students." *Journal of Projective Techniques* 20(1956):70–77.

13. Davis, J. A. *Education for Positive Mental Health*. Chicago: Aldine, 1965.

14. Dunn, H. L. *High-Level Wellness*. Arlington, Va.: R. W. Beatty Co., 1961.

15. Fiedler, F. E.; Dodge, J. S.; Jones R. E.; and Hutchins, E. B. "Interrelations Among Measures of Personality Adjustment in Non-Clinical Populations." *Journal of Abnormal and Social Psychology* 56(1958):345–351.

16. Gaitz, C. M., and Scott, J. "Age and the Measurement of Mental Health." *Journal of Health and Social Behavior* 13(1972):55–67.

17. Grinker, R. R., Sr.; Grinker, R. R., Jr.; and Timberlake, J. "Mentally Healthy Young Males (Homoclites)." *Archives of General Psychiatry* 6(1962):405–453.

18. Gurin, G.; Veroff, J.; and Feld, S. *Americans View Their Mental Health*. New York: Basic Books, 1960.

19. Hamburg, D. A., and Adams, J. E. "A Perspective on Coping Behavior." *Archives of General Psychiatry* 17(1967):277–284.

20. Heath, D. H., *Explorations of Maturity*. New York: Appleton-Century Crofts, 1965.

21. Jahoda, M. *Current Concepts of Positive Mental Health*. New York: Basic Books, 1958.

22. Leighton, D. C.; Harding, F. S.; Macklin, D. B.; Macmillan, A. M.; and Leighton, A. H. *The Character of Danger*. The Stirling County Study of Psychiatric Disorder and Sociocul-tural Environment, Psychiatric Symptoms in Selected Communities, volume 3. New York: Basic Books, 1963.

23. Maitlin, N. *The Demography of Happiness*. Puerto Rico Master Sample Survey of Health and Welfare, ser. 2, no. 3. Rio Piedras: University of Puerto Rico School of Medicine, 1966.

24. Offer, D. *The Psychological World of the Teen-Ager: A Study of Normal Adolescent Boys*. New York: Basic Books, 1969.

25. Parsons, T. "Definitions of Health and Illness in the Light of American Values and Social Structure." In *Patients, Physicians and Illness*, edited by E. G. Jaco. New York: Free Press, 1958.

26. ———. "An Approach to Psychological Theory in Terms of the Theory of Action." in *Psychology: A Study of a Science*, edited by S. Koch. New York: McGraw-Hill, 1959.

27. Phillips, D. L. "Social Participation and Happiness." *American Journal of Social Psychia-try* 72(1967):479–488.

28. Rosenberg, M. *Society and the Adolescent Self-Image*. Princeton, N.J.: Princeton Univer-sity Press, 1965.

29. Seeman, J. "Toward a Concept of Personality Integration," *American Psychologist* 14(1959):633–637.

30. Silber, E., et al. "Adaptive Behavior in Competent Adolescents." *Archives of General Psy-chiatry* 5(1961):354–365.

31. ———. "Competent Adolescents Coping with College Decisions." *Archives General Psy-chiatry* 5(1961):517–528.

32. Smith, M. B. "Explorations in Competence: A Study of Peace Corps Teachers in Ghana." *American Journal of Psychology* 21(1966):555–566.

33. Srole, L.; Langner, T. S.; Michael, S. T.; Opler, M. K.; and Rennie, T. A. C. *Mental Health in the Metropolis*. New York: McGraw-Hill, 1962.

34. Wallace, A. F. C. *Culture and Personality*. New York: Random House, 1961.

35. Winton, F. R., and Baylis, L. E. *Human Physiology*. 4th ed. Boston: Little, Brown, 1955.

Editorial Note

Robert White's development of the concept of competence in a clinical psychological framework stresses that the desire to be efficacious is a natural part of the process of growing and learning. That is, the young child, if provided with at least a modicum of stimulation from the human and physical environment, reaches out for experience and tries to manipulate and master the world around him. The healthy or well-organized community may conceivably show some comparable tendency to assert a collective efficacy, but the evidence, in American cities at least, suggests that community competence is far from an inherent propensity, and must rather be intentionally fostered with a good deal of patience and sophistication. In this chapter Cottrell tries both to specify the characteristics of a competent community and to sketch some of the ways in which collective competence may be nurtured.

Just as the study of individual competence emphasizes a concern for mental health, for identifying and cultivating personal assets, so the study of community is directed to the promotion of effective community action or "wellness." We are not so much interested in repairing a "sick" city or keeping it from disintegrating as in encouraging the community to be more adept and energetic in resolving its problems—and, ultimately, in affording the opportunity for the development and utilization of community structures for satisfying individual lives. Our absorption in community organization and the processes of community action is perhaps the most cogent illustration of the greatly expanded scope of social psychiatric thinking in the last two decades. As this entire volume testifies, it is no longer enough to think of the social environment as a significant background for the occurrence of individual health and illness; instead, we seek to understand the ways in which intrapsychic, interpersonal, and interinstitutional processes are conjointly implicated in shaping the quality of life.

There would appear to be important parallels between competent individual functioning and competent communal functioning. For example, the capacity to mobilize resources, to be flexible in moving from problem to problem (perhaps to "learn," or possess a capacity to generalize or transfer skills), and the mounting of a coherent communications network among systemic components all apply to either unit of analysis. But one dramatic difference between the two lies in the nature of executive capacity or regnant processes: The politics of individual coherence are presumably subject to a single directive agency, the brain, while communities as such have no analogue to the brain, no central nervous system. Totalitarian communities apparently come closer to the model of singular control than do democratic ones, although even here the organismic analogy is overwrought. In any event, Cottrell is explicitly addressing the issue of collective competence in a democratic polity.

In the absence of a single authoritative control center, the thrust toward competence in the community requires that numerous elements of the population—representatives of groups, agencies, and offices—be brought together in a sustained dialogue. This chapter describes certain conditions that must be achieved if participatory decision making is to be generated and continued. It underscores the difficulty and complexity of community action, and properly focuses on planning as the typecase of democratic decision processes. One might venture the proposition that planning is genotypical to effective community action, whatever the immediate substantive concern: Experience in the planning process begets competence, and a plan that is agreed upon and can be carried out is in turn perhaps the best proof of collective capacity.

Finally, it is important to identify several issues that deserve further analysis:

1. *What is the relation between Cottrell's competent community and the well-integrated community described by Leighton? There is surely significant convergence in the two formulations.*
2. *How does participation in a competent community articulate with the dimension of social participation in Chapter 16 on a health index?*
3. *What might Cottrell's account of the structure of collective efficacy contribute to our knowledge of personality and leadership styles? Is the gifted community leader one who is particularly acute in self-other awareness?*
4. *Can it be demonstrated that population mental health levels in a competent community exceed those in a less effective city?*
5. *What is the relation among the several levels or scopes involved in varying definitions of "the community"? How, for instance, does the individual's "personal" community of intimates articulate with the community as neighborhood, city, occupational grouping, region, and nation-state?*

R. N. W.

CHAPTER 11

The Competent Community

LEONARD S. COTTRELL, JR.

ONE OF the more obvious characteristics of the average American local community is the presence in it of a multiplicity of agencies and organizations directed to nourishing some interest, meeting some need, or rendering some service. Even in the more impoverished areas of the inner city there are usually an impressive array of so-called service agencies supported by outside sources, in addition to numerous indigenous organized groups.

A second pervasive condition becomes evident only when an attempt is made to mobilize and coordinate the resources of a community for a focused attack on some problem. Such an attempt quickly reveals such a welter of institutional rivalries, jurisdictional disputes, doctrinal differences, and lack of communication that effective joint action seems well beyond practical possibility. And the problem of original concern begins to appear relatively simple compared with that of rendering the community capable of coordinated collective action.

A less frequently noted but nevertheless equally real feature is that the majority of those organizations designed to render service or cope with particular problems are so constituted that the recipients of services or targets of problem-solving efforts—i.e., clients—have little or nothing to do or say concerning setting policy or making decisions concerning goals and operations of these institutions.

When the President's Committee on Juvenile Delinquency and Youth Crime undertook to organize programs to test the feasibility and utility of coordinated comprehensive community-based attacks on the problems of juvenile delinquency and youth crime, it made initial grants to a number of communities. The grants were intended to assist the communities in developing a coordinated plan based upon a careful diagnosis of the critical problems of their youth, and in projecting a new program of action in which the agencies and institutions would closely integrate their operations in such a way as to produce a coherent focused attack on all aspects of the youth problem. The effort to produce such a plan with the kinds of commitments, institutional changes, and accommodations it required was exhausting, frustrating, and sometimes exhilarating. No community achieved the perfect plan. Most were only able to put together an uneasy and rather half-hearted accommodation that in several instances collapsed under the strain of actual operation.

As the planning efforts continued and action phases were initiated, it became increasingly evident to the staff and consultants of the president's committee that the impact of programs, regardless of how good their content, would be relatively minor unless the indigenous populations of the communities themselves were involved in all phases of their development and operation. It is hardly necessary to point out that for professional agency personnel, trained to provide services for clients and to operate programs for people, the requirement that they work with their clients in identifying what the problems are, deciding on priorities as to goals, and working out ways of implementing them, was an enormous complication. Some simply refused to attempt the task; others tried and failed. Most achieved at least some degree of participation of community members— sometimes with startling results, gratifying as well as painful.

This is not the place to recount the exciting history of the brief but highly significant and instructive experience of the president's committee. (Knapp and Polk [7] have written an excellent history and a highly illuminating analysis of this experience.) It is sufficient for purposes of this chapter to report that the staff and consultants early began to recognize that they were involved in much more than a program to control juvenile delinquency. What they found themselves doing was attempting to aid the demonstration communities in the novel and complicated task of upgrading their capabilities to function as communities in coping with a wide range of problems, including those of youth. It was in this broadening of perspective and through the rich empirical experience of trying to aid communities to evolve feasible and effective programs that the notion of a competent community emerged.*

* The general concept of competence as applied to the interpretation and evaluation of human behavior has been used by various writers since it was first explicitly suggested by Harry Stack Sullivan in 1947. Foote and Cottrell [2,5] proposed six component elements of what they defined as interpersonal competence. They elaborated hypotheses concerning the interaction processes in the family and other socializing agencies that determined the degree of development of the components of interpersonal competence. Later White [12,13] used the term primarily as a motivational concept positing

The concept of a competent community still is far from precise definition. However, as communities were observed from the perspective of evaluating their competence and as further thought and discussion were devoted to the attempt to determine what appeared to differentiate the more competent from the less competent, some tentative defining characteristics and essential conditions were identified. These will be discussed later in this chapter. For our present discussion, a competent community is here conceived as one in which the various component parts of the community: (1) are able to collaborate effectively in identifying the problems and needs of the community; (2) can achieve a working consensus on goals and priorities; (3) can agree on ways and means to implement the agreed-upon goals; and (4) can collaborate effectively in the required actions. It is proposed here that a community that can provide the conditions and generate the capabilities required to meet the above performance tests will be competent to cope with the problems of its collective life.

It is recognized, of course, that conditions imposed by larger political, economic, and social contexts provide resources as well as intrude problems with which the local community cannot cope, regardless of how competent it may be. This we shall have to consider later in our discussion. But it should be noted here that a competent community in our terms can go a long way in coping with problems, even when they arise from larger external conditions.

When beginning to consider whether problems arise from conditions inside or outside the community, one immediately runs into the difficult question: What is the community? What are its boundaries? The semantic problem of giving a precise and unambiguous definition of the term "community" need not detain us here. The term applies to collectivities ranging from a tiny mountain village to the "world community" that mankind must achieve if it is to survive.

the presence in the organism of a drive toward effectiveness in interaction with the environment. Inkeles [6] uses the concept with primary emphasis on the socialization of the person to meet the role requirements in a given social structure. M. Brewster Smith [10] published a very useful review of the literature on competence and kindred concepts, with special reference to the problem of the socialization of the child for competent behavior. In this review he proposes his own conception of the core characteristics of "the competent self." Prior to the present chapter, Cottrell [3,4] has used the term in describing the performance of communities. While there is no clear theoretical continuity between the concept of competence as applied to the behavior of the person and as applied to a collectivity such as the community, readers who have reviewed the six components of interpersonal competence proposed by Foote and Cottrell [5] will detect a certain kinship between some of those components of interpersonal competence and certain of the proposed components of community competence, e.g., empathic or role-taking ability of the person and communicative competence in the community, or autonomy of the person and self-other awareness in community relations. Furthermore, those familiar with the conceptualizations of the processes of interaction by George H. Mead [8] will see that both the concepts of personal and community competence are rooted in the Meadian tradition. Virginia Boardman [1] has made the most explicit use of the concept of competence of a collectivity thus far reported. Adapting the proposed components of community competence, she constructed an index of family competence and found that this index correlated significantly in the negative direction with school attendance records of the children in the family.

The range of meaning includes limited interest groups as well as the usually conceived population living in a local area and conducting overlapping and interdependent life activities that are perceived to bind the residents into a collective entity with which they are identified and to which they give a name. It is this more usual type of local community with which we are primarily concerned in this discussion. Such local groups will be found to vary in the degree to which they see themselves as community entities, and the degrees of "communityness" can be indexed in various ways. For practical purposes, it is not too difficult to determine the boundaries of a self-aware community. Once the boundaries are determined, the practical questions with which we are concerned are as follows. What conditions are necessary and what specific capabilities must be developed to enable the community to function competently as a community? What operations are required to provide the necessary conditions and capabilities?

So far as I know, there are presently no systematic, logically complete, empirically tested answers to these questions. The best we can do at the moment is to make a start by drawing on fragments of practical experience, observation, and relevant conceptualization to identify what appear to be essential conditions that must obtain to a substantial degree in the community if it is to function effectively as such. The conditions I shall discuss below represent just such a pragmatic distillation. No claim can be made that the list is exhaustive. The categories are not mutually exclusive and are heavily interrelated. For present purposes, the most useful way to regard them is as aspects of community functioning that could be the objects of concrete practical effort in a program designed to enhance community competence. Measures of change in these variables could well provide an index of the level of overall competence. Here then are some proposed essential conditions of community competence.

Commitment

Commitment to the community as a valued relationship that is worthy of substantial effort to sustain and enhance is an essential condition of the capability of the community to act effectively. And the extent to which such commitment exists among constituents of the community is an important part of any measure of its competence. Precise identification of conditions that encourage and intensify commitment has not been made, but it does appear that people become genuinely committed to a community when: (1) they see that what it does and what happens to it has a vital impact on their own lives and values they cherish; (2) they find that they have a recognized significant role in it; and (3) they see positive results from their efforts to participate in its life. No ready-made general prescriptions for specific actions aimed to optimize commitment exist, but it is clear that this component will yield a range of specific targets for concrete programs. It is also clear that pseudocommitment based on empty slogans and artificial "boosting" campaigns will have little durable effect. It is encouraging that whatever the causes, people of all ranks and conditions often show that they are capable of becoming deeply committed to things of which they are a part, even under the most demanding and unpromising circumstances. It is a universal tendency to be attached in many ways to one's own locality, "be it ever so humble," but cheap exploitative, manipulative use of this sentiment can turn into bitter rejection.

If commitment is based in part on consciousness of the degree to which one's interests and welfare are vitally involved in the functioning of the community, then programs directed to sharpening this awareness should affect commitment. However, such efforts will certainly backfire if the negative and inimical aspects of the community are denied or glossed over. The negative aspects can be frankly dealt with as challenges and conditions that can be realistically attacked. Proposed remedies, of course, must be honest, and not make-believe promises that never get implemented.

Commitment comes with genuine involvement. Increasing the awareness of members of the significant roles they have in the collective life should enhance the sense of commitment. Here again, honesty in appraisal of the extent to which various segments have a vital share in the collective life is indispensable. Where appraisals reveal lack of significant roles, analyses of the barriers and programs in order to discover potential significant roles are indicated.

Commitment grows with realization that what one does makes a difference. People may be encouraged and helped to achieve what appear to be significant roles in the community, but if they do not find that they are actually making a significant impact on community processes and problems, the activity becomes meaningless. They then fall victims to that chronic sense of individual impotence peculiar to modern life. Alienation and reduced commitment result.

The reader will quickly perceive that the kinds of efforts suggested above to generate and enhance commitment will themselves, if successful, have substantial impact on the character of the community. The direction of this impact will, as we shall show later, be toward greater competence. Thus, in seeking to create committed people, the community itself may become created.

Other lines of endeavor can be suggested, but enough has been said to indicate this is no easy undertaking that can be accomplished by a few "civic parades," TV booster programs, and pious slogans by the local chamber of commerce and other promotional organizations. Nor can reliance be placed on a multiplicity of "services" devised by outside "experts" and dropped on the community.

Self-Other Awareness and Clarity
of Situational Definitions

Those who seek to control and exploit or to reduce the capacity of a community or some segments of it to act effectively will strive to blur identities and control perceptions of the situation in order to induce alignments and attitudes consonant with their special goals and interests. In our conception, a working hypothesis is that the degree to which communities can cope realistically with their problems is determined in considerable part by the clarity with which each component perceives its own identity and position on issues in the community context in relation to that of the other component parts. This includes awareness by each segment of its own interests and how these relate to the interests of the other elements—the degree of conflict or compatibility of interests as perceived, for example. Communities are unlikely to be very effective in identifying their real problems or in finding constructive working accommodations among their various groups if they try to work with blurred identities and conflicts, or communality of interests that are wittingly or unwittingly concealed. In the discussions, debates, and political struggles through which the community strives to arrive at working accommodations and to develop consensus on goals, policies, and programs, competence will increase to the degree that identities and their realistic positions are matters of clear self-other awareness. If such awareness is permitted to lead merely to confrontation and "nonnegotiable demands," then progress toward competent functioning is impeded.

The processes of increasing the realism and clarity of awareness of self and other and of their realistic situational positioning, and of controlling and utilizing constructively the resulting intensification of discord and conflict, is the most misunderstood and hazardous phase of community development. It was this aspect of the work of the president's committee and later of the Office of Economic Opportunity that generated the most opposition from the local "Establishment" and the Congress, and was the cause of the most determined efforts to scuttle the whole community development movement.* The technology of helping people learn to make creative use of conflict is an undeveloped field, and is indispensable for the development of competence of communities.

Difficult learning and unlearning is involved in achieving competence in realistic perception of self and other, and in the realistic appraisal of situations. People will have to unlearn habits of uncritical swallowing of whatever is dished out. They have to develop a healthy skepticism and skills in critical weighing of

* See in this connection Huey Perry [9]—an excellent parallel reading for this chapter and a must for those interested in community development.

information, and at the same time retain a sensitivity to fresh ideas and perspectives. Conversion to doctrinaire ideologies is no substitute for the skills considered here. Practice in down-to-earth, realistic situational analyses of each concrete issue is the surest way of developing the capabilities called for.

Articulateness

Closely related to clarification of identity and interests is the ability of each segment of the community to articulate its views, attitudes, needs, and intentions, and further, to articulate its perception of the relation of its position to that of the other segments of the community. Ordinarily the different groups in a community will vary widely in facility for articulate statement of a situation. Action programs aimed at increasing competence of the community will frequently have to include, for some groups, elementary training in communicative skills, speaking to an audience, conducting committee discussions, and formulating clear statements of a position on various issues.

Communication

The factors of awareness and articulateness are reciprocally influential, and both are intimately related to capacity to communicate. As used here, communication refers to much more than mere emission and reception of oral or written symbols or indicative gestures and acts. Meaningful communication requires that the sender of the message take the role of the recipient and respond covertly, i.e., incipiently, to his own message in the way he anticipates that the other will respond. Unless he can do this, he literally does not know what he is saying, since the meaning of his message is given in the anticipated imagined response of the other. To be sure, his interpretation of the role of the other may be erroneous and his anticipation may not be fulfilled, but if interaction continues, erroneous perceptions will be corrected and the participants will become more accurate in their role taking. In this way the interacting population amasses its supply of common meanings upon which efficient communication must rest. This is what is meant when we remark that participants in a common enterprise learn to "speak the same language." The population of a community may speak the same language in a formal linguistic sense, but lack the communality of meanings referred to here. Communicative effectiveness and the accumulation of common meanings obviously depends on the ability to listen, to receive, quite as much as it does on the ability to send. To listen, to hear what the other is actually saying, also requires accuracy in taking his role and seeing the situation from his position. In an era of shouting and confrontation and din of mass media, it is increasingly rare to find competent listening with comprehension of what the other is saying. It is no accident that our words common, community, and communication stem from the same root, and the capability of a community to function effectively as such emerges with its skills and facilities for genuine two-way communication.

Adequate development of communicative skills and facilities should do much to aid in the identification and clarification of real issues and to facilitate productive discussion and debate. Such a development should aid greatly in reducing the bootless shouting, name calling, and obfuscating nondiscussion that so frequently passes for "community action." Enhancement of genuine communication is greatly aided by the design of effective channels of expression and discussion that are simple and readily accessible. The usual ones of press, politics, and other existing organizational channels are frequently inadequate, but could be greatly improved by deliberate effort. A network of connective, functional local forums and other discussional devices that actually aid discussion and crystallization of opinion, and funnel it undistorted to decision-making bodies, is badly needed in most communities. Some already established institutions can, by taking thought, be made to serve this function.

It is important at this point to take note of the fact that skill and accuracy in role taking do not necessarily lead to constructive "understanding" and collaborative effort. Accurate perception of the other's position and intentions can be used to outwit and exploit him, as skillful propagandists well know. These skills increase community competence only when they are used in an honest search for bases for collaborative endeavors to define common goals and collaborative means of implementing them.

Conflict Containment and Accommodation

Skills and capabilities implicit in the foregoing component conditions of competence do not ensure an absence of conflict. Indeed, as commitment increases, identities and situations become clarified, positions on issues become articulated, and communication becomes more effective, conflict may and frequently does become intensified. Furthermore, as conflict emerges, the interacting elements become less and less able to communicate effectively. What is required is a repertoire of procedures whereby open conflicts may be accommodated. All conflict tends to move toward some form of accommodated relation that enables the antagonists to live in relative peace, even though the bases for conflict may not be resolved.

The desideratum here is inventiveness in the development of procedures for working out accommodations that will keep conflict within bounds, while enabling the participants to continue efforts at resolutions of the sources of the conflict. Conflict is not something to be avoided or suppressed at all costs. Where it exists, it should be recognized and its sources made explicit. The competence required is that of accommodation and restoration of genuine communication, and a continued realistic search for resolution and rapprochement. Arbitration, civil procedures, and voting are forms of accommodative procedure. Labor contracts, segregation, and peace treaties can be seen as forms of accommodation in that they operate to reduce open conflict. Some forms of accommodation will obviously facilitate continued interaction more readily than others. The competent community will show a versatility and inventiveness in the use of established procedures and in development of new procedures that will produce forms conducive to continued and flexible interaction.

Participation

If we pause at this point and look back over the alleged components of community competence just discussed, we can see that they are not clearly separable independent factors but do in fact exercise a good deal of reciprocal influence on one another. In particular, effective communication quite obviously depends upon articulateness and self-other clarity, and they in turn are dependent upon communication. Or perhaps it is more accurate to say that all these emerge in a process of interaction in which they are both process and product. In any case, they and the motivational factors we have grouped and called commitment are essential to participation in the processes of community life. Participation in the sense we are using that term is not the equivalent of competence, but it is an indispensable element of community competence. It is a developing process in which the person commits himself to a community in which he contributes to the definition of goals as well as to ways and means for their implementation and enjoyment. As a capability it develops with the development of the components described above, and participation in turn is a significant condition for their growth.

Management of Relations with the Larger Society

The foregoing conditions may be optimally present, but our community could nevertheless be rendered less than competent by conditions impinging upon it from the outside. No local community, of course, can be entirely autonomous. It is therefore necessary for a community to be aware of the context of relations in which it exists and to develop its capacity to adapt to those conditions—to utilize resources and supports which the larger social system makes possible and to act to reduce the threats to its life posed by larger social processes inimical to it. Any community can be mortally crippled or completely destroyed by overwhelming natural catastrophes or cultural, social, political, or economic forces too massive for it to cope with or adapt to. But, within a wide range of situations, knowledge of the social processes surrounding it and skill in utilizing them or managing their impact is possible with even modest understanding and technical talent directed to these factors. Upgrading these capabilities is an essential part of achieving competence.

It is in this area of problems that all elements of a community need to be especially alert and well informed. All too frequently, a community has accepted advice and decisions of various local, state, and federal "planning and development experts," only to discover that it has been sold down the river for exploitation by special interests which control these alleged public agencies, or by the self-perpetuating bureaucratic concerns of the agencies themselves.

Communities must learn to make full use of specialists who command technical knowledge and expertise. They will find it necessary to participate in continued planning to meet changing conditions and new problems generated both inside and outside the community. This need imposes the further necessity of learning how to use experts and specialists without being controlled by them. One important device is to structure the situation so that the experts are clearly subordinate to a broadly representative, tough-minded citizens' group which can be trusted to see that the technical issues are translated into terms the community can understand, and widely communicated and discussed in the framework of the long-run values and welfare of the whole community. No community can trust even the best-intentioned specialists to perform this function for it.

Machinery for Facilitating Participant Interaction and Decision Making

The processes of interaction required for achieving consensus and making decisions require rules and regularized modes of procedure. In small communities these may be quite simple and informal. As size increases, direct face-to-face participation in all phases of consensus building and decision making become less and less feasible. More formal means for debate, discussion, and representative procedures are required. This means increased risk of inadequate communication and the development of rigid and unresponsive institutional machinery that frequently impedes the processes it is ostensibly designed to facilitate. Competent community performance requires constant scrutiny and review of procedures to insure optimal communication and interaction among all parts of the community's structure. Mere verbal assurances that our traditional institutions provide these necessary functions is not enough. Evidence of actual performance is necessary.

Some General Observations

Some general comments may be of help at this point.

1. The component conditions presented as essential to the development of a competently functioning local community are not logical derivatives of a systematic general theory. Rather they emerged from observations of practical efforts of local populations to develop capabilities necessary to function as communities in coping with local problems. Actually, the categories appeared as designations of types of tasks that had to be addressed by staffs which sought to help the localities identify problems, define goals, and mobilize resources to cope and implement. At this state of development of theory and practice, it is probably wiser to continue to regard these and other potential categories as indicating things to do with and to local groups by way of increasing their capacity to act effectively as collective entities, rather than attempt to determine whether or not they can be encompassed in a general theory. These categories can also be used tentatively as criteria by which to measure progress toward improved competence. With increasing empirical experience, a more coherent and systematic conceptualization should emerge, thus providing a more incisive analysis of the critical processes involved.

2. No claim is made that the present tentative list of essential conditions is

exhaustive. But action based on the present list should reveal other essential components. There are factors such as material resources, geographic location, population characteristics, cultural and political conditions, and so on, that certainly bear on the effectiveness with which a community can act as such. However, the ones we have selected here appear to be relevant under any condition under which the community may exist. They apply to a materially impoverished fishing community as well as to an affluent suburb. It is not a foregone conclusion that the high-consumption community would be found to be the more competent; it is quite possible for the fishing village to be highly competent. The other conditions just suggested may, in some sense, be viewed as modifiers of the tentative "essentials" we have proposed.

3. Obviously the categories are not mutually exclusive. Indeed, they are for the most part inextricably interrelated. The justification of attempting a separation is primarily to give practical handles for taking hold of and working with a complex phenomenon. Thus, instead of undertaking vague ad hoc and relatively unfocused efforts to increase the community's competence in general, specific concrete programs can be mounted to increase genuine communicative capabilities and institutional devices for facilitating communication; promote greater clarity of analysis of the actual lines of interest cleavage and acting perspectives; encourage more participation in discussion, decision making, and action; and so on.

4. We reiterate that the conceptualizations attempted here are directed to the enhancement of competent functioning within a participant democratic framework. It is quite possible that a very different cultural context would require a different set of conditions for effective collective action. It would be interesting and useful for clarifying ideas about competence as here conceived to analyze the requirements for community competence under an authoritarian system.

5. It should be apparent to anyone reasonably familiar with a specific community that changes induced by efforts to enhance competence along lines suggested here would frequently be accompanied by a good deal of social and political turbulence. Indeed, unless great care, discretion, and skill are exercised and extended preparatory work is done, the situation can readily become explosive. In communities with longstanding hostilities, deprivations, and repressed unresolved conflicts, progress toward greater awareness and articulateness frequently results in premature and destructive confrontations and violence. These situations may be precipitated by segments who see their power position threatened, or by disadvantaged groups who see no way of gaining power except by violent means. In this connection the reader is again referred to Huey Perry's excellent chronicle of the experience of Mingo County, West Virginia.[9] The experiences recounted in that work do not cover all conditions here regarded as essential to competent functioning, but do illustrate the enormous productivity of, as well as intense reaction to, even partial efforts in the development of competence.

The grave risks involved in the kinds of programs suggested should not, indeed must not, be allowed to inhibit attempts to create competent communities if democracy itself is to survive.

6. Ideas and conceptualizations are useful to give structure and direction to action. But they must eventually rest on pragmatically tested operations for their implementation. The space limitations of a single chapter preclude any attempt to consider the "how-to-do-it" aspects of our problem. This must be left to later communications and to the gleanings of experience in community development practices that may be of relevance, even though not enjoying the focus provided by the present analysis.

However, a thoughtful consideration of each of the suggested component conditions of competence will readily suggest possible concrete steps that might be taken in any attempt to enhance the particular capability. These suggestions will occur especially to those who have engaged in even a limited amount of actual community development effort. Furthermore, experience indicates that when one line of action is undertaken with people (not imposed upon them), new possibilities emerge and can be evaluated and tried out.

Another encouraging word is that communities frequently demonstrate that they can learn from the experience of attempting to increase their abilities to function as such, provided, of course, that the experience is not too traumatic for the community to assimilate and continue to function, and also provided that the experience can be articulated and its significant components and "lessons" perceived by the participants.

7. Finally, it should be noted that in most instances communities will need assistance from personnel who are perceptive, skillful, and courageous, and who can work with and facilitate various community groups in developing the relevant capabilities without attempting to become the "leaders" or to become agents for imposing programs and services on the community. This partnership must be genuine and not a "slick trick" for putting something over on one or another group or on the community as a whole. If the latter is the case, the community will be left less competent than it was before it was exploited.

The Competent Community and Mental Health

The relevance of the development of community competence for mental health may be viewed from the broad perspective of how the general level of competence of the community can condition the mental health of its population. Another perspective is that of considering the relevance of the competence level for the development of specific programs considered to be aids to improving mental health.

From the more general perspective, it could with substantial justification be claimed that development of the competence of the community as conceived here would itself be a program of mental health. (I have discussed elsewhere certain aspects of this approach at greater length.[3]) There can be little doubt that the conditions of modern mass technological society tend increasingly to depersonalize and dehumanize much of our collective life. Persons perceive themselves to be living in an environment of enormous social, economic, and political forces that vitally affect their lives, yet over which they feel they have no control. The resulting alienation, devaluation of the self, and accompanying passivity, apathy, and loss of a sense of significance form a profound handicap to achieving a vigorous sturdy mental health and to functioning as parents in developing mentally healthy children. The discovery that they and their neighbors can take effective collective action to cope with their common problems, that they can become meaningful and effective actors in the life of the community, is frequently found to be a powerful stimulus. Certainly, the recapture of at least some share in the determination of one's fate and a new sense of worth and potency should provide some of the necessary basis for mentally healthy development. To the extent that a community provides the arena for effective participation by the individual in the vital processes of his society, it is a significant factor in his mental health.

If the problem is viewed from a more specific perspective, it is clear that the level of competence of the community is highly relevant to the effectiveness of specific programs aimed at improving its mental health. Anyone who has sought to provide mental health facilities, services, promotional campaigns of information and education, and so on, knows that such enterprises require vigorous participation by the community itself in their development. If such participation is lacking, the program will subside into a relatively minor enterprise that falls far short of its potential. It may seem wasteful of time and effort to try to establish a mental health program by going through the hard work and sometimes stormy episodes of involving the significant elements of the community in the laborious task of looking at their situations, assessing their needs, identifying problems, achieving consensus on goals, and making hard decisions of what action to undertake with what priorities—all of which is attended by high risks of failure or at least some severe setbacks. It is especially embarrassing when some government bureaucratic funding agency is breathing down one's neck and demanding proof of RESULTS. It is of some comfort, however, to recognize that these apparently irrelevant operations and crises can themselves be part of the mental health-producing processes of building the competence of the community. For mental health is not a matter of the condition of that abstraction, the isolated individual. It is essentially the quality of and is inextricably bound up with the relations of the person with himself and with his fellows as individuals and as groups. The capacity for effective functioning in those intrapersonal, interpersonal, and intergroup relations is a measure of his mental health.

REFERENCES

1. Boardman, V. "School Absences, Illness and Family Competence." Ph.D. dissertation, University of North Carolina, 1972.
2. Cottrell, L. S., Jr. "New Directions for Research on the American Family." *Social Casework* 34(1953):54–60.
3. ———. "Social Planning, the Competent Community and Mental Health." In *Urban America and the Planning of Mental Health Services*, Symposium No. 10, pp. 391–402. New York: Group for the Advancement of Psychiatry, 1964.
4. ———. "The Competent Community—A Long-Range View." Address to the Houston Community Leaders Forum, Houston, Texas, October 29, 1967. Mimeographed.
5. Foote, N. N., and Cottrell, L. S., Jr. *Identity and Interpersonal Competence.* Chicago: University of Chicago Press, 1955.
6. Inkeles, A. "Social Structure and the Socialization of Competence." *Harvard Educational Review* 36(1966):265–283.
7. Knapp, D., and Polk, K. *Scouting the War on Poverty.* Lexington, Mass.; D. C. Heath, 1971.
8. Meade, G. H., *Mind, Self and Society.* Chicago: University of Chicago Press, 1934.
9. Perry, H. *They'll Cut Off Your Project.* New York: Praeger, 1972.
10. Smith, M. B. "Competence and Socialization." In *Socialization and Society*, edited by John A. Clausen, pp. 270–320. Boston: Little, Brown, 1968.
11. Sullivan, H. S. "Tensions Interpersonal and International: A Psychiatrist's View. In *Tensions that Cause Wars*, edited by Hadley Cantril, pp. 79–138. Urbana: University of Illinois Press, 1950.
12. White, R. W. "Motivation Reconsidered: The Concept of Competence." *Psychological Review* 66(1959):297–333.
13. ———. *Competence and the Psychosexual Stages of Development.* Nebraska Symposium on Motivation, edited by M. Jones, pp. 97–141. Lincoln: University of Nebraska Press, 1960.

Editorial Note

Cardoza, Ackerly, and Leighton offer here a comprehensive exercise in applied social psychiatry. Starting from an explicit theoretical base in community process, epidemiology, and styles of intervention, they develop a scheme for action and proceed to subject that scheme to an empirical test. It has been frequently and accurately observed that the social sciences are not sufficiently attuned to the cumulative accretion of knowledge; important learnings are seldom replicated. Yet, although the authors conclude with a plea for more rigorous testing of the model they advance, this chapter is itself a significant replication: Can the lessons derived from long immersion in local affairs in rural Nova Scotia be transferred to urban Massachusetts? The tentative and heartening conclusion is that they can.

The authors' program in Somerville is in several senses a concrete illustration of the principles of the "competent community" enunciated by Cottrell in Chapter 11. The investigators worked independently of one another, but their findings are remarkably convergent. They are at one, for example, in insisting that effective local action cannot be founded solely, or even principally, on the executive activities of outside experts; rather, it depends on putting local resources into effect. Each also emphasizes the key element of communication skills as these skills relate to authentic self-other awareness. And each is frank to recognize intergroup and interpersonal conflict as realities of community life, to be understood and worked with rather than shunned.

The fundamental modesty and sense of proportion displayed by Cardoza and his colleagues is perhaps central to their success. They asserted no grandiose aims of reforming or transforming the community. Instead, the program began where Somerville was at that point in its collective history; the action to be promoted was characterized by selective targeting of a population at risk, the setting of achievable goals, and the use of accessible strengths already at hand in the community.

Cardoza's role as catalytic agent in inducing increased attention to the needs of the elderly population merits careful analysis. Unobtrusive but highly skilled, he combined the talents of the observer-interviewer-researcher with those of the change agent. Basically, he served the function of the catalyst-as-communicator; he was the switchboard for a flow of community information and sentiment. In this guise, the "outsider" helping agent might be said to energize the local social system by bringing diverse parts of the institutional network together and fostering a heightened community dialogue. The increased circulation of ideas and attitudes among individuals and agencies is probably a necessary, if not sufficient, condition of social change. Cottrell, of course, stresses this, and it has also been found integral to viable health planning on the local level.[32]

One might ask how the model of action set forth in this chapter bears on Hollister's discussion of the community psychiatrist in his diverse "interventionist" roles (Chapter 13). The attempt to enhance the psychological health of older people, to arrest the grim deterioration of isolated men and women, to spur agency responsiveness and public awareness—all these would appear to represent a blend of consultation, education, and prevention. Cardoza's conception of the change agent's role is avowedly that of a generalist; he is not a psychiatric professional, but rather a politician, leader, and community consultant. His achievements in Somerville would lead us to reinforce the suggestion that the psychiatrist is not always the helper of choice in these matters. The generalist can collaborate effectively with mental health specialists without being himself clinically trained. Indeed, it may well be that the traditional mental health professional is ill-equipped educationally, experientially, and temperamentally to feel comfortable with the "bridesmaid principle" of unobtrusive and nondirective intervention.

R. N. W.

CHAPTER 12

Improving Mental Health
Through Community Action*

VICTOR G. CARDOZA
WILLIAM C. ACKERLY
ALEXANDER H. LEIGHTON

THIS CHAPTER reviews briefly the theoretical ideas and empirical findings which support the notion that societal processes which produce stress may lead to psychiatric disorder.† Based on this, a conceptual model for improving mental health through community action is outlined, and the results of applying the model in an urban mental health center are described.

* This chapter appeared in the Community Mental Health Journal, Vol. 11, Number 2, June 1975.

The background studies in Stirling County on the feasibility of community intervention by a mental health center were supported by the Milbank Memorial Fund and the National Institute of Mental Health.

† The authors wish to acknowledge with sincere thanks the editorial assistance given by Margaret B. Schworm.

The Nature of the Problem

The question of trying to improve the mental health of a population by changing social patterns arises from both theoretical and empirical considerations. Theory states that psychological and psychophysiological disorder will occur when an individual is placed in a position of severe and/or prolonged psychological stress. This is a widespread idea that enters a number of different bodies of theory, and one of us has attempted a summary and synthesis.[12] For another overview, see Levine.[19]

Heredity and psychodynamic factors of early life are not ruled out by this orientation. Rather, it is held that they may influence the degree of individual susceptibility to a stress reaction. Using a cardiac analogy, one can say that in many instances the effect of stress is to produce decompensation, and so render manifest an underlying potential for malfunction.

A second theoretical point is that conditions stressful to individuals frequently derive from the social characteristics of communities. In thinking about this, it is useful to regard communities as systems with component subsystems, and, further, to visualize these systems as having two dimensions. One takes the form of regular patterns of interaction among people, often called "structure" and exemplified in such phenomena as social stratification, kinship networks, and leadership hierarchy. The other consists in shared feelings, attitudes, values, and opinions which, taken together, govern the behaviors that make up the structure and which may be labeled shared "sentiments." The extent of sharing in a community varies according to topic, some sentiments pervading the whole system, while others are limited to one or a few subsystems.

These two dimensions—structure and sentiments—interact so as to constitute a community's functioning in the interests of its survival. Communities often differ from each other in the way this functioning is conducted because of differences in current situations and differences in past history, that is, cultural development. These variations can result in different degrees of stress in one community as compared to another, and, within a particular community, in some parts of the system as compared to others. Those parts of communities that are poor or which occupy minority status are familiar examples.[10,33]

The theory, however, does not limit stress to such categories, even though they are perhaps at present the most discussed. It suggests, rather, that there may be other groups in a community also subject to harmful degrees of stress due to their particular locus in the system. For example, certain jobs that pay well enough may be stressful because of uncertainties and conflicts inherent in them (college presidents), or because the shared sentiments of the community place them in low esteem (garbage collectors). Other prejudicial sentiments relating to age and sex may adversely affect large numbers of people scattered in a variety of places throughout the system. Exposure to rapid alteration of normative values due to migration, technological change, or cultural shifts often produces stress in the form of disorientation and fear, and this may occur more in one part of a community population than another. There are also events in the arc of life, such as bereavement or retirement, which happen to most people and constitute a "crisis" period of stress.[4,20]

Finally, but still within the framework of social stress theory, it is to be noted that whole communities sometimes become demoralized or "disintegrated." By this we mean that there is general failure of community functioning such that almost everyone in the population is exposed to stress.[14,15]

To sum up: Theory supports a commonsense notion that the societal processes of communities are apt to produce situations of psychological stress, which in turn are apt to evoke manifestations of psychiatric disorder. It is to be expected that as stress varies among communities, or within a given community, so will the frequency of individuals with psychiatric disorder. Implicit in this theory is the idea that the reduction of situations that produce stress will reduce the frequency of manifest psychiatric disorder in the population.

Turning now to empirical findings, epidemiological surveys conducted during the last several decades have indicated a distribution of psychiatric disorders in populations that is in keeping with the above theory.* The findings point to some communities having greater frequencies than others, and they show that within communities there are major variations according to socioeconomic condition, social role, age, sex, and so on.

Empirical results also indicate that there are very large numbers of people who suffer from impairing psychological and psychophysiological disorders. This hovers around 20 percent for adults in many of the populations so far examined. It is evident, therefore, that psychiatric services, as they are now constituted, are able to cope with only a small part of such numbers—especially when one realizes that in many communities, and in some parts of most communities, the percentage figures are much higher. There is thus an obvious and practical need of some urgency to search out ways for supplementing clinical service with programs for reducing common forms of socially induced stress.

For a number of years two of the authors (Cardoza and Leighton) have been conducting such explorations. The problem became defined in their thinking as: Is it feasible and desirable for a community mental health center to attempt social change as a means of reducing stress and so improving mental health? There are, of course, large ethical and political issues implicit in this question. In the present chapter, however, we shall confine ourselves to an inquiry regarding the feasibility of one approach.

* See references 5, 6, 9, 11, 17, 18, and 29.

The organizational base from which the possibility of community change was explored consisted in the mental health center that had been developed as part of the Stirling County Study. This outpatient facility serves a small town and rural area in which there has been much research and a good deal learned about the distribution of social stress and about the existence of resources for coping with it.

The work took shape in a number of trials and quasi-experiments that ranged through such activities as the formation of co-ops and social clubs to projects in land reclamation. An operating frame of reference was developed that drew in part on applied anthropology * and on human relations in industry.† In particular a debt was felt to the concepts of the late M. L. Wilson.[26] Both authors were influenced by previous experience, one (Leighton) having worked as a social scientist in problems of the American Indian, the forced relocation of Japanese Americans, and human relations in industry, while the other (Cardoza) had been active in politics for fifteen years as an elected representative.

After some years of exploratory studies, Cardoza and Leighton decided that the answer to the feasibility question (Can a mental health center initiate social change?) was a qualified "yes," and they believed they had evolved some useful guidelines and principles.[13,16,23] The question then arose as to whether these were limited to Stirling County, or could be applied in a quite different kind of setting. In particular, Cardoza was anxious to find out if they could be made to work in an environment in which he had no previous connections of any kind. It seemed that if such could be demonstrated, the principles and methods might have some general applicability for mental health centers. In what follows we shall first outline the conceptual scheme, or model, and then recount the results of its application in an urban mental health center.

A Catalytic Model

Our model rests on the view, already noted, that every community is a system with component subsystems, all interrelated and playing parts in the functioning of the whole. We anticipate that some parts of the system will generate serious stress for the incumbents, and we shall refer to such people as "high-risk groups," meaning by this a high risk of developing manifest psychiatric disorders.

Among the sentiments in the community, there will be some—more and less widely shared—that have a focus on desired changes. These constitute feel-

* See references 1, 3, 8, 24, 27, and 28.
† See references 2, 7, 21, 22, 25, 30, and 31.

ings that something is wrong and should be corrected, or that something positive should be achieved. We shall refer to these as "felt needs."

Three points are important in connection with felt needs. One is that communities very often have unused resources (both material and informational) for meeting many of their felt needs. This happens when those who have the needs are unaware of the resources, while those with the resources are unaware of places where they would be useful. It is as if the needs and the resources were lying about in a network, but with their strands unconnected.

Second, some felt needs appear incompatible with others; since by definition they are shared among at least some persons in the community, this creates a situation of actual or potential conflict. The mainsprings of the conflict may be inherent in the needs and, therefore, fairly resistant to efforts at modification. Different groups of people often have different interests. On the other hand, the conflict may be largely in perceptions, or in apprehensions about ways and means, and so lie open to amelioration.

Finally, there are questions of reality. Some felt needs may be based on misconceptions regarding matters of fact (e.g., Krebezin will cure cancer), or on failure to take into account the consequences of attainment (e.g., taxes no one wants to pay), or on misreadings as to what is attainable from a practical point of view (e.g., individual psychiatric treatment should be available to everyone).

Putting all this together with the notion of high-risk groups, it is to be expected that there will be felt needs pertinent to reducing the stress that bears on such groups, and that in some instances, but not all, the felt needs can become motivational forces toward constructive change. The requirement is that something happen to bring resources and needs together in a way that avoids both the paralysis of conflict and the disappointment of pursuing illusory goals.

An aspect of community structure which is obviously important from the viewpoint of inducing change is the pattern of leadership. As studies have shown, it is to be expected that there will be both formal leaders and informal leaders, or opinion setters—that is, people who exert influence without occupying a named position of leadership. It is also to be anticipated that the political process will contain a number of competing groups that have both manifest and hidden goals, and that the relationships among these groups will involve a range from cooperation with various trade-offs, through neutrality, to longstanding, intransigent hostility. All of which means that any effort to reduce the social stress affecting high-risk groups has to be guided by some knowledge of this complex of relationships.

While all of the above has been cast in terms of community functioning, our model takes account of the fact that the actual process is carried out by individuals. Hence, the approach to understanding the processes in a particular community is partly a matter of identifying individuals who play key roles, ascertaining their sentiments and capabilities, and discovering how they fit into the workings of the community, both formally and informally.

Against this sketch of high-risk groups, felt needs, and community process, let us attempt to sum up our notion of the catalytic approach. A first step is scanning the selected community in order to understand the main points about its structure and sentiments, and in the process identifying groups that are high risk from a mental health point of view. There should then follow an assessment of relevant felt needs, with a view to identifying those which show promise of being a basis for action. The criteria for judging this promise include such matters as appropriateness of a felt need in terms of what is known about mental health and mental illness, the presence of resources in or available to the community, and at least a sporting chance of being able to overcome or get around the inevitable obstacles. The total process of bringing together felt needs and resources (including informational resources) often means a working through and reformulation of the felt needs in terms of specific goals and plans for action.

There are a number of points to be made about the application of this model—items which might be called "principles of action." We shall introduce them in the course of reporting the case history.

One comment, however, is in order at this point, and pertains to our use of the word "catalytic." The analogy to a chemical catalyst is far from perfect. In a chemical reaction the catalyst gets the process going and intensifies its effectiveness, but is not itself changed. In any human activity, no participant in the process can remain unaffected or unchanged. Furthermore, while in this model the human agent of change does parallel the chemical analogue in that he gets the participation of the community going in a selected activity and intensifies it, he then withdraws, expecting it to continue without him.

The Mental Health Center

Before beginning our case report on the application of the catalytic model, it is appropriate to outline briefly the history of the Somerville Mental Health Center, the base of operations. The center was started by one of the authors (Ackerly) in 1964 as a clinic for children. Although overwhelmed with demands at first, the staff, after a period of about five years, achieved a sense of being in control of the situation and was able to think of expanding into adult services.

While from the beginning the group had an orientation toward the community, it was not with prevention in mind. Ackerly wanted the staff to get close to where people lived in order to make it more possible for families to enter the treatment system. He also wanted the staff to become involved in community programs so that community people would learn about the center and become interested in its activities and potentiality. In particular, he hoped that such people would help by undertaking community actions that would improve the effective utilization of treatment facilities; in short, he wanted to take steps that went beyond the scope of the mental health professional. Thus he spent some years working in the direction of community acceptance of the center and became acquainted with much of the community's social and political characteristics.

Somerville is a nonacademic, concrete-minded place, uncertain as to what mental health is all about. The first problem, therefore, was to develop understanding among potential clients regarding what the center could do, and from this, create a willingness to try the services. Outreaches made to priests, family doctors, and school personnel (people already trusted in the community) succeeded in establishing a number of bridges for enhancing the service capabilities.

As a result of these activities, the clinical staff of the center underwent a change in style of action. In the beginning, Ackerly and others had a tendency to think of themselves as "experts" who would instruct the people in the community regarding what they should know about psychiatry. This approach, it was found, rarely, if ever, worked. As a result, the staff abandoned the idea of "teaching" and instead tried to work collaboratively with the community's leaders and opinion setters. For example, when a probation officer referred a young person to the center, he was urged to come, together with the family, and join with them, the offender, and the staff in a mutual effort to find a solution.

As a result of all this, Ackerly and his staff gradually moved toward the idea of preventing mental illness and began thinking in terms of high-risk groups. It seemed possible that some changes in the community and its goals could provide more lasting improvement than an approach solely through treatment. Some of the metaphors they began to use were "vaccinate rather than cure" and "build fences at the top of the cliff rather than keep an ambulance at the bottom."

The Case Report

The project had its origin when the authors met at a monthly workshop on preventive psychiatry sponsored jointly by the Harvard School of Public Health and the Department of Mental Health of Massachusetts. With goals agreed upon as outlined earlier in this chapter, collaboration started and Cardoza undertook a demonstration of the catalytic model. His time in Somerville was on an intermittent basis—usually several days a month—since he continued with his responsibilities in Stirling Country.

The scanning operation began with a focus on the Mental Health Center itself. Cardoza thought it essential to understand the structure, sentiments, and functioning of the center, with particular reference to the team's own range of felt needs. In order to accomplish this, he avoided the isolation of an office and had himself placed in a corridor next to the coffee machine. Here he was both visible and accessible to everyone, from the director to the cleaning lady. This open and conversational rather than "expert" approach constituted a nonthreatening position from which to gather information and to initiate explanation, and it also served to rouse interest in some members of the center team and to make all members accepting toward the project.

In turning his attention to the community, Cardoza at first conducted his explorations through introductions provided by the center, but then soon branched into contacts he developed for himself. Attending selected meetings, studying the physical layout of the community, and reading about it were other activities that contributed to the development of his orientation.

One of the first organizations whose meetings he attended was a neighborhood group, essentially a storefront cooperative, that was in the process of organizing. By chance, an event occurred which provided an opportunity to show the center and some community members what the approach looked like in action. At one of the meetings, discussion came up about a local political leader, a long-term resident of the district, who had been well-known and well-liked until he had been elected to public office. At that time it seemed he had undergone a marked alteration for the worse. There was talk of organizing a protest march on City Hall to demand that he change what was seen as a high-handed attitude toward community affairs. When Cardoza was asked his views concerning this, he replied: "Like Will Rogers, I only know what I read in the newspaper, so I'm not really qualified to say anything. But, tell me a little more about this man, what he was like before the election, what sort of problems he faces now. Has anyone sat down with him and asked why he is doing these things?"

Members of the organization took the implied suggestion and, when they did talk matters over with the politician, discovered the existence of numerous facts they had not taken into consideration. The man was under pressures which they had not realized and was more open to changing his conduct than they had supposed. It was then decided to work out a compromise solution to the problems which all faced.

Important to note here is what may be called the principle of the "Fully Open Approach." Cardoza did not begin with any a priori idea or recommendation regarding compromise. His foremost assumption was the desirability of finding out the facts and the reasons behind them; when this was done, the solution (in this case to compromise) emerged from the situation.

Of course, one cannot expect that things will always work so easily. The fact that in this instance they did was a considerable aid to the development of the kind of procedure Cardoza was talking about.

Simultaneous with his study of the formal and informal organization of the community and the characteristics of its shared sentiments, Cardoza also searched for identifiable high-risk groups. This was done in conversations with center staff, members of the Social Agencies Executive, people active in the O.E.O. programs, and clergymen, and also through attending meetings of the Community Council and the Mental Health Association. While many topics passed in review, the elderly gradually emerged as a high-risk group concerning which there was a marked and somewhat widely shared felt need in the community.

It is appropriate at this point to note that here again the Fully Open Approach is illustrated. Cardoza did not enter Somerville with the elderly already in view as the high-risk group to which he wanted to give attention. He began with the question, "What high-risk groups are here?" and, in the course of time, identified numbers of them. Through applying the criteria mentioned earlier, he came to the conclusion that the elderly would constitute a suitable project. Although there were other groups that might also have been chosen (children in problem families, youth exposed to the drug culture, the unemployed), both community and center appeared particularly ready for action involving the elderly.

The Fully Open Approach may be so obvious as to make calling it a principle and giving it a title seem a little absurd. We do so, however, because utilization of this principle appears to be relatively rare in practice. The structure and sentiment patterns of agencies, the training of professionals in categorical disciplines, and the nature of the political process through which public money is obtained and distributed gnerally combine in such a way that the service professional enters a community with preconceived assumptions about just what groups are high risk, and with preformulated plans as to just what should be done for them.

Once serious attention had become focused on the elderly, it became important to assemble as much factual information as possible. This was aided by a survey that had been conducted by the local government in 1970. From this it appeared that of the 87,000 people in Somerville, 15,237 were over sixty, and of these 10,788 were over sixty-five years of age; there were large numbers of single elderly persons (mostly widows and widowers) living alone, and 540 were in nursing homes or institutions for the aged.

Cardoza looked for the opportunity to do field work, that is, make some direct observations, and this was afforded in part at a cafeteria where he often had breakfast. He noticed that numbers of elderly persons were there in the early hours, and engaged some of them in conversation. A typical story was that of a man who lived alone nearby: He said it was not very warm in his room, he had poor eyesight and could not read, and hence he went to bed early. He also woke early, and so had nothing to do but wait until he could get up and go out to the cafeteria for breakfast. He tried to stretch his money, he said, so that he could have something to eat, but toward the end of the month his allotment check tended to run out and he was reduced to having just coffee. Lunch and dinner were better because there was a senior citizens' assistance program at another restaurant.

The center team, after discussion with Cardoza, began studying those resources in the community which were or might become available to programs for the elderly. A number were identified: church organizations, such as the Legion of Mary, and different sodalities; the Visiting Nurses' Association; the Board of Health; the Somerville Council on Aging; Family Service; Sisters of the Poor; the Home for the Aged; the Somerville Recreation Department; the Girl Scouts; the Mayor's office; the O.E.O. programs; VISTA; the Special Legislative Council on the Aging; and the several nursing homes. It soon became apparent that while many of these were doing excellent work, there was little coordination among them, nor any clearly defined set of priorities.

The head of the recreation department, which operated tours and clubs, had more experience with the elderly than virtually anyone else in the city. He knew their prejudices and their pride, and the practical difficulties they faced, particularly that of getting around in wintertime. Most of his experience, however, was with the mobile elderly, those who were able to get out to church, to golden age clubs, to drop-in centers, and to visit their families.

Our orientation was, of course, to look for high risk as defined by social factors that create stress. Many of the elderly, it seemed, had programs that were doing a good deal to protect them from stress and hence from reacting with psychiatric disorders. Clearly, if an elderly person were in satisfactory physical condition—alert, had a good memory, and was fairly vigorous—he could utilize the services, retain contact with his friends, and stay mentally healthy. There was, in short, a circular set of relationships which can be summed up by: "The healthier he is, the healthier he stays."

There were other elderly persons, however, in whom socially induced stress was evident, in the form of isolation. The social patterns of the community were not geared for looking after individuals whose vigor had begun to fail in a significant way. It seemed probable that the isolation in which they found themselves would lead to depression, and this, in turn, to more isolation, and so on, in a downward spiral to confusions and disorientations. Cardoza and the staff concluded that social isolation was a key stress in Somerville for this population, and that there was a considerable number of people exposed to it. Thus, within the total elderly group, we identifed the "withdrawn elderly" as our specific high-risk focus.

Individual cases that became known to the center provided illustrations of the kind of thing that was happening—persons discovered in a severe state of agitated deterioration and requiring commitment. One woman reported finding an eighty-year-old man alone in his room who had not eaten for three days, had bed sores, a severe cough, was disoriented, and had no one to do anything for him. She had great difficulty in finding any community service (police, hospitals, physician) that would assume responsibility.

The clergy constituted one of the few groups in the community aware of the withdrawn elderly, and it seemed to some of these men that depression was a problem. This possibility was made vivid for us when a seventy-five-year-old retired school teacher jumped to her death less than a block from the center.

In turning to the problem of connecting up resources and needs, we discovered an obstacle in the form of certain views that were shared even among some of those who had a major concern for the elderly. A visiting nurse, for example, at first maintained that she had never known of a suicide among them. As discussion with her continued, however, she began to reflect more about the matter and eventually recalled that this person did not eat, that one refused physical attention, and in the end she concluded that depression and suicide were indeed actual problems.

With others, however, resistant sentiments were greater, and there was a certain amount of stereotypic thinking. One man, active in work for older people, raised questions as to whether they desired to have people visit them. He thought that the average elderly person, unable to keep up his home in the manner he wished, would not want anyone to call. The individual who said this did not have any factual evidence for his point of view, but he was nonetheless quite sure he was right.

There was also a rather strong feeling in the community that "a great deal" (by implication "enough," or "too much") was already being done for older people, and this raised barriers to perceiving needs that were not being met. One of the women who ran a drop-in center was very possessive about "my" elderly and very proud of a visiting program she had, but we found after a little persistence that most of this was on paper. Some visiting did occur on a casual, friendly basis among the elderly themselves, but there was little involvement of other groups.

Let us pause here to note what has happened thus far in terms of our model: The felt needs and formal-informal structure of the Mental Health Center have been mapped, and acceptance achieved for the general idea of our project and for the person who is to implement it. The formal and informal structure and felt needs in the community have also been explored. Further, a range of high-risk groups have been reviewed and a selection made regarding one—the withdrawn elderly. Taking this as the focal point, further study has been conducted regarding interaction patterns, felt needs, and background sentiments. Areas of conflicting sentiments and misinformation have been identified. There also has been a review of the resources in the community that might be brought to bear on helping the withdrawn elderly, accomplished in the course of reviewing social organization and sentiments.

Having thus, in a sense, made a "diagnosis," Cardoza began to carry out a plan of "treatment" by weaving networks of communication between resources and people who knew about the problem. This was done through conversations, through traveling back and forth between individuals and groups, and through bringing them together for discussions. The work began with people already identified as having high concern and low resistance, and then gradually drew in others in a way designed to inform them and to alter some of their resistance by having them interact with people who held different views. Various members of the center staff joined with Cardoza in these efforts.

At the end of about a year, the outcome had taken a number of forms. One was a visiting program carried out by several groups of high school students, primarily for people in nursing homes. Another consisted in a group of thirty to thirty-five elderly persons who undertook visiting others living outside these homes.

Programs of instruction were also established for the visitors. The purpose here was to sensitize the visitors to problems they might encounter and to prepare them for handling these. Each visitor was assigned a resource person to whom he or she could turn for advice or help.

The Somerville Community Council, a coordinating group, became much interested in the project and took a leading part in the implementation of the goals. Other agencies that participated were the Mayor's Council on Aging, the Somerville Welfare Department, the Somerville Housing Authority, the Eastern Middlesex Opportunities Council, the Recreation Commission, the Visiting Nurses' Association, and the Somerville Hospital.

The planning associate of the community council established a special task force, consisting of the various agencies and interested elderly, to clarify the problems and set up connecting links between agencies. Because many services already existed, a decision was made not to establish a new agency for the elderly, but to form an administrative body called the Core Agency Services for coordination, fiscal policies, record keeping, research, and planning. A comprehensive

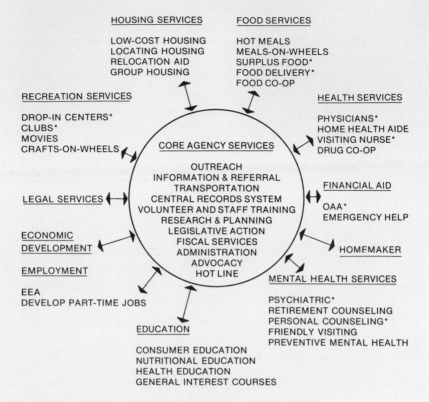

MODEL FOR SOMERVILLE ELDERLY PROGRAM

HOUSING SERVICES

LOW-COST HOUSING
LOCATING HOUSING
RELOCATION AID
GROUP HOUSING

FOOD SERVICES

HOT MEALS
MEALS-ON-WHEELS
SURPLUS FOOD*
FOOD DELIVERY*
FOOD CO-OP

RECREATION SERVICES

DROP-IN CENTERS*
CLUBS*
MOVIES
CRAFTS-ON-WHEELS

HEALTH SERVICES

PHYSICIANS*
HOME HEALTH AIDE
VISITING NURSE*
DRUG CO-OP

CORE AGENCY SERVICES

OUTREACH
INFORMATION & REFERRAL
TRANSPORTATION
CENTRAL RECORDS SYSTEM
VOLUNTEER AND STAFF TRAINING
RESEARCH & PLANNING
LEGISLATIVE ACTION
FISCAL SERVICES
ADMINISTRATION
ADVOCACY
HOT LINE

LEGAL SERVICES

FINANCIAL AID

OAA*
EMERGENCY HELP

ECONOMIC
DEVELOPMENT

HOMEMAKER

EMPLOYMENT

EEA
DEVELOP PART-TIME JOBS

MENTAL HEALTH SERVICES

PSYCHIATRIC*
RETIREMENT COUNSELING
PERSONAL COUNSELING*
FRIENDLY VISITING
PREVENTIVE MENTAL HEALTH

EDUCATION

CONSUMER EDUCATION
NUTRITIONAL EDUCATION
HEALTH EDUCATION
GENERAL INTEREST COURSES

*SERVICES WHICH ARE CURRENTLY PROVIDED TO SOME EXTENT

FIGURE 12.1

plan then evolved very rapidly, and this is illustrated in Figure 12.1. A number of services, identified by the asterisks, came into being almost at once, and others followed afterward.

A point to note in Figure 12.1 is that the Mental Health Center is not the coordinating agency. On the contrary, it is one of the contributors to the Core Agency Services along with numerous others. Having played its catalytic role in initiating the process represented in Figure 12.1, it makes its further contributions mainly in terms of its regular clinical service role. Similarly, Cardoza and Ackerly as individuals refrained from assuming any administrative part in the program for the elderly. In doing this, they were following an operating principle which we have called "Always the bridesmaid, never the bride."

The "Bridesmaid Principle" states that the catalytic agent should never assume an executive position in the change program he is trying to bring about. He should rather take an attending and facilitating role. If a committee is formed, for example, he should resolutely decline to be chairman, but willingly accept the post of secretary and work very hard running errands, collecting information, and serving as resource person and advisor to the chairman and members.

There are several reasons for this principle, of which two may be noted here. One is that if the catalyst assumes an executive position, he ceases to be a catalyst and becomes a protagonist. His capacity for objectivity and considered judgment is thus greatly compromised. In short, the catalytic model is abandoned and some other process takes over. Furthermore, the position of protagonist is apt to lead a person into being a member of a faction and so developing not only friends but also enemies, and becoming embroiled in political issues of the community that have little to do with such goals as reducing isolation for the elderly. If the catalyst represents a mental health center, much political involvement can, in the long run, have negative effects on the center's functions as the power of the different factions shifts in the course of time. One can readily see here problems that are parallel to those often experienced by the church in the world of politics.

The second reason for the principle is that assumption of an executive position by a catalyst makes it very difficult for him to pull away later without the whole program collapsing. This is especially true if the catalyst is an outsider to the community. Although the program may be favorably viewed in the community, it is apt to be considered his project and so may not really become a part of the community's structure and functioning.

At the time of present writing, two years after initiation, the project is still going forward. The Somerville Community Council has become more involved, and with help from the United Community Services of Greater Boston has developed an Elderly Planning Committee. The Massachusetts Department of Elderly Affairs is interested in having Somerville join with Cambridge in setting up a joint home-care organization. After the first year, Cardoza gradually withdrew from the program until at the present time he no longer has any connection. The way is thus open for the Mental Health Center to begin again with a different high-risk group.

Next Steps

On the basis of this exploratory study and its predecessors in Stirling County, it seems to us that the next steps should include research that is quantitative and which approximates an experimental design. Three primary questions stand in need of attention.

The first is, does the catalyst really make any difference? Would there be essentially the same results if he never appeared at all? It could be argued that all our procedure amounts to is detecting a trend that is headed for a desirable outcome and then climbing on board, much as politicians sometimes do. Obviously, we do not think that this is what has been happening, but something more than opinion is needed. Hence, although there are serious methodological difficulties, due to the fact that it is never possible to match two communities with much accuracy, a series of comparative studies should be undertaken with a view to ascertaining whether the catalytic approach makes a difference, and if so, how much in terms of time, costs, and effectiveness.

The second question is whether a change aimed at relieving stress does in fact have this effect. The approach to this will require operational definitions of stress and the development of indicators that can be treated quantitatively, a difficult business, but by no means impossible. One could, for example, set up indicators which would show changes in the numbers of isolated elderly.

The third question is whether the relief of stress has any effect on the frequency of illness in the population. Attacking this problem requires not only indicators and comparative studies of well-selected communities, but also a series of measurements at different points in time. Such a study would be exceedingly complex, yet we think it would be feasible through the adaptation of epidemiological survey techniques such as those that have been employed in Stirling County, Midtown Manhattan, and elsewhere.

REFERENCES

1. Arensberg, C. M., and Niehoff, A. H. *Introducing Social Change: A Manual for Americans Overseas*. Chicago: Aldine, 1964.

2. Barnard, C. I. *The Function of the Executive*. Cambridge: Harvard University Press, 1968.

3. Bunker, R., and Adair, J. *The First Look at Strangers*. New Brunswick: Rutgers University Press, 1959.

4. Caplan, G. *Principles of Preventive Psychiatry*. New York: Basic Books, 1964.

5. Dohrenwend, B. P., and Dohrenwend, B. S. *Social Status and Psychological Disorder*. New York: Wiley-Interscience, 1969.

6. Essen-Möller, E. "Individual Traits and Morbidity in a Swedish Rural Population." *Acta Psychiatrica et Neurologica Scandinavica*, Supplementum 100 (1956):1–160.

7. Gardner, B. B. *Human Relations in Industry*. Chicago: Richard D. Irwin, 1945.

8. Goodenough, W. H. *Cooperation in Change*. New York: Russell Sage Foundation, 1963.

9. Hagnell, O. *A Prospective Study of the Incidence of Mental Disorder*. New York: Humanities Press, 1966.

10 Hughes, C. C.; Tremblay, M. A.; Rapoport, R. N.; and Leighton, A. H. *People of Cove*

and Woodlot: Communities from the Viewpoint of Social Psychiatry. The Stirling County Study of Psychiatric Disorder and Sociocultural Environment, vol. 2. New York: Basic Books, 1960

11. Langner, T. S., and Michael, S. T. *Life Stress and Mental Health.* The Midtown Manhattan Study, vol. 2. New York: Free Press, 1963.

12. Leighton, A. H., *My Name is Legion: Foundations for a Theory of Man in Relation to Culture.* The Stirling Country Study of Psychiatric Disorder and Sociocultural Environment, vol. 1. New York: Basic Books, 1959.

13. ———. "Poverty and Social Change." *Scientific American* 212(1965):21–27.

14. ———. "Some Propositions Regarding the Relationship of Sociocultural Integration and Disintegration to Mental Health." In *Social Psychiatry,* edited by J. Zubin and F. A. Freyhan, pp. 1–7. New York: Grune & Stratton, 1968.

15. ———. "Cosmos in the Gallup City Dump." In *Psychiatric Disorder and the Urban Environment,* edited by B. H., Kaplan. pp. 4–12. New York: Behavioral Publication, 1971.

16. ———, and Murphy, J. M. "Behavioral Sciences and Health." *Mount Sinai Journal of Medicine* 40(1973):551–561.

17. Leighton, A. H.; Lambo, T. A.; Hughes, C. C.; Leighton, D. C.; Murphy, J. M.; and Macklin, D. B. *Psychiatric Disorder Among the Yoruba: A Report from the Cornell-Aro Mental Health Research Project.* Ithaca, N.Y.: Cornell University Press, 1963.

18. Leighton, D. C.; Harding, J. S.; Macklin, D. B.; Macmillan, A. M.; and Leighton, A. H. *The Character of Danger: Psychiatric Symptoms in Selected Communities.* The Stirling County Study of Psychiatric Disorder and Sociocultural Environment, vol. 3. New York: Basic Books, 1963.

19. Levine, S., and Scotch, N., eds. *Social Stress.* Chicago: Aldine, 1970.

20. Lindemann, E. "Symptomatology and Management of Acute Grief." *American Journal of Psychiatry* 101 (1944):141–146.

21. Mayo, E. *The Human Problems of an Industrial Civilization.* New York: Macmillan, 1933.

22. ———. *The Social Problems of an Industrial Civilization.* Boston: Harvard School of Business Administration, 1946.

23. Nangeroni, A. "Social Action in Preventive Psychiatry." *Canada's Mental Health* 16 (1968):19–24.

24. Paul, B. D., ed. *Health, Culture, and Community.* New York: Russell Sage Foundation, 1955.

25. Roethlisberger, F. J., and Dickson, W. J. *Management and the Worker.* Cambridge, Mass.: Harvard University Press, 1939.

26. Sanders, I. T., et al. *Experience with Human Factors in Agricultural Areas of the World.* Washington, D.C.: Extension Service and Office of Foreign Agricultural Relations, U.S. Dept. of Agriculture, 1949.

27. Sasaki, T. T. *Fruitland, New Mexico: A Navaho Community in Transition.* Ithaca, N.Y.: Cornell University Press, 1960.

28. Spicer, E. H., ed. *Human Problems in Technological Change.* New York: Russell Sage Foundation, 1952.

29. Srole, L.; Langner, T. S.; Michael, S. T.; Opler, M. K.; and Rennie, T. A. C. *Mental Health in the Metropolis,* The Midtown Manhattan Study. New York: McGraw-Hill, 1962.

30. Whyte, W. F. *Street Corner Society.* Chicago: University of Chicago Press, 1943.

31. ———. *Industry and Society.* New York: McGraw-Hill, 1946.

32. Wilson, R. N. *Community Structure and Health Action.* Washington, D.C.: Public Affairs Press, 1968.

33. Wittkower, E. D., and Dubreuil, G. "Psychocultural Stress in Relation to Mental Illness." *Social Science and Medicine* 7 (1973):691–704.

Editorial Note

In the following contribution Hollister scrutinizes the triad of community mental health strategies that attempt to go beyond clinical therapeutic ministrations to the distressed individual. Consultation, education, and prevention are the prongs of psychiatric outreach into the social environment, the extension of the helping agent's concern beyond hospital or clinic walls. The relation of these strategies to our fundamental propositions is clear: They represent patterns of intervention into processes of social disintegration, with concomitant efforts to strengthen the resources of individuals and groups most vulnerable to the stress of life. This chapter also addresses several of the key issues set forth in Chapter 1, notably the debate over the proper role of community psychiatry and the problem of linking local agencies to provide coordination and continuity of care.

Hollister is particularly acute in his consideration of the gulf between our presumptive understanding of these extended strategies, and our operational capacity to translate them into action. He counsels moderation and humility; we should, he contends, forsake grandiose promises and concentrate on modest, readily accessible forms of helping. In the field of primary prevention, for example, we currently lack the knowledge to forestall the development of schizophrenia, or even of severe neuroses. But through programs of early detection and special education we do have the means to reduce sharply the incidence of early school failure, and should energetically pursue this goal.

Drawing analogies with physical medicine and public health, Hollister suggests that there are many ways for community psychiatry to foster the well-being of populations, short of dramatic "cures" for mental illness. His argument parallels that of psychologist Bernard Bloom,[3] who set forth a "miasma" theory of public mental health: Just as nineteenth-century sanitarians were able to lessen the rates of infectious disease by cleaning up the physical environment, even working under the vague and incorrect causal theory of miasma, so we in community psychiatry can tackle elements of the social environment that have been identified as noxious to psychological health. In the absence of an airtight etiological theory, it is still possible—indeed mandatory—to mount an assault on poverty, school failure, loneliness, and many other psychologically deleterious social processes.

This chapter's emphasis on prevention for individuals and the altering of stressful interpersonal situations reinforces the contributions of Hamburg, Adams, and Brodie on coping behavior (Chapter 9) and of Cardoza, Ackerly, and Leighton on the promotion of community action (Chapter 12).

R. N. W.

CHAPTER 13

Programing Consultation, Education, and Prevention: Unfulfilled Strategies

WILLIAM G. HOLLISTER

PROPONENTS of the use of consultative, preventive, and educative strategies find themselves squarely in the middle of the battleground between the major forces contending for predominance and resources in the mental health field— those upholding the model of clinical treatment versus those supporting the model of social system intervention. Each of these points of view seeks to define and control the consultative, education, and prevention areas of mental health programing in line with their respective values and goals. This continuing contention, as well as other factors, leaves these program areas relatively underdeveloped and even neglected.

Underdeveloped Consultation Program Strategies: Clinical and Social System Approaches

The clinically minded school sees consultation programs as a supplement to direct clinical services, a logical outreach of therapeutic interventions. Its most orthodox wing principally endorses case-centered consultation as a way to extend psychiatric-like services to more of the unserved population. The more liberal-minded clinicians have moved on into using "consultee-centered consultation"(Gerald Caplan's definitions) [9] as a necessary tool to meet wider population coverage. Dr. DuPuy's [10] preliminary reports on his current surveys of the U.S. population by the National Bureau of Health Statistics show that 16.9 percent of our people have psychological disabilities, but only 2 percent are using psychiatric and psychological resources. These facts, plus the alarming levels of pathology in the population revealed in the recent series of population surveys, have convinced many that the passive receptive services model of "you come to me" programs is not enough. Any reasonably comprehensive provision of service to all or most persons in need requires active outreach. This will mean less insistence that each person in need be willing to: (1) declare himself sick; and (2) decide to accept patienthood and dependently place himself in medical or other hands. This means greater recognition that most people in need of mental health care do not accept patienthood, do not define their problem in medical terms, and will not come to named mental health facilities. Actionwise, it portends that mental health care must be extended beyond the mental health center or office, and be provided within other helping frameworks, most of them nonmedical, where most people are willing to take their problems, defining them in their own way. Thus those clinicians who wish to serve the bulk of the epidemic we have will soon find themselves having to do most of their diagnostic studies, disposition recommendations, case consultations, and consultee consultations within social services and public health departments, schools, courts, and correctional and other human service agencies, as well as with general medical practitioners, ministers, and industrial personnel staff. Most often, their motivating concept and goal will be mainly to provide some form of reparative ameliorative intervention to people in trouble, hopefully at an early stage of the person's disability.

Once clinicians equipped with knowledge about human behavior and skills in behavior change move out into new and varied settings, they encounter new sets of problems and are cast into roles that raise self-doubts. Caplan,[9] Bindman,[3] Klein,[15] Beisser and Green,[2] and others have documented the many vicissitudes experienced in outreach and consultation services, so they will not be reviewed here. For instance, physicians, whose power has been granted them out of patients' willing dependence in critical life-death-disability situations, often experience difficulty fulfilling their legal, ethical, and therapeutic responsibilities when they find they have no control over their consultee and his client. Consultation calls for a shift from a dominant responsible power position to solve a problem into a collaborative, confidential exploration and mutual problem-solving approach in which the consultee alone holds the continuing responsibility for the person or problem under discussion and is free to reject the consultant's ideas and recommendations.

Most difficult of all, the plan mutually evolved must be one that fits the personality, competencies, and work realities of the consultee, who is to turn around and help someone in need. This means that the consultant must not only be able to bring clinical understandings about a person whom he often does not personally see, he must translate these clinical insights into role functions and behaviors well within the competency of the child welfare worker, teacher, public health nurse, parole worker, rehabilitation counselor, medical practitioner, or other helping discipline member. Together, in discussing the possible ways of helping the person in need, they must evolve plans that fit the consultee's setting, agency, and its program, fit the personality of the consultee who is to give the help, and fit the person to be helped. This is often a considerable task. The consultant, to do his job well, cannot use some general consultative interpersonal process, but must spend some time learning about the resources, mission, limitations, and staff relationships in the consultee agency framework, as well as learning about the roles, competencies, behavior codes, goals, limits, and relationships of the consultee and his or her discipline. Unfortunately, many clinician consultants fail to invest in extra study of these settings and roles; they prefer to fall back on a general relationship process that often leaves the insights they provide untranslated into the consultee's competencies and job realities.

These problems of the consultant in power and collaboration, in fitting solutions to the resources, often are compounded by dissimilarities between the consultant system (the mental health center) and the "consultee system" (i.e., school, court, and so on). Many "consultee systems" still resist foreign professionals who come in "to help them." Some still deny the existence of emotional problems in their clientele, decline any responsibility or need to deal with their clients' mental health problems or behaviors, or may insist on their own competency and, therefore, deny any need for consultation. Entering consultants may get "walled off" or extruded like foreign bodies, be perceived as threats to staff, be clung to dependently, be neglected, be misused as pseudotherapists or pseudosupervisors, or even become tools for subgroup power struggles. Successful consultation programing requires continued efforts to resolve the constant stream of interpersonal and interagency problems that emerge.

In summary, the concept of expanding the range and coverage of community mental health care by erecting a confederation of helping agencies, a circle of cooperating agencies whose staffs are to be strengthened by in-service education and consultation provided by the mental health centers, is a bold conceptual leap forward over an awesome canyon of difficulties. To date, few mental health centers have chosen to commit the extensive staff time and money required to go out to meet and work even partially with other disciplines and agencies, to try to serve the seven-eighths of the people with problems who do not and may never come to the center itself. Because of biases and values built in during preservice training, most clinicians prefer the classical clinical work in the center over the more difficult consultative work away from the center, where "one never knows who, how many, or how well he has helped" and where "one can too easily be seduced out of role." In short, the clinical schools' concept of the role of consultation programing has rarely had an adequate demonstration, and so it is still an unconsummated bold leap forward.

In contrast, while the clinical model proponents have been struggling with the technological, logistical, social resistance, and economic problems of launching wider personal care through consultation networks, the standard-bearers of the social system model of intervention have been fumbling to get a foothold on the slippery ground of social system level consultation. Persons of this school see clinical repair services as necessary but eventually futile in stemming the tide of psychological disorders, unless they are complemented with a direct attempt to change the group interactions or other social forces that contribute to these disabilities. They see psychological accidents happening faster than the repair shops can ever mend them. They cite Albee's prediction that our manpower resources are and will be inadequate for a clinical attack on the problems in our population. They cite public health's experience that major endemics are not conquered by clinical care alone, that attacks on the causative stresses and their vectors are also essential.

The social system intervention-oriented leaders draw strength from Gruenberg [12] and others who have substantiated that some of our therapeutic institutions produce iatrogenic disabilities, and from the host of studies that seek to show that deleterious social environment is an operative factor in poor personality development and maladjustments. Spokesmen such as Donald Klein [14] suggest that consultation might best be directed to effecting changes in the family, work group, school, or organizational relationship networks that may be stressing people. They draw converts from clinicians who do group and family therapy, and they borrow tool ideas and intervention patterns from the fields of public health, group process, social psychology, and, more recently, organizational development.

Here again our ideological and theoretical concepts of what is possible have been exceedingly difficult to translate into practical program application.

Whether a consultant is appointed or assumes the role of change agent for a group, an organization, or a community, there is almost always an eventual challenge to that consultant's mandate. Who are you to try to change the system? Can you prove the group is hurting this person? Soon the consultant receives challenges or competition from other disciplines such as law, politics, economics, and business, which claim prior or higher rights to control how a system or organization might be changed for the better. Soon the effort to diminish the way a group or agency is "grinding up people" becomes a group-wide ethical and/or administrative problem, involving dimensions and issues of doubtful relevance to the mental health consultant's profession, background, training, area of responsibility, and mandate. Efforts to build a healthier group environment, a more competent community along the lines Cottrell outlines in Chapter 11, may eventually involve activities and a continuity of effort far beyond the usual mandate given a mental health program by the taxpayers and their governing boards.

Systems-oriented consultants have achieved some success in changing organization policies or helping set up "exception mechanisms" when individuals are "hurt" by a policy. They have helped families, school groups, business managers, and groups of workers build more mutually supportive interactions, develop decisions and procedures on a participatory basis, and learn how to decrease stresses. But here again the task has only begun. The technology is evolving, but the public trust and mandate that mental health professionals should be paid for and allowed to change pathogenic groups has not yet been fully given, even though these professionals try to justify such a responsibility by predicting that social system interventions might decrease psychological disability and increase personal competency. Thus another programing potential is relatively untried. As of 1975, it appears that neither the clinician's hope to extend more care over consultation networks nor the environmentalist's hope to mount social system interventions have been given extensive enough implementation to really evaluate their potential as strategies of mental health programing.

Mental Health Education Programing: Will It Go Commercial or Professional?

Like consultation, mental health education is remarkable for its programatic underdevelopment. Its development has similarly been retarded by a polemic between those professionals who label it "unproductive activity" and those who call it "essential." As usual, when a service the public wants gets bogged down in interprofessional argument, other forces move in and take over, further compounding the problems of technology, the mandate to perform, and professional acceptability.

As of 1975, very few public mental health programs devote more than minimal resources to operating a mental health education program. Of those that do, most of the effort goes into public relations news releases or into "education about mental illness." Films, lectures, pamphlets, and other media are used to transmit messages about the prevalence of problems, the various kinds of disorders, the need for resources, and possible solutions or treatments. Better still, some "resource use" educational efforts communicate about the kinds of care available, the various kinds of care givers, and the costs of care, as well as how to use such resources and how families can be helpful. Certainly such education helps to build a baseline of public understanding, which hopefully leads to better utilization of services and increased citizen support of our expensive and poorly understood programs. Some professionals complain that such education only builds up unrealizable expectations and lures more people with unmet needs for care into joining the waiting lists of our sadly overburdened clinical care providers.

Very few public mental health programs venture any extensive commitment into an "education to produce mental health." In fact, professional polarization over the value of this has led to general neglect and abandonment of this kind of education by many mental health professionals, with consequent takeover by commercial and group process partisans.

Why this abandonment? Mainly because "education for mental health" is beset by goal-setting problems. For example, here are some of the difficult questions frequently used to "shoot down" program development in this area.

What is mental health? Is it the same for all people? Who has the right to decide what is mentally healthy and set the goals for a program? Would such a program only impose WASP (White Anglo-Saxon Protestant) values on other social groups?

Add to these trials some clinicians making trenchant comments such as "We don't know enough yet about personality development and human behavior to tell anybody what behavior is best" or "Educational impacts are too ephemeral and superficial to change behavior." Frequently such professional opinion has become a rationale for withholding commitment of funds and staff.

It is right in this vacuum of professional noncommitment to an education for mental health that others, not all of whom are fools, walk in where professional "angels" fear to tread. For instance, the commercial literary world has discovered that the "psychological era" has arrived and the public is avid for behavior and relationship information. As a result, almost every magazine on the newsstands features on its cover articles on child behavior guidance, sex, interpersonal relationships, and the behavior problems of everyday living. A hundred "soap operas" explore the vicissitudes of human stress. Writers comb through professional articles and interview behavioral specialists to abstract messages or experiences to feed to an insatiable public demand, attested to by the public's willingness to spend its money for such information. Too much of it (not all) is specious, trumped-up distortion, incomplete pictures, or oversimplistic pat formulas of questionable general applicability. Some of it represents the best that the behavioral sciences know and are willing to share. Some clinicians have discovered the public interest in such education and have reaped a bonanza for such writings. In brief, there is no such thing as no "education for mental health." Whether well or poorly done, it is being carried out by commercial, volunteer, and group process organizations. It is rarely being done by professional or public mental health service organizations backed with research, evaluation, an adequate budget, and competent full-time staff. With few exceptions, notably in voluntary mental health-related agencies, mental health education has not won status as an essential component of public mental health programs.

In face of this paradoxical situation, another professional group has recently undertaken the cause of promoting personality development education. The rise of behavioral conditioning therapies, as well as the deepening of group process theory and practice, has led to a more comprehensive redefinition of education. Whereas education was formerly looked upon as a completely cognitive experience entailing the transmission of ideas that would have only slight impact on powerful internal psychodynamics, the tide has changed and education is conceptualized as both a cognitive and an affective process. These days we speak more of emotional reeducation, of group interactions for providing experiences that change people's feelings about themselves and others or build willingness to explore new relationships and behaviors. Some theorists now conceptualize psychotherapy as a special intensive learning experience. Focus on fostering ego functioning as well as the unlearning or learning of behaviors has helped to legitimate educational approaches to behavior change. Specially structured life-space learning experiences like token economies, patient governments, remotivation sessions, or therapeutic communities are now used as components of therapy and rehabilitation programs for the mentally ill.

In summary, mental health education for clinical purposes as well as for personal growth purposes for nonpatients has arrived. Now people seeking growth in sensitivity, relationship skills, self-understanding, and other insights are flocking to personal growth or encounter groups, to human relations skill labs, or to other kinds of interactional or coactional experiences that are labeled as educational, not therapeutic, activities. Charlatanism has reared its ugly head, but there are many serious, professionally led attempts, and a modicum of research to underwrite scientifically and professionally the quality of these

235

various behavior education and group process endeavors. New theories of human transactions, ego functioning, and game theory are helping to map additional inroads into this new psychological territory. This is becoming a kind of "education for mental health" that does not impose a behavioral formula, but that attempts to catalyze the processes of self-development and relationship building. Again, it is a mental health education movement that in the main arises from professional and agency resources outside of the public mental health programs.

It is to be hoped that the various emotional reeducation, behavioral change education, ego psychology, and group process contributions that are making possible a "process enrichment" education for mental health will help to dissolve some of the professional paralysis now retarding this field. Hopefully we will begin an era in which public mental health programs will serve patients, their families, and nonpatients with carefully organized, professionally staffed, well-evaluated programs that are a permanent and essential component of the program. (For further evaluations see Goldston [11] and Jacoby [13].)

Prevention: A Program Pariah or a Potential?

This trilogy of unfulfilled strategies in mental health consultation, education, and prevention concludes with an examinatiom of some of the forces preventing prevention programing. At a recent legislative hearing in North Carolina, citizen group after citizen group called for more attention to mental health prevention efforts. Finally a legislator turned to a panel of testifying mental health experts to ask: "Everyone seems to talk prevention, but can you give me the name of a single state mental health program that has a well-organized prevention program?" The embarrassing silence was long, finally broken by hesitant comments about bits and pieces of prevention programing being scattered all over the country. However, no one state had, as yet, pulled it all together into a balanced and well-staffed program.

In prevention, as in consultation and education, a polarization of professional opinion seems to defuse the commitment of funds and staff. On one hand, most of the clinical treatment-oriented people tend to give highest priority to the intensive and expensive task of caring for people already ill. Although many admit that prevention should be pursued, they are reluctant to commit mental health's limited resources to it. The stereotypical comments run: "We have not yet learned how to prevent mental illness, and furthermore, we have no proof that prevention works!" Their antagonists, the socioenvironmentalist health development-minded people, often reply: "Stop applying unfair yardsticks and premature scientific demands. It is extremely difficult to prove conclusively why something did not happen. You will never learn how to practice prevention until you try it. Give us as many years and as much money to develop a prevention technology as you had to develop psychotherapy. Give the prevention seed a chance to sprout and mature before you evaluate its eventual potential."

At first this dialogue appears to be a head-on debate, but then one begins to sense that the protagonists are talking past each other. They are often not talking about the same facets of prevention or the same target groups to be served. The controversy becomes muddled in deciding what is to be prevented. This is compounded by confusion over what kind of prevention is being talked about. Some people use the word "prevention" to mean primary prevention, stopping a process before it affects an individual. Others use the word to mean secondary prevention, arresting a disabling process early, and some think in terms of tertiary prevention, the prevention of relapses and disability. If there were some clearer communication, some of the dissonance might shift to a more harmonious integration.

What is to be prevented? Some of the answers to this key issue have led us to unrealistic expectation, while other answers have been more humble and feasible. Before sorting out what is achievable, some cues can be provided by examining what we already have successfully prevented. Oddly enough, despite the current programatic paralysis, the mental health field has already experienced some spectacular victories of prevention. Paresis, which took up 12 percent of the nation's mental hospital beds, is about gone. It responded not just to treatment but to a nation-wide VD education, contact-tracing system, plus blood and spinal fluid-screening programs. Pellagrous psychoses, which once filled 25 percent of our Southern mental hospital beds, surrendered, not to bedside care but to laws requiring vitamin-enriched flour. Lead psychoses and their deliria responded to the environmental change of eliminating lead pipe. Hysteria, a purely psychological disability, seems to have responded to public education and change in sex mores. Much has also been learned by clinicians and others about screening for, detecting, and intervening early enough for secondary prevention of emotional disabilities. Slowly our arsenal of procedures for rehabilitation and the prevention of relapse, tertiary prevention, is growing.

What have we learned from such victories? First, it is easier to mount a prevention attack when you can isolate one etiological agent and/or its carrier. Second, victory more frequently comes with giving not just clinical care but also by using environmental change, education, and the interventions of nonmedical colleagues. Third, it is easier to perform secondary and tertiary prevention than to program primary prevention. These positive learnings were unfortunately accompanied by the rise of some illogical expectations that seem currently unattainable. These relatively direct single-etiology victories raised hopes that other mental diseases could soon be prevented. Because so many of the mental disabilities listed as diseases in medical books arise from unknown or multiple etiologies or from poorly understood processes, our hopes of preventing diseases have in the main not been fulfilled. We have learned some ways to prevent some of the disability or progression of certain conditions, but the hoped-for preventive breakthrough for pathological entities such as schizophrenia, mania-depressive psychosis, and other mental disorders has not yet come.

The issue of "What is to be prevented?" has become "What *can* be prevented?" In the darkness of today's limited knowledge, we may well have to climb down from our high expectations of being able to initiate programs to prevent the major psychoses, most neuroses, or character disorders. Perhaps we need to be more humble in our goals. After all, the preventive efforts for physical disease did not start by learning how to prevent major diseases like cancer or heart disease. Preventive care here started with the more humble and simple goals of preventing: (1) symptoms, i.e., pain, spasm, fever; (2) injuries, i.e., to eyes, bones, soft tissues; (3) the consequences of deprivation of air, water, clean food, and vitamins; and (4) too much body defense response to toxins and allergens, i.e., ephedrine for a facial bee sting. Perhaps the mental health field also needs to start with the more humble goals of preventing: (1) symptoms like fear, anxiety, and rage; (2) traumas or stresses that impair personality development or break up interpersonal relationships; (3) the consequences of emotional deprivation; and (4) undue stress and/or inappropriate behavioral responses, i.e., flight, fight, introjection, blaming others, displaced anger, and other noncoping behaviors.

This more humble set of prevention goals brings us to the task of learning how to prevent self-defeating or harmful behaviors in order to prevent role failures in school, on the job, or as parents. It challenges us to focus on ways to prevent parent-child, husband-wife, or boss-employee relationship breakdowns, and on learning how to abort some of the stress reactions so many people are having. Hopefully, in the next decade both clinicians and environmentalists will find common ground and a complementary relationship in attempting to pursue these less heroic and more feasible goals of prevention. The clinicians can bring their pathology, diagnosis and repair knowledges to bear to increase the effectiveness of the early detection, and early treatment, that is secondary prevention, and to provide more widespread aftercare that will be a tertiary prevention. In addition, they might contribute their clinical data to help foster retrospective studies that will sort out what stresses, deprivations, relationship breakdowns, and behaviors have led to their patients' decompensations. Such studies should feed directly into the hands of the environmentalists' information on what stresses are the most injurious and should be eliminated or decreased, as well as data on what personality types are vulnerable to what stresses.

In this area of pinpointing critical stresses, identifying coping mechanisms, and delineating the insights basic to self-control of overreactions, the clinicians can be contributing key tools to the environmentalists as the latter seek to modify the groups, organizations, relationships, and situations that overwhelm certain vulnerable individuals. This emerging technology can then be linked to newly developed methods of detecting vulnerable people, like Dr. Eli M. Bower's methods to detect which primary-age school children are likely to become behavior problems, emotionally handicapped, or school failures before the breakdown actually occurs.[6,7] Once we can detect the vulnerables and know which kind of stresses might disable them, the stage is set for specific primary prevention by programs to decrease stress that are directed to specific target groups of susceptibles. Such efforts will lend themselves to research and evaluation.

The hypothesis is that once clinicians and environmentalists abandon temporarily the goals of preventing specific disease entities and begin to pool their efforts to prevent certain behaviors, interpersonal transactions, and emotionally depriving experiences, they may find more common cause. They can then begin to collaborate in developing and programing achievable and supportable primary prevention programs. They will not be without models and tools. As reported at the legislative hearing mentioned above, there are bits and pieces of prevention programs throughout the country, some not operating under mental health auspices, that can serve as guideposts and nuclei. There are programs like the one in Sumter, South Carolina, to detect emotional unreadiness for school and do a preschool preventive intervention that cuts first-grade failures in half. Without attempting a review of programs, there are planned *interventions to cut down the stresses* that create job failure, parenthood failure, and many other kinds of role failure or self-image destruction. There are programs to rescue vulnerable, scapegoated, low pecking-order employees or students from noxious group situations and move them to a new, more supportive environment. This is *moving people out of the path of stress.* There are other programs that seek to *fortify people against a stress they must face,* such as anticipatory guidance education of those about to endure an expected crisis or a new anxiety-provoking situation. Even the lowly fire drill is a group panic prevention technique that uses the paradigm of *cutting down overreactions to stress* in a situation in which the behavioral overreaction has proven many times more destructive than the stress impact. Finally, there are interventions that bring critically needed emotional support and coping *assistance* to people confronted with a personal crisis, like grieving over a loss.

The program models exist, but too often their imaginative use and implementation awaits a resolution of the clinical versus environmentalist controversies over goals and resources. Instead of competition, we need the creation of clinician-environmentalist collaboration, adventurous leadership, and a reasonable period of time to grow and mature before being made rigorously accountable to cost benefit analysts. Under these conditions, more state mental health programs could begin to pull the bits and pieces of prevention programing together into a more comprehensive approach. Perhaps then the public could be made aware of the extensive amounts of secondary and tertiary prevention already being done. The public could be better informed about the need to implement a collaborative clinician-environmentalist approach to a primary prevention with more humble and achievable goals. Hopefully, then the legislators, hearing the public's concern for preventive services and assured by seeing that clinicians and environmentalists are working together as complementary partners, will give the mandate and the funds to develop this long unfulfilled strategy.[7,16,17]

Summary

All three of the fields of mental health programing reviewed, consultation, education, and prevention, are stalemated or held back by differing points of view, some vigorously held by the clinically centered proponents as contrasted with the viewpoints of environmentalists. Some of the controversy is over genuine dilemmas. Some of the dichotomies are the products of a situation in which both groups are right, both approaches are needed to serve the public and personal needs of our citizens, but the conflict arises over competition for public recognition and mandate, for access to scarce funds, because resources are still too limited to meet the total range of mental health needs. Most unfortunate of all is that some of the polemics are unnecessary. Some of them are caused by lack of communication and lack of study of the other side's point of view, goals, values, and experience.

The organization of this book, in attempting to draw together the best of the clinical and environmental viewpoints and technologies, sets the model for what needs to happen in the fields of mental health consultation, education, and prevention to bring their as yet unfulfilled strategies to fruition.

REFERENCES

1. Albec, George W., *Mental Health Manpower Trends.* New York: Basic Books, 1959.
2. Beisser, A., and Green, R. *Mental Health Consultation and Education.* Palo Alto, Calif.: National Press Books, 1972.

3. Bindman, A. J. "Mental Health Consultation: Theory and Practice." *Journal of Counseling Psychology* 23 (1959):473–482.

4. Bloom, Bernard L. " 'The Medical Model,' Miasma Theory, and Community Mental Health." *Community Mental Health Journal* 1 (1965):333–338.

5. Bower, E. M. "Primary Prevention in a School Setting." In *Prevention of Mental Disorder in Children*. New York: Basic Books, 1961.

6. ———. In *Principles of Preventive Psychiatry*, edited by G. Caplan. New York: Basic Books, 1964.

7. ———. "K.I.S.S. and Kids: A Mandate for Prevention." *American Journal of Orthopsychiatry* 4 (1972):556–565.

8. Brandon, S., and Gruenberg, E. M. "Measurement of the Incidence of Chronic Severe Social Breakdown Syndrome." *Milbank Memorial Fund Quarterly* 41, suppl. (1966):129–149.

9. Caplan, G. *The Theory of Mental Health Consultation*. New York: Basic Books, 1970.

10. DuPuy, H. Personal communication.

11. Goldston, S. E. "Mental Health Education in a Community Mental Health Center." *American Journal of Public Health* 58 (1968):693–699.

12. Gruenberg, E. M.; Branden, S.; and Kasins, R. V. "Identifying Cases of the Social Breakdown Syndrome." *Milbank Memorial Fund Quarterly* 41, suppl. (1966):150–155.

13. Jacoby, A. "Mental Health Education." *Canada's Mental Health* 17 (1969):26–31.

14. Klein, D. C. "Consultation Processes as a Method for Improving Teaching." In *Behavioral Science Frontiers in Education*. New York: Wiley, 1967.

15. ———. *Community Dynamics and Mental Health*. New York: Wiley, 1968.

16. VanAntwerp, M. "The Route to Primary Prevention." *Community Mental Health Journal* 7 (1971):183–188.

17. Wagenfeld, M. O. "The Primary Prevention of Mental Illness: A Sociological Perspective." *Journal of Health and Social Behavior* 13 (1972):195–203.

Editorial Note

Several contributions in the present volume address themselves to the mental health implications of extremely rapid social and technological change. Kiev, for example, discusses in Chapter 8 the psychiatric issues confronting the developing countries; Farnsworth in Chapter 15 analyzes the role of the adolescent in a swiftly moving American society. Mertens is concerned in the following selection with an especially critical type of social change in the densely interdependent industrial societies, namely, organizational change. In our era, when so much of human activity, particularly in the occupational sphere, occurs in the framework of the large organization, the capacity of the organization to accommodate innovations assumes central significance. This capacity is not only important to the success of the organization as a collective enterprise, but is also vitally implicated in the psychological well-being of individual members. The occupational role is patently a key one for the individual, since it is the potential source of satisfaction (or dissatisfaction) of so many of the essential human strivings. For instance, the world of work may be the stage for the exercise of volition, for securing a sense of one's place in society, and for the enjoyment of group membership. On the community level, excellence of organizational functioning—and of the relations among organizations—bears directly on the quality of social integration.

There are perhaps two features of contemporary change processes that render Mertens's argument fundamental. The first is surely their pervasiveness and pace, the atmosphere of swirling change captured by such phrases as Toffler's "future shock" [78] or Bennis and Slater's "temporary society." [5] That is, we apprehend that swift and far-reaching change must come to be regarded as the normal condition, the accepted environment of our lives. It follows that the effort to prepare people to feel comfortable with change is a chief task of social psychiatry. The second feature is man's increasing propensity to plan for change, to shape its course and bring it under a modicum of deliberate control. One might argue that planning, trying to subject change processes to some version of executive rationality, is in a way the organizational analogue of Freud's goal for individual rationality: "Where id was, there shall ego be."

In any event, Mertens sets forth a clear prescription for the psychiatrist's role in helping to induce innovation in organizations. In this account, the sociotherapist is not so much the agent of change as the facilitator of change, the one who prepares the ground of group readiness to be aware and to cope. He promotes an organizational model of the "anticipatory guidance" discussed by Hamburg, Adams, and Brodie (Chapter 9) on the level of the individual. The sociotherapist's activity is also strikingly reminiscent of the catalytic role advanced by Cardoza, Ackerly, and Leighton (Chapter 12). Thus Mertens notes: "The sociotherapist is a temporary consultant. His definitive integration into the organization that consults him often indicates the failure of his intervention."

Sociotherapy's core is defined as the overcoming of a group's resistance to change. In this endeavor we find a reaffirmation of some principles threaded throughout Part III. Two that are of special moment are the emphases on the communications/information patterns of groups, and on the extension of the mental health professional's role(s). Mertens asserts that the change agent induces a change in the amount of information available to the group (the message) and in the system for exchanging information (the medium). This effort to improve the circulation of ideas appears once again to constitute a basic premise for intervention in the community structure, at whatever level. It underlies the social psychiatric approach to a system of relationships, rather than to single persons.

The professional's extended role is sharply depicted here. Akin to the roles of consultant and educator as Hollister poses them (Chapter 13), the sociotherapist moves far beyond the clinical setting. The psychiatrist's bold outreach is evidenced in a complex two-stage process of: (1) group change per se among the small immediate target population; and (2) group-inspired organizational change in the "back-home application" of the sociotherapist's teachings and the small group's learnings. The professional's acceptance of such a subtle, attenuated outcome recalls the sage's definition of the good man—one who plants trees under whose shade he will never sit.

R. N. W.

CHAPTER 14

From Theory to Practice:
The Meaning of Sociotherapy

CHARLES J. MERTENS[*]

ONE OF the major objectives of social psychiatry is the modification of social organizations. These organizations are diverse in nature. They may be industrial enterprises, schools, churches, professional groups, or groups of those who are sick (alcoholics, the handicapped, those who have had coronary heart disease, and so on). They may be urban, rural, ethnic, or economic communities. They may occasionally be entire regions of a country.

These examples show how the institutions to be modified may be either structured or free form, formal or informal, and conscious or unconscious of a need for change. They show how much the procedure of any intervention may be adapted to the characteristics of the group, and to the circumstances which call for change.

The development of the human sciences permits us to envisage such an intervention as a clinical act. The term *sociotherapy* [55,75] seems to be the most adequate one for designating that intervention. It calls attention to the circumspect, programed nature of the act, and defines its spirit, purpose, and method.

This chapter sets forward the principles governing that clinical act. It is

* Translated by Stephen M. Isaacs.

based on clinical observation of groups treated, and on certain experimental givens.

We begin with the principle that sociotherapy is practiced on groups of limited size (primary groups),[76] which are representative of a population (parent institution) whose organization is to be modified. Sociotherapy is never applied directly to a large group. It deals with a few individuals (ten to thirty) grouped together: key members, or those who set the norms, or a random sample from one hierarchic level of the institution. Only rarely (especially at the beginning of clinical involvement) does one bring together subjects belonging to different hierarchic levels. Sociotherapy aids a *small* group in resolving its problem. Thus, sociotherapy aims at modifying the entire organization, by means of action on a group that has been kept small, and that has been separated from the parent institution. This is done either by repeating the action on an increasing number of new samples, or by preparing the subjects treated to carry on, in the environment from which they came, an action that is similar to the one from which they themselves have benefited.

The effects that one expects from such intervention are varied. In principle, sociotherapy brings an increase in efficiency, and a decrease in organizational stress, in an enterprise; an easing of prejudices among races; advances in the struggle against poverty of a certain region; the fostering of healthful habits (or ones conducive to the early detection of cancer and cardiovascular ailments); the institution of new techniques (such as water fluoridation); improvement of the managerial procedures and human relations at the core of an organization; and resolution of interpersonal and intergroup tensions and conflicts. Sociotherapy has as its goal the changing of the *behavior* and the *attitudes* of a few individuals who meet for several hours or days, in order to discover their *needs*, analyze their *problems*, work out a *strategy* for change, and formulate *criteria* which can be used to evaluate the progress of their action. The role of sociotherapy ends with these four immediate objectives. Changes which occur outside the group, and which operate at the level of the *structure* and the *culture* of the parent institution, are not an immediate goal. Those changes are the ultimate objective of sociotherapy, but result exclusively from its immediate effects on small groups. The sociotherapeutic approach is roundabout, both because of its target (it addresses itself not to the institution to be changed, but to representative samples of that institution), and because of its method (it does not produce the change, but renders a group capable of choosing and achieving an option).

Sivadon [75] defines sociotherapy as the artificial modification of a social milieu for the purpose of adapting that milieu to a mental patient. We give the term a much wider meaning. The objective cited by Sivadon is, by our definition, only a special case. Sociotherapy includes, for us, all forms of intervention

245

which aim at improving the degree of integration of a group, by acting on the way the members of a group relate.

Sociotherapy makes a group more functional; by this we mean more normative, more inceptive, and more perceptive.

1. A normative group is able to define its goals, i.e., its raison d'être, and to express these objectives in terms of measurable norms, thus making possible an evaluation of the results of the action.
2. An inceptive group is capable of coordinating action taken in view of its objectives, i.e., of searching for and implementing the means necessary for achievement of the objectives.
3. A perceptive group is prone to search for information and to analyze the circumstances, or to analyze itself for the purpose of adapting its means to its goals (or to give up its goals and dissolve).

Thus, a readiness to change is not an immediate goal of sociotherapy; it is the consequence and the benefit of that therapy. The immediate goal of all sociotherapy is the *functionality* of the primary group.

Socioanalysis (better known as group dynamics or T-group) is only one of the forms of sociotherapy; it is to sociotherapy what psychoanalysis is to psychotherapy. Van Bockstaele,[80] in introducing the term socioanalysis, designates by it those groups which try to improve their system of relations by analyzing the *mental constructs* (unconscious collective fantasies) and *individual motivations* which give rise to the dynamics of their group. Socioanalysis is a very developed and often counterindicated form of sociotherapy. It takes its inspiration largely from psychoanalysis.

Sociotherapy does not limit itself to the analysis of collective fantasies and individual motivation, but also analyzes the *structure* and the *culture* of the treated group. By structure we mean:

1. The processes of interaction.
2. The systems of communication.
3. The ways that roles are distributed.[54]

Structure develops spontaneously in all groups.

By culture we mean the norms (laws, usage, customs, beliefs) which grow up in all groups, and which govern them. We also mean the symbols (statutes, myths, folklore) which reinforce these norms, and which announce the gratifications or punishments that sanction observance of or deviance from the model.

Finally, sociotherapy analyzes the significance that groups give to circumstances (economic, sociocultural, or ecological) which bear upon group survival and upon the group functions. When a group analyzes its structure or its culture, one talks about the *maintenance* functions of the group. When a group aims at its object or goal, one talks about *production* or action.

14 / From Theory to Practice: The Meaning of Sociotherapy

The role of the sociotherapist [15] is to remove the resistance which is present in the small group he treats. This resistance consists of various forms of behavior, described by Bion,[7] that hinder group decision making. It is manifested at several points in the decision-making process, from difficulty in obtaining group consensus to systematic failure to back up the consensus with action. Difficulty in forming a decision, or in testing the perceptiveness and inceptiveness of a decision, is indicative of resistance which the group manifests at the thought of change. The resistance permits the group to avoid analysis of troubling problems, and at the same time keep a clear conscience. Analysis of group resistance leads inevitably to analysis of interpersonal perceptions, and, from there, to analysis of motivations, fantasies, social structures, culture, and external circumstances that condition the interpersonal perceptions. One observes in all sociotherapeutic groups the same beginning of collective thinking, and the same succession of topics of discussion. Figure 14.1 shows this pattern.

Skillfully controlled by the sociotherapist, the sociotherapeutic process normally leads to progressive abandonment of the group's resistance, to development of a more functional system of relations, and to the capacity of the group to resolve its problems and tensions. The schematic (Figure 14.1) shows that the sociotherapist never advocates a particular solution or a particular philosophical or political attitude. If he did so, he would leave his role and go beyond his field of competence. Moreover, he would lose his therapeutic power. The sociotherapist contents himself with removing the resistance which hampers group process. This he does by making the members of a group more interdependent, and more likely to envisage—for and by themselves—the possibility of change and the strategy necessary for introduction of the change in the organization which they represent. The therapist can, at the very most, aid the members of a group in finding the logistical support needed for the change, *after* taking away the resistance to the change.

This description shows that sociotherapy is not linked to any one theory, school, or even branch of the behavioral sciences. It draws upon all valid teaching or learning theories. In the domain of theory, it attempts to understand how social relationships allow for a system of apprenticeship. In the domain of technique, it attempts to eliminate the resistance that hampers normal functioning of the group. Sociotherapy is not tied to any political or philosophical stance. Rather, it makes groups more likely to choose freely, in awareness of their reasons, a political or philosophical stance to which they wish to adhere. This last aspect gives sociotherapy its moral value.

Sociotherapy is didactic when it modifies the structure or the culture of a group. It becomes therapeutic when it takes away group resistance to modifying its structure or its culture. A functional group is able to understand and to feel why it is referring to a certain norm or why it is afraid to change that norm.

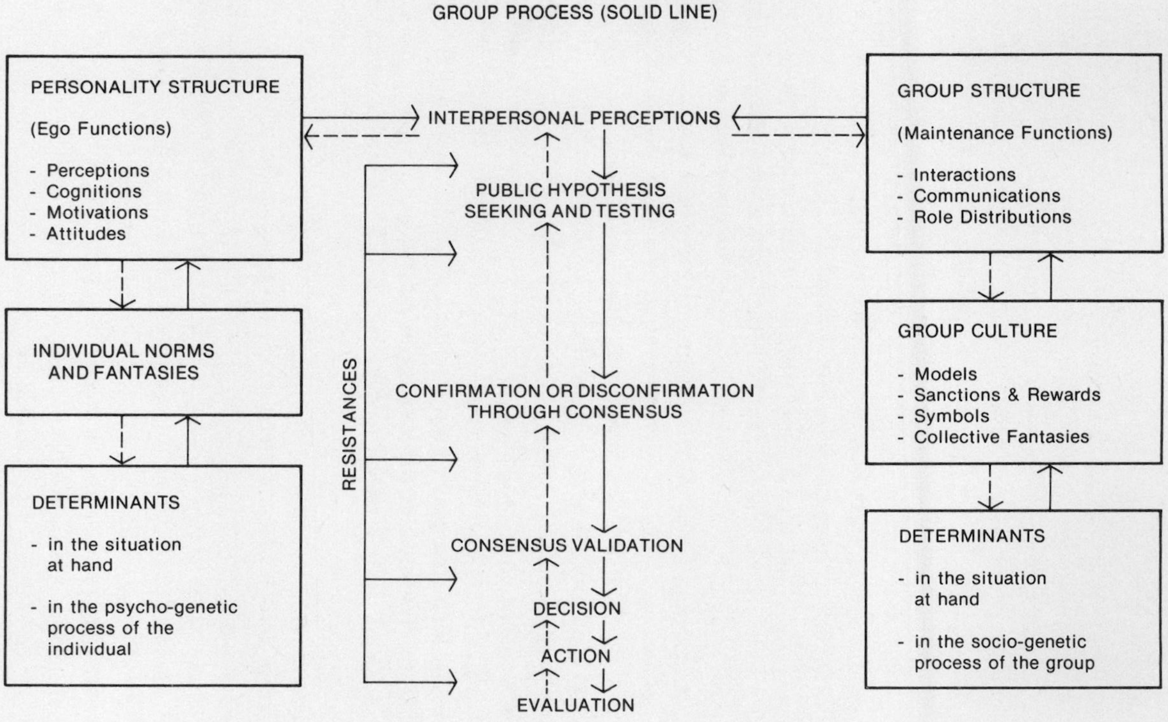

GROUP PROCESS (SOLID LINE)

GROUP STRUCTURE
(Maintenance Functions)

- Interactions
- Communications
- Role Distributions

GROUP CULTURE

- Models
- Sanctions & Rewards
- Symbols
- Collective Fantasies

DETERMINANTS

- in the situation
  at hand

- in the socio-genetic
  process of the group

INTERPERSONAL PERCEPTIONS

PUBLIC HYPOTHESIS
SEEKING AND TESTING

CONFIRMATION OR DISCONFIRMATION
THROUGH CONSENSUS

CONSENSUS VALIDATION

DECISION

ACTION

EVALUATION

RESISTANCES

PERSONALITY STRUCTURE
(Ego Functions)

- Perceptions
- Cognitions
- Motivations
- Attitudes

INDIVIDUAL NORMS
AND FANTASIES

DETERMINANTS

- in the situation
  at hand

- in the psycho-genetic
  process of the
  individual

THE SOCIOTHERAPEUTIC PROCESS

FIGURE 14.1.

Sociotherapy takes its inspiration from the theories of psychopathology that describe the origin of anxiety in relationships and the ego-defense mechanisms which attenuate anxiety but distort perceptiveness, inceptiveness, and normativeness.

Sociotherapy As a Clinical Science

Like any clinical act, sociotherapy proceeds from diagnosis to treatment. But sociotherapy does not proceed exclusively to the diagnosis, prognosis, and treatment of a problem. It attempts to institute this mode of clinical thought in the treated group, and, by constant elucidation of the resistance to it, to train the group in using it. By definition, sociotherapy addresses itself to the processes that give rise to a certain pattern of relations. Sociotherapy does not address itself to the members of a group. That is an error that would-be sociotherapists often commit. In so doing, they personalize their intervention, and pose a danger to the cohesion of the group. They change both the object and the objective of their intervention.

The object of sociotherapy is the organization of the system of relations, the system of interdependence (p. 399),[15] the way of being together or "manière-d'être-en-commun" of individuals who act collectively. In T-groups—which are, as we have said, only one of the possible methods of sociotherapy—the collective action has as its sole goal the analysis of the group's maintenance functions. In technical terms, we say that in a T-group the maintenance functions and the action are merged. This unity of the two functions of maintenance and action defines the T-group and gives it its unique character. In all other organizations, the two functions alternate; they do not coincide.

The reasons that lead an organization to consult a sociotherapist are often obscure and indirect. This situation very much complicates the role of the sociotherapist. He becomes, during his intervention, the object of the resistance of the group. The group rejects him, or worships him, in order to avoid taking its own responsibility. Things become even harder when the intervention of the sociotherapist is solicited by the management of an organization, but is directed at their subordinates. These difficulties are adequate reason for the sociotherapist to limit himself exclusively to analyzing group resistance, and to have with those who solicit his intervention a very clear agreement about the nature of his mandate before that mandate begins.

Sociotherapy runs into another problem. A lot of therapists (especially the young) are tempted to force or accelerate the process illustrated in Figure 14.1. They quickly form interpretations that conform to their own theoretical schema (often a psychoanalytical one), but which have no link to the reality of relations in the group. When the sociotherapist abandons the phenomenological point of view, and ceases to perceive or to live the relations of the group in the same spirit as its members, his observations become brutal. They arrive before the group can test out their soundness. They put the group, or some members, up for debate, and are disabling rather than therapeutic. They accentuate group anxiety and reinforce group resistance, instead of dissolving them. They often serve as a screen on which the group and therapist project their own neurotic compulsions. Thus, they turn the intervention away from its objective. One is justified in calling such behavior *wild introspection*. It is the type of intervention characteristic of the therapist who is not able to analyze the deeper motives that lead him to treat a group. Similarly, it characterizes the therapist who is ignorant of the elementary rules governing all psychotherapy. So often, one intervenes in a group for secondary reasons, without searching out the real causes that motivate the client, the subjects, or the therapist; without justifying the techniques that one uses; and without anticipating the effects of the intervention for the client organization. The practice of sociotherapy involves an experimental theory of change (p. 117); [20] "There is a need to elaborate . . . a theory of social change and a methodology of psychosociological action," says Pages (pp. 170, 196).[64] He adds that it must be "precise enough to be experimentally controlled." Frank said it clearly: "Ultimate elucidation of the effects of psychotherapy depends on the success in conceptualizing human interaction, at both personal and social levels" (p. 230).[20]

Sociotherapy involves understanding the group processes, analyzing the efficiency of the group's maintenance functions and action, learning the mechanisms that govern group change, sensing the individual and group resistance to change, and knowing the effects of the different techniques to the needs of the group in the situation that it faces. It involves comprehension of contemporary sociocultural conditions which affect the organizations that it treats.

We will take up the last point first. Then we will study the process of change, both at the individual level and at the level of the group. To conclude, we will consider the effects of the various techniques used in sociotherapy.

Sociocultural Factors Underlying the Demand for Sociotherapy

The progress of science generated the development of technology and the expansion of industrialization. Industrialization cannot be achieved without a high degree of labor division. This high degree of specialization forces society to become more complex and increasingly based on highly interdependent relationships. Profound social and psychological changes are always pressed on the people who benefit from technological progress. If these people are not well prepared for these changes and cannot cope with the demands of the new industrial society, they may react to progress by becoming inflexible, uncooperative, and increasingly hostile to any form of industrialization. In some countries resistance to change has effectively halted the improvement of the economy.[57]

The major obstacles to technological progress are unawareness of the sociopsychological processes underlying social change, and lack of skill in managing that change. The main difference between developed and developing countries is the ability to set up organizations that provide for specialization and successful interdependent relationships.

A Central African still takes care of most of his needs himself; he hunts, cooks, builds his house, makes his tools, raises and stores his food supply, and practices his own medicine. Although interaction with others within the tribal community is frequent, trade within—and to a greater extent without—the kinship is restricted. A native of New York City, on the other hand, depends for his slightest need on an extended and complex network of specialists; safety, transportation, food, clothing, shelter, entertainment, and equipment and maintenance are provided by many different people.

Industrialization brings into existence a new philosophy of man and society. It causes a permanent change in values and models, in behavior and communication patterns, in roles and expectations, in leadership styles and group decision-making processes. When a society moves from a kinship and rural system, based on subsistence economy, to an industrial and urbanized setting, based on consumption economy, the cultural values shift away from tradition. Tradition is considered valuable in a primitive community, but in an industrialized society it is looked on as irrelevant: A child who does as his father did is "old fashioned," and a company that does not keep modifying its product loses business.

As a result, technical progress presents a major problem. For although most persons pay lip service to innovation, when the necessary changes affect them, they, too, look for reasons to escape that innovation. We are all eager for innovation as far as immediate rewards are concerned, but we are reluctant to accept the personal upheaval required by it. We do not want to accept social change as a permanent feature of our lives, even though we may see a need for it if progress is to continue.

The United Nations conferences on the applications of science and technology to underdeveloped areas, held in Geneva in 1964 and New Delhi in 1968, showed clearly that the gap between the powerless countries and the developed countries will increase if the latter do not teach the former how to adapt to the social and psychological requirements of an industrial civilization.

Most people, especially those in power, are inclined to believe that man and societies are usually ready for change. However, psychology and sociology increasingly demonstrate that men are highly conditioned by their past and tend to stereotype their actions. People resist social and psychological changes. Managers, community leaders, engineers, public service administrators, and economists are all eager to plan, program, budget, and control on the technical and financial levels. They believe that the people and social systems involved in the industrialization must understand, accept, follow, and even be creative in their wake. They become upset when they meet resistance, or depressed when they encounter disapproval. They tend to solve conflicts through power equalization procedures (such as bargaining) or law enforcement. We all forget that change, because it implies the unknown, is threatening. We lose sight of the fact that any relationship which imposes blind obedience, and which is unprepared for shifts in values and unexpected actions, is especially paternalistic and induces disinvolvement.

If a father remains a father when his child grows, his child will remain a child and never become a partner. We must remember that anything imposed from above inspires submissiveness rather than responsible cooperation, and increases the risk of aggressive retaliation.

Generating social change is a major task for any industrial promoter and a major concern for our age. When French essayist Alexis Carrel spoke thirty years ago of "l'obsession social de notre temps," [12] he was expressing the predominant fear of man facing his unexpected and growing technological power. Existentialism, phenomenology, and psychoanalysis are attempts to refocus attention on human concerns as man feels threatened by a loss of identity, a loss effected by the unpredictable changes initiated by science. It is possible that university students were so restless a few years ago because they felt insecure and unable to foresee their roles in modern life. They are growing up in a turmoil of cultural changes created by technological progress and its related socioeconomical reforms. They lack stable behavior models. No wonder the young long for peace, demand participation in the decision-making processes, and reject a consumption economy by exhibiting a "don't care" attitude. Change will never take place smoothly if the related fears cannot be overcome. Science will never open the way to prosperity and peace if the social and psychological problems it arouses are not resolved by those persons actually affected. Industrialization of any kind is not going to be successful if the human side is not managed with the same forethought as is given the technical side.

The main cause for resistance to change lies in man's fear of losing his familiar status. Anyone who faces technological change fears losing his job, feels inadequate to cope with an altered setting, apprehends a change in roles, resents having to struggle with the increased complexity of new assignments, condemns any reranking of his present priorities, and is bewildered when his values are questioned or his habits upset. Loss of status and role modification are threatening because they are part of losing one's identity. Persons who do not feel as though they belong to a stable community, and no longer have a familiar frame of reference, are unable to see ahead. Instead, they become passive and helpless, feel depressed, and are angry. They resist any and all suggestions.

In *Managerial Psychology*, Leavitt points out four areas in which change can be induced (Figure 14.2).

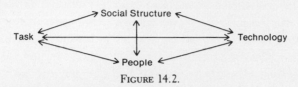

FIGURE 14.2.

If change occurs in one area, it immediately affects the others. Students of social change have learned that it is almost useless to focus on the area of technology first; instead, they have found it more fruitful to begin at the human level. Social and psychological changes can only be induced by making the *people*, exposed to industrialization and technological progress, disclose their own needs, fears, and expectations.

The people facing social change have to discover their own new behavior models. They should be made capable of analyzing their own resistance to change. Those affected by innovation should become actively involved in its design, and should consider themselves part of this design. This process of self-analysis is a necessary step toward social change, and is even more essential when industrialization precipitates migration or acculturation (i.e., a change in the culture, such as a shift of values or symbols).

The Processes Involved in Sociotherapy

THE AGENT, THE SUBJECT, AND THE OBJECT
OF SOCIOTHERAPY

To facilitate our discussion of the sociotherapeutic process, we will speak from now on of the agent, the subject, and the object of the intervention. The agent of an intervention is the therapist. He is the one who animates the treated group, and furnishes it the concepts and theories that are indispensable to an understanding of the processes of the group. It is he who stirs up the resistance of the group, and who induces insight. It is with him that the group identifies, and upon him that the group transfers its fears, aggressiveness, love, and conflicts. He becomes the screen on which the group projects its problems.

The subjects of an intervention are the members of the treated group, those whose attitudes and behavior one wants to change. The subjects of an intervention are not necessarily the clients (i.e., those who solicit the intervention). When the two are not the same, the intervention often begins with an analysis of the attitudes that differentiate the subjects and the clients.

The object of an intervention is the purpose of that intervention: the change that is foreseen. This change comes about through change in the group's consciousness of its past experience. The change occurs when the members of the group begin to anticipate, collectively, a new type of behavior that is more gratifying, and that makes them feel more secure, than the customary behavior. The change comes about during the process of analyzing the resistance that impedes the group from making decisions that permit it to anticipate the change. It is thus easy to see that the immediate object of sociotherapy—the topic discussed—is the resistance which shows up during the group process, or, in other words, during the process of collective decision making.

For greater clarity, we will now distinguish between two levels at which sociotherapy makes this analysis of resistance.

THE TWO LEVELS OF SOCIOTHERAPY

Every organization has a system of relations (a structure and a culture) among individuals who already possess their own personality structure; thus, social change occurs at two levels: [59]

1. An individual pairs with another individual, or integrates himself into a group whose cultures differ from his own. In these two cases, one helps a subject to identify with another individual who personifies a different cultural model.
2. A group integrates a stranger, or evolves a model with which it identifies collectively. In these two cases, one helps a group to conceive models that are different from the customary ones.

If the change occurs on the individual level, it affects one or all of the phases of individual conduct (p. 144): [20,41] the perception of objects, the cognitive significance accorded to those objects, the affective connotation that the objects evoke, and the behavior that follows. Intervention at the level of the individual gives rise to new habits, changes and conditionings (both classical and operant) which bear upon conduct, and modifies motivation.

If the change occurs on the group level, it affects one or all of the phases of the group process: [54] its maintenance functions and its production.

The distinction between the individual level and the group level can be used to separate intervention *in* the group (sociotherapy) from intervention *by* the group (psychotherapy). It goes without saying that the modifications that have taken place at one level always bring about modifications at the other level (p. 36).[20] All sociotherapy has psychotherapeutic effects, and vice versa. The object of sociotherapy is group process, but even so one must from time to time deviate from strict sociotherapeutic procedure in order to conserve the psychotherapeutic effects of the intervention. For this reason, a group's intervention progresses at the speed of its most resistant member.

THE BASIC EFFECTS OF SOCIOTHERAPY

The result of a successful intervention is always to increase the capacity of a group to be perceptive, inceptive, and normative. A therapeutic intervention shapes the course of a group's decision-making process toward the anticipation of change. As long as a group has not learned to cope with the fears or anxiety associated with the "changing process," it will, consciously or unconsciously, avoid bringing any matter related to the change under discussion. Fears of change have many roots. A member of the group may be afraid to lose his status or to experience (from a psychogenetic point of view), during the changing process, the revival of earlier conflicts.[17] He may even be afraid to identify with the therapist or with his fellow members. A group may apprehend to impair its cohesion or to rekindle (from a sociogenetic point of view) former tensions, rooted in the history of the group.[14] At the level of the individual or at the level of the group, anxiety may be concealed in unconscious fantasies, deeply rooted in the past experience of the individual or in the history of the group. The unfolding of these fantasies can only be achieved through identification, as will be shown later in this chapter.

As the intervention progresses, the subjects tend to become more interdependent (pp. 397–419);[13] they become more able to achieve reciprocal identification.[8] Bit by bit, the group alleviates its anxiety and allows for a more truthful analysis of its resistance, or its own group process and the determinants of this process, as shown in Figure 14.1. Clinical experience points to the similarity[82] of the stages of this unfolding process in all the groups undergoing sociotherapy. Gibb[21] and others[8,23,44] rightfully use the term "maturation" to designate this process. The end point of this maturation is group functionality and receptivity to change. Intervention always consists in creating a relation whose maturation brings about—with minimal delay and maximal capacity to cope with anxiety— a functional, interdependent group, between the subjects and the agent first, and among the subjects last.

To understand more completely the effects of an intervention in an organization, it is necessary to consider the nature of the change produced, first at the level of the individual and then at the level of the organization.

CHANGE AT THE LEVEL OF THE INDIVIDUAL

An individual changes his behavior *when his identification with an* external *source of information about an object is more gratifying,*[56] *and makes him feel more secure, than his* internal *replaying of past experience of the same object.*

When a person feels more satisfied and more secure in *anticipating* a glass of beer (which he has never tasted) than in *remembering* a glass of Coke (which is what he has drunk in the past), obviously he will abandon the Coke for the beer. If he has never had beer, he can anticipate its effects only by *identifying* with someone who is drinking beer. His change is then brought about by the satisfaction and the feeling of security that the identification creates in him. Change comes about when the *sensations* that come with a fantasy about an object, or about the agent, are more gratifying, and lead to greater feelings of security, than the sensations that come with some other, more customary fantasy.

In the course of an indirect intervention, the fantasy evoked is of the *change* (e.g., the drink of beer). In a direct intervention, the fantasy evoked is of the *agent* (the model for identification). A change of attitude is always produced by direct intervention.[69] The change never shows itself immediately in the behavior of the person, except in cases of imitation. Rather, it shows up in a change of attitude, in a decision to change behavior, in an attempt to bring about what Frank calls a new "assumptive world" (p. 144).[20]

Proceeding to the act, or stabilizing the acquired behavior, are not the same things as acquiring the attitude. In a large part they depend on circumstances that have nothing to do with the therapeutic situation. Wolfe [85,86] showed, by studying the placebo effect, and Frank (p. 67) [20] insisted upon the fact that *the subject's relation to the agent modifies his expectations; the expectations bring about physiological changes, and those changes constitute a predisposition to the occurrence in reality of what the subject has expected, i.e., the attitude.*

In examining the essential points of the numerous works which have a bearing on the taking up of an attitude [77,79] or on therapy,[32] we notice that change is facilitated by four conditions:

1. Identification without restraint.
2. Experience of the effect of the change, and of the effect of the identification.
3. Introspection or insight, and analysis of the determinants of conduct.
4. Putting into practice the acquired behavior, and making it habit.

It is the job of the agent to create these conditions in the course of his clinical interventions.

Identification. The foundation of all change (pp. 486–489) [4,59] is identification, with its alternation of projection (you are me) and introjection (I am you). Identification makes possible the *transference* through which the subject experiences in his relation with the agent the uselessness of his defenses, and the benefit to be had from a new existential position vis-à-vis the agent, first of all, and vis-à-vis the object (presented by the agent), second of all. Identification creates a "corrective experience" [1] which is the groundwork of change. Every obstacle to identification creates ambivalence, and causes the change to deviate from the model.

There are two kinds of obstacles. The first kind of defense comes from fear of being like the model. The second kind of defense comes from fear of parting from the current collective model.

If the agent is perceived as a powerful model, willing to share his power, he will be followed blindly. Many organizations, or even nations, have profoundly changed their way of life in a very short span of time under the influence of such a leader. Such leaders appear as magic, apostolic, and charismatic identification models. One may think of Christ, Mohammed, Luther, or even Caesar, Napoleon, or Hitler; they always elicit love or hate. If the agent is not able to assume that role—which is generally the case—each of his corrective interventions will induce some degree of ambivalence. This ambivalence is transferred to the object of the intervention and induces conflicting or unstable attitudes and behaviors.[40] For this reason, the different schools of therapeutic thought agree in defining the role of the agent:

1. He should refrain from value judgments [19] but remain available as a source of information.[67,68,72]
2. He should focus attention to the transference relation,[5,61] which provides an opportunity for the subjects to experience their resistance or anxiety and to abandon their defense mechanisms.
3. He should stimulate active, but freely given, participation of the subjects (p. 124),[20] and induce improvisation,[33] free association,[22] the projection of conflicts, and the introspective analysis of the determinants of conduct.[59]

These roles cannot be assumed without the induction of certain attitudes within the relationship between agent and subject. At the start of any intervention the subject will manifest his independence from the agent; during the identification process, he will become dependent. Little by little the subject will manifest his counterdependence before he is able to shape a functional interdependence between himself and the therapist. Clinical experience repeatedly demonstrates this same sequence in any therapeutic relationship.

Nevertheless, the relation that associates the agent with the subject must remain free, in order to remain conducive to feelings of security. The subject of the intervention must be able to break it off at any time without damage. Also, the end of the intervention must be marked by the autonomy of the subject. The subject must be able to do for himself and by himself what, during the intervention, he did with the agent and often for the agent.[55] The sociotherapist is a temporary consultant. His definitive integration into the organization that consults him often indicates the failure of his intervention.

Research carried on by our laboratory [57,66] has shown that the identification of the subject with the agent takes place most easily when the power of the agent, and the social distance between the subject and the agent as perceived by the subject, are neither too great nor too small. Identification comes about most easily when the model is socially close, but powerful.

Experience of the Effect of the Change. An attitude is stabilized by experiencing the effects of a new form of behavior. There is no stable change without experience. Behavioral change precedes attitudinal change. At the beginning of an intervention, the new behavior is often unconceived of, unachievable, or feared. Experience of its effects can occur only in the imagination. By fantasizing about the new behavior, the subject feels the effects of the behavior. Identification considerably reinforces this activity of fantasizing. Identification provides the model (that other me) that makes it possible for the subject to observe, or to feel inside himself, the effects of a form of behavior before he has himself been able to adopt that form of behavior in his outside life. This is the case of the subject we cited above, who was used to drinking Coke, who had never drunk beer, and who *changed* his attitudes.

The more a subject can anticipate the effects of a form of behavior, the greater are the chances that he will adopt that form of behavior. It is therefore advantageous to encourage verbalization of the feelings that accompany a new attitude: the verbalization stimulates the fantasizing. That is the principle behind "synectics" methods, such as brainstorming. It is also the reason that sociotherapy creates an atmosphere favoring the transference of feeling onto the person or the agent: the transference focuses traditional attitudes, stimulates fantasy, and leads to the subject's experiencing the uselessness of the defenses that he puts up against the identification that will start his change of attitude. By transferring his attitudes in his relation to the therapist, the subject can experience the effects of his resistance to the agent.

If experience of the effects of a change can be anticipated in a way that gratifies and leads to feelings of security, the subject goes on to the act. The act reinforces the new behavior by operant conditioning. This is the principle behind such methods as business games, role-playing, and the case method.

The works of Hilgard [29] on operant conditioning, and of Greenspoon [24,25] and Krasner [39] on the influence of approval on variations in language; the principles set forth by Thorndike as explained by Nuttin [60] and by Zeigarnik; [34] and a great many other studies [72,83,85] have shown that social approval regulates conduct. An attitude or a decision to change one's behavior is always fashioned according to *the image of a social model*. This model is an object of identification, since, as Krasner showed,[40] the effects of the conditioning vary according to the person who brought that conditioning into being.

It is important to note in passing that the above works also called attention to the often unconscious nature of conditioning.[39] Change can occur without the subject's being conscious of the changes in himself—even when the change is not a case of imitation. Introspection provides a fertile soil for conditioning only when that introspection leads to feelings of security; that is, when the introspection comes about through identification.

Introspection and Insight. Introspection, consciousness, and verbalization all indubitably contribute to making a changed attitude more precise and more stable. Nevertheless, they do not *constitute* the change (p. 220).[20] They can even retard the change if they are simply an imitation of the therapist, and are more a defense against a change of attitude than an attitude themselves. Frank expresses this idea very clearly: "Insight or ability to verbalize self-understanding may be mistaken for genuine attitude change" (p. 220).[20]

Frank has also summed up extremely well the role of insight in change: "To change a person's image of himself today, it is necessary to change his view of his future. But the future is not here yet, so his view of it can only be changed by a re-interpretation of his past" (p. 161).[20] The subject, as a result of identification with a model that is corrective and makes him feel secure, can modify the signification[46] of his past, and develop, through his relation with a model, a decision to change his behavior.

Putting into Practice. Practicing contributes to change, as it makes the effects of behavior concrete. The context becomes content, and the behavior becomes habit.[31] Through practice, external sources of information are internalized. Through conditioning, a subject introjects the spatio-temporal organization of his behavior[62] and the norms or values which sanction his behavior.[10] Typing, parallel parking of a car, toilet training, and acculturating to the customs of a country illustrate this process of introjection.

CHANGE AT THE LEVEL OF THE ORGANIZATION

Since every organization should be a functional system of interdependences (the efficient way of exchanging information), change can affect:

1. The *content* of the information exchanged. In this case we will speak of change in the message.
2. The *system* of exchange. In this case we will speak of change in the medium.

In the first case, the modification affects the object of the change. By this we mean the amount of information available to the group or the way the group perceives the object. Is prevention of coronary diseases really useful? What does delegation of power imply? How costly is water fluoridation? In the second case, the modification affects the structure and the culture of the group. Why is there a lack of communication between production and research in our enterprise? Is there any way to deal with deviance in our city other than through law enforcement? Why do Jim and John fight with each other all the time in this group?

An organization begins to change at the instant one of its members changes. The model for this change is the agent. At the level of the group, the problem is not one of change; this always remains an individual problem. The problem to be solved at the group level is the simultaneity of change among the different members of the group. The problem under consideration is thus the cohesion of the group or the coherence of the information available to the group. The role of the agent is to teach the group how to seek and coordinate information efficiently. Improving the coordination of information in a group can only be achieved through a modification of the group's structure or culture. However, each modification of the group's structure or culture brings to bear the revival of its socially rooted conflicts.[37,38] Therefore, the only condition favorable to change in a group is the analysis of its resistance to solve these conflicts. The key to the induction of social change lies in the analysis of this resistance, carried on while members of the group are experiencing, through identification with the agent, a way of relating to one another which is corrective (leading to a functional use of available information) and induces greater feelings of security (less fear to unfold the group's conflicts). In those instances, functional interdependence develops in the group; intersubjectivity [28] appears. The group's model becomes a safe object of identification.[12] The group creates the medium which enables it to tackle the message. From that instant on, the agent can withdraw from the group. Self-regulation is on its way.

The Techniques Employed in Sociotherapy

There are numerous techniques used in sociotherapy. The following list notes some of them.

1. Lectures, dogmatic teaching, tutoring, coaching.
2. Modeling, audio-visual aids.
3. Observations.
4. Demonstrations.
5. Reading assignments.
6. Programed learning.
7. Panels.

8. Seminars, discussion groups.
9. Consultation groups.
10. Criss-cross panels.
11. Case study.
12. Study of actual cases, live cases, critical incidents.
13. Balint's groups.
14. In-basket exercises.
15. Action mazes.
16. Business games.
17. Simulations.
18. Operation interlock.
19. Audit.
20. Need analysis.
21. Evaluation.
22. Brainstorming, synectic groups.
23. Leaderless groups.
24. Encounter groups.
25. Role-playing, psychodrama.
26. Junior boards.
27. Sociocentric exercises.
28. Sensitivity training.
29. Group counseling.
30. Group therapy.
31. Intergroup games.
32. Triad groups.
33. Process analysis (Bales).
34. Individual counseling.
35. Individual psychotherapy.
36. Self-linking tests.
37. Psychoanalysis.

The choice of technique depends on the needs of the group. The therapist must pass skillfully from one technique to the other, constantly adapting his role to the stage of the group in the change process described previously. It is up to the therapist to sense whether theoretical support, case analysis, a lived experience, or an introspective analysis of relations best enables the group to overcome the resistance it is showing at any given moment. In saying "best," we recall that any intervention must strive, above all else, to maintain the possibility of an identification first between the subjects and the agent, and then among the subjects themselves. For outside such an identification, the group will never reach the functional interdependence that is the goal of all sociotherapy. Moreover, the therapist must guard against the ever-present risk of wild introspection.

To respect this fundamental principle and to adapt his role to the needs of the group at a particular moment, the sociotherapist needs to understand the change process. In addition, he must understand the applicability of the various techniques available. To do so, one must first understand their *nature,* and second, their *impact.* Keeping this in mind, we now explain the techniques.

THE NATURE OF THE TECHNIQUES

Intervention in a group can be *direct* or *indirect.* It is indirect when it modifies the objects or the milieu to which the group must adapt. One is referred to Figure 14.2. In an indirect intervention, sociotherapy consists exclusively in bringing about verbal expression of the emotions felt by the members of the group, in view of the change.

However, sociotherapy usually proceeds by *direct* intervention. It changes the system of relations of a team. It weakens the resistance of the group, adds to the potential for interdependence of the members of the group, and makes the group capable of considering change. A direct intervention can be either message-centered or medium-centered. We will call it *message-centered* when it takes up a question that does not directly concern the group treated. Presentation of an abstract theory, bringing up concepts about operations, and the playing of a business game would fall into this category. A *medium-centered* intervention puts up for discussion the group itself. We will say that a medium-centered intervention is *deferred* when it discusses the resistance of the group in general, that is, after the fact. We will say that it is *instantaneous* when it illustrates this resistance at the very moment that the resistance acts. Instantaneous intervention gives no quarter. It forces the group and its members to ask themselves about the real reasons for their acts.

To discuss the organization chart of a business is to proceed by the indirect route. To discuss with the group the advantages and disadvantages of an organization chart, as these can be seen in a particular case, is to carry on an intervention that is direct, but message-centered. To analyze with some of the members of the business the system of relations among them is to carry on a medium-centered deferred intervention. To do so at the very moment that these relations are in evidence, to proceed to an analysis of the causes (individual and sociocultural determinants) and effects (on interpersonal perceptions, on group consensus, on consensus validation, and on the functionality of the group) of this system of relations, is to perform a medium-centered instantaneous intervention.

The changes brought about by an intervention have a greater chance of being stable when the intervention is instantaneous. But the anxiety aroused by an instantaneous intervention runs the risk of provoking much sharper resistance in the group. The anxiety is compensated for by a temporary accentuation of the identification (or aggression) directed at the agent of the intervention, or at one subject by another.

The nature of a technique can be more fully understood when one analyzes in sequence the *content* of the technique, the *topics* it treats, the degree of *verbal expression* it employs, the mode of *reflection* to which it gives rise. All of these are interrelated, and each one has implications for all of the others.

The content. Every technique used in intervention uses at least one of the following: (1) concepts: symbols or models; (2) theories: knowledge, values, beliefs, hypotheses; (3) logic: strategy, procedures, methods; and (4) actions. The resistance of a group increases as one moves from concepts to actions. The choice of an appropriate content is therefore one of the aspects of sociotherapeutic procedure.

The topics treated. The topics treated by a group are often *abstract*. Development of an abstract theory *can* make it easier to solve a problem, but often does not. Groups frequently rationalize, which serves as a form of resistance, allowing the group to avoid the interpersonal tensions that could give rise to a pragmatic anticipation of change. Rationalization also allows the group not to change its system of relations. One often sees groups confronted with change get tangled up in long theoretical discussions that contribute next to nothing to the solution of their problems, and that delay action or the analysis of group resistance.

The topics treated can be *fictional* or imaginary, such as those used in case study. This procedure rarely gives rise to resistance.

On the other hand, the topics treated can be *true*, that is, taken from the actual past experience of the organization to which the subjects of the intervention belong. This is the situation with live cases and certain kinds of role-playing. It is even possible to *live* the topics in an instantaneous manner; such techniques include T-groups, sociocentric exercises, and self-linking tests.

Theoretical and abstract information is indispensable; it furnishes a useful logistical support to collective thought. But it also can be a form of resistance to change. From the moment it prevents the group from progressing toward techniques that are more immediate, and give rise to more anxiety, it constitutes resistence. If the group is not capable of handling the anxiety that is inherent in an analysis of its own resistance and motivations, we may expect that it will not yet confront change.

The degree of verbal expression. Certain techniques encourage *verbal expression* of the attitudes and sentiments that give rise to the behavior of the group. This is the goal of synectic procedures, discussion groups, and role-playing. In principle, the expression of feeling (conscious or unconscious) leads to an understanding of group resistance. Nevertheless, it can also reinforce resistance. This is particularly the case when projection or dramatization of a feeling (as in role-playing) allows the group to avoid consideration of this feeling in a real situation. It is also the case when a group avoids considering its real problems by regressing toward a state of group euphoria. The collective love of the group can become so exalted that it serves as an excuse to deny the hate and aggressiveness also present in the group. Such denials are frequent. The group avoids change by giving itself the illusion that all problems are resolved, or adopts a procedure for change that ignores the difficulties to which the change gives rise.

The mode of reflection. Some techniques encourage logical *reflection.* Reflection is just as indispensable as verbalization. However, like verbalization, it also can set in motion new forms of resistance to change. Some of these are:

1. Rationalization.
2. The splitting of the group into cliques, which avoid crucial problems with each other for the sake of fighting. These cliques displace the aggressiveness that comes from change, directing it at an "evil object", the other clique.
3. The banding together of certain members of the group who feel the same sexual, political, or philosophical affinities, and who flee to a narcissistic, collective isolation.

All these effects of group reflection bring what Bion calls a flight from group reality.[7]

The degree of introspection. Several techniques encourage introspection. We have already spoken of them.

These diverse categories define the *nature* of the techniques employed in sociotherapy. From them the therapist will make a program that is fitted to the cognitive and effective needs of the group, and to its ability to face the anxiety inherent in change. We now examine the impact of these techniques.

THE IMPACT OF THE TECHNIQUES

The techniques of intervention in organizations can be best understood and used when the agent of the intervention tries to analyze for each specific case: the *role* that he plays in the enterprise in which he intervenes; the *phase* in which his intervention is located; the *type of relation* established in the intervention; the *topic of discussion* of the intervention; the *style of learning* involved in the intervention; the *focus* of the intervention; and the *processes* toward which the agent of the intervention directs the attention of the subjects. This analysis will make it possible for the agent not only to decide what technique he ought to use, but also what therapeutic attitude he ought to assume.

The role of the therapist. The essential role of the therapist is to be a model for identification that is gratifying and leads to feelings of security. This model makes it possible for the members of a group to look for the precise determinants that retard the exchange of information among themselves that is necessary to anticipate the change. It is by learning from the therapist how to look at their own group processes that the subjects overcome their resistance to change. In other words, through identification with a new social model, their group becomes more functional and their relations more interdependent. Through this experience the therapeutic relationship modifies not only the expectations of the subjects with regard to the therapist, but also with regard to the object. Through his intervention, the therapist places an object into the group's experience. The subjects project ôn that object not only their own experience regarding that object, but their feelings about each other and their feelings toward the therapist. If they have already learned how to analyze these projections, they will, as a group, be receptive to changing their attitudes toward the therapist and toward their own group; henceforth, they will start to anticipate the change process collectively. The decision to change will already be in progress.

If an advisor teaches a group how to apply a cholesterol-free diet, or how to adopt a new managerial attitude (e.g., delegation of power), the group will start to consider these matters only after its members have learned how to exchange information regarding their resistance to diet or delegation of power.

The phases of the intervention. Functional organizations, when confronted with the need for change, always assimilate the change in three phases: (1) getting information; (2) organizing the information; and (3) internalizing the information. In the first phase the therapist integrates himself in the group. He will expose the group to an object; in other words, he will suggest a change. Henceforth he will not be concerned about the object as such, but will help the group to seek information and overcome its resistance to change. Therefore he will provide the group with concepts or reference theories, but above all he will help the group to analyze its own group process. He will teach the members of the group to express their tensions, fears, and anger, to elucidate their interpersonal perceptions, and to analyze their group decision-making process and its determinants. Through this exercise he will prepare the group to engage in the second phase.

During the second phase the group learns to proceed by itself; it will build a new organizational structure and shape a new cultural model. The group will venture to test its hypotheses regarding the object and it will take the risk of considering a change.

In the last phase the group internalizes the new model. It will now be motivated for the change; it will start considering the change process and evaluating its effects. At this point, the therapist's intervention has come to an end.[52]

One cannot forget that this entire evolution takes place in a sample. During the sociotherapy this sample is away from its customary sociocultural surroundings. It is taken from the organization to which it belongs to make the assimilation of change easier for it. The sociotherapeutic situation is necessarily of a temporary and artificial nature—as are all situations in which something is taught. Transfer of the behavior and the attitudes acquired to the real environment presents numerous difficulties for which the subjects must be prepared *during* the intervention. The Bethel school has often raised this problem by speaking of the "back home application." [8] Subjects who participate in sociotherapy, and who change their attitudes and their behavior, must realize that the organization may be accompanied by signs of hostility or false pleasantries. Those who did not participate in the sociotherapy are jealous, feel threatened, and closed-mindedly defend themselves against any change that one might suggest to them. If the subjects of the sociotherapy are not able to do at home, with the members of their parent organization, what the therapist did with them, the intervention remains without effect. All sociotherapy should end with an initiation into sociotherapeutic techniques. Without that instruction, application of sociotherapy back home in the parent organization may be more damaging than beneficial.

The type of relation established in the intervention. During the intervention, the therapist is repeatedly bringing about three types of relations. One distinguishes:

1. The *demonstrative* relation, which is an *agent-object* relation.
2. The *transference* relation, which is an *agent-subject* relation.
3. The *experimental* relation, which is a *subject-object* relation.

In the first type of relation the therapist explains a theory, presents a model, illustrates a case, poses a problem, provokes expression, or brings about consciousness of certain needs. In the second type of relation he brings out, then analyzes, the resistance and the defenses that the thought of change arouses. The subjects of the intervention transfer all their apprehensions, all their aggressiveness, and all their needs for dependence to their relation with the therapist and their teammates. Once these difficulties have been overcome, the therapist brings into being the third type of relation. In this relation the subjects, freed from their apprehensions and resistance, can find out by themselves and for themselves the usefulness of change.

Interventions run into a lot of difficulties when the therapist is unaware of the type of relation he is establishing with the subjects of his intervention. The therapist must allow for the fact that resistance is always more pronounced when the transference relation is approached, and when he takes as its topic of discussion the transference relation with the therapist. Much attempted sociotherapy is wild, unproductive, and full of jolts, because the therapist is confused about the type of relation present in his intervention.

The topic of discussion of the intervention. The therapist can, at his own discretion, present physical objects or psychic realities; advance terms, concepts, theories, or values; or talk about behavior, attitudes, sentiments, or motivation. In every case, the resistance that he arouses grows when he moves from concrete reality to the subjective experience of that reality. This phenomenon is quite clear when he moves in the course of an intervention from a case study, to the

266

analysis of a live case, to the elucidation of the interpersonal relations actively at play in the situation at hand. Here, too, the therapist must be careful to avoid confusion.

The style of learning involved in the intervention.   We distinguish four styles of learning (p. 491): [4] (1) imitation; (2) experimentation; (3) reflection; and (4) introspection. While the first of these may be conscious or unconscious, the last is necessarily conscious. Here, as elsewhere, resistance increases when one uses the kinds of intervention that are more conscious.

The focus of the intervention.   Much the same is true for the focus of the intervention.[45] The group may focus on: (1) perceptions; (2) conceptions; (3) motivations; or (4) behavior. Each of these can be either more or less conscious. The progressive involvement of the subject as the focus shifts toward behavior is opposed by ever-stiffer resistance.

The processes put up for consideration.   As we have pointed out, the topic of an intervention can be either message-centered or medium-centered. In the second case the group learns to analyze either: (1) its own (formal or informal) group process; (2) its interpersonal perceptions; or (3) the motivations of its members.

The first approach leads to socioanalysis, the last to psychoanalysis. Clinical experience indicates that it is often impairing for a group to shift brusquely from a message-centered topic to a medium-oriented one, or from a socioanalytic introspection to a psychoanalytic one. The therapist should never overrule the expectations of a group. He should help the group to cope with the anxiety induced by the prospect of a change or by the insight gained into the motives for resistance to change. He should not impose change or insight. Insight never modifies a behavior; rather, it is often damaging and increases anxiety and resistance. The capacity to deal with the anxiety induced by the insight shapes new behavioral patterns. This capacity develops when the group learns to disclose the motives of its resistance without threatening the group's cohesion or the self-images of its members. The stability of a behavioral modification increases in proportion to the resistance that the therapist succeeds in overcoming without damage.

It is in light of the considerations just discussed that the therapist will choose among the many techniques which presently constitute the arsenal of sociotherapy. In deciding upon dogmatic teaching, demonstrations, case study, live cases, role-playing, or socioanalysis, the therapist *should not concern himself with technique alone,* but with the way in which that technique can facilitate a corrective identification.

The same is true for his choice of therapeutic attitude. It is not directivism or nondirectivism, deferred analysis or instantaneous analysis, message-centered or medium-centered, fictional or true, that is important. What *is* important is the *result* of the therapeutic attitude on the identification of the group with the therapist.

By remaining conscious of the role that he assumes in an organization, the sociotherapist can be a corrective model. To do any more is to do too much. It is to use the client organization for purposes that are narcissistic, or related to the therapist's own defense structure. To do any less is to cause harm. It is to fail to achieve with the members of the client organization the relations that make it possible for them to reach their goals by themselves and for themselves. Gaston Berger once said: "L'objectivité de monde apparait comme un intersubjectivité transcendenté"—*The objectivity of the world manifests itself as a transcendent intersubjectivity*. It is the role of the therapist to achieve that transcendent intersubjectivity by applying, with intelligence and foresight, the techniques which he has at his disposal.

REFERENCES

1. Alexander, F., and French, T. M. *Psychoanalytic Therapy: Principles and Apllications*. New York: Ronald Press, 1946.

2. Argyris, C. *Interpersonal Competence and Organizational Effectiveness*. Homewood, Ill.: Dorsey Press, 1962.

3. Barnett, H. G. *Innovation. The Basis of Cultural Change*. New York: McGraw-Hill, 1953.

4. Bennis, W. G.; Benne, K. D., and Chin, R. *The Planning of Change*. New York: Holt, Rinehart, 1961.

5. Bennis, W. G., and Slater, P. E. *The Temporary Society*. New York: Harper & Row, 1968.

6. Berman, L. "Countertransferences and Attitudes of the Analyst in the Therapeutic Process." *Psychiatry* 12 (1949):159–166.

7. Bion, W. R. *Experiences in Groups*. New York: Basic Books, 1959.

8. Bradford, L. P.; Gibb, J. R., and Benne, K. D., eds. *T-group Theory and Laboratory Method: Innovation in Re-education*. New York: Wiley, 1964.

9. Bronfenbrenner, U. "The Study of Identification Through Interpersonal Behavior." In *Person Perception and Interpersonal Behavior*, edited by R. Tagiuri and L. Petrullo. Stanford, Calif.: Stanford University Press, 1962.

10. Cantril, H. *The Why of Man's Experience*. New York: Macmillan, 1950.

11. Carrel, A. *Man the Unknown*. New York: Harper, 1935.

12. De Cock, G. *De invloed van de groepschohesie de groeps norm, en de informatie op met aantal arbeids ongevallen*. Leuven: P.M.S.S.C., 1964.

13. Dill, W. R.; Hilton, T. L.; and Reitman, W. R. *The New Managers—Patterns of Behavior and Development*. Englewood Cliffs, N.J.: Prentice-Hall. 1962.

14. Ey, H. *Manuel de Psychiatrie*. Paris: Masson, 1960.

15. Faucheux, C. "Théorie et Technique du Groupe de Diagnostic." *Bulletin de Psychologie* 12(1959):6–9.

16. Fenichel, O. "Problems of Psychoanalytic Technique." *Psychoanalytic Quarterly*, 14(1941):222.

14 / From Theory to Practice: The Meaning of Sociotherapy

17. ———. *La Théorie Psychanalytique des Névroses*. Paris: P.U.F. 1953.

18. Ferenczi, S. "Introjection and Transference." In *Contributions to Psychoanalysis*, edited by Richard C. Badger, p. 318. Boston: 1916.

19. Finesinger, J. E., and Kellam, S. G. "Permissiveness—Its Definition, Usefulness and Application in Psychotherapy." *American Journal of Psychiatry* 115(1959):992–996.

20. Frank, J. D. *Persuasion and Healing*. Baltimore: Johns Hopkins Press, 1961.

21. Gibb, J. "Group Growth Criteria." Unpublished memo. Washington D.C.: National Training Laboratories, 1956.

22. Glover, E. "The Therapeutic Effect of Inexact Interpretation: A Contribution to the Theory of Suggestion." *International Journal of Psychoanalysis* 12(1931):397–411.

23. Golembiewski, R. L., and Blumberg, A. *Sensitivity Training and the Laboratory Approach*. Itasca: Peabock, 1970.

24. Greenspoon, J. "The Effect of Two Non-verbal Stimuli on the Frequency of Members of Two Verbal Response Classes." *American Psychologist* 9(1954):384.

25. ———. "The Reinforcing Effect of Two Spoken Sounds on the Frequency of Two Responses." *American Psychologist* 68(1955):409–416.

26. Guest, R. H. *Organizational Change. The Effect of Successful Leadership*. Homewood, Ill.: Dorsey Press, 1962.

27. Hebb, D. O. "Drives and the Conceptual Nervous System." *Psychological Review* 62(1955):243–254.

28. Hesnard, P. *La psychanalyse du lien interhumain*. Paris: P.U.F., 1954.

29. Hilgard, E. R. *Theories of Learning*. New York: Appleton-Century-Crofts, 1948.

30. ———. "Methods and Procedures in the Study of Learning." In *Handbook of Experimental Psychology*, edited by S. S. Stevens. New York: Wiley, 1951.

31. Holmberg, A. R. "The Research and Development Approach to Change: Participant Intervention in the Field. In *Human Organization Research*, edited by R. N. Adams and J. J. Preis, pp. 76–89. Homewood, Ill.: Dorsey Press, 1960.

32. Hornstein, H. A.; Bunker, B. B.; Burke, W. W.; Gindes, M.; and Lewicki, R. J. *Social Intervention: A Behavioral Science Approach*. New York: Free Press, 1971.

33. Hovland, C. I.; Janis, I. L.; and Kelley, H. H. *Communication and Persuasion: Psychological Studies of Opinion Change*. New Haven: Yale University Press, 1953.

34. Jacobs, A., and Spradlin, W. W. *The Group as Agent of Change*. New York Behavioral Publications, 1974.

35. Janis, I.L., and King, B. "The Influence of Role-playing on Opinion Change." *Journal of Abnormal Social Psychology* 49(1954):211–218.

36. Jaques, E. *The Changing Culture of a Factory*. London: Tavistock, 1951.

37. Kelman, H. C. "Attitude Change as a Function of Response Restriction." *Human Relations* 6(1953):185–214.

38. King, B., and Janis, I. "Comparison of the Effectiveness of Improvised versus Nonimprovised Role Playing in Producing Opinion Changes." *Human Relations* 9(1956):177–186.

39. Krasner, L. "Studies of the Conditioning." *Psychological Bulletin* 55 (1958):148–170.

40. ———; Weiss, R. L.; Ullmann, L. P. "Responsivity to Verbal Conditioning as a Function of Two Different Measures of Awareness." *American Psychologist*. 14(1959):388.

41. Krech, D., and Crutchfield, R. S. *Elements of Psychology*. New York: Knopf, 1962.

42. Lawrence, P. R. *The Changing of Organizational Behavior Patterns*. Boston: Harvard University Press, 1958.

43. Leavitt, H. J. "Applied Organizational Change in Industry. Structural, Technical, and Human Approaches." Paper presented at O.N.R. Conference on Organizations, 1962, Carnegie Institute of Technology, Pittsburgh, Penna., and *Managerial Psychology. Introduction to Individuals, Pairs, and Groups in Organizations*. Chicago: University of Chicago Press, 1972, p. 161.

44. Leighton, A. H.; Clausen, J. A.; and Wilson, R. N. *Explorations in Social Psychiatry*. New York: Basic Books, 1957.

45. Lewin, K., and Grabbe, P. "Conduct, Knowledge and Acceptance of New Values." *Journal of Social Issues* 3(1945):56–64.

46. Lidz, T. "Some Unsolved Problems of Psychoanalytic Psychotherapy." In *Progress in Psychotherapy*, edited by Fromm-Reichmann, Frieda, R., and Moreno, J. L., pp. 102–107. New York: Grune & Stratton, 1956.

47. Likert, R. *New Patterns of Management*. New York: McGraw-Hill, 1961.

48. Lippit, R.; Watson, J.; and Westley, B. *The Dynamics of Planned Change*. New York: Harcourt, Brace, 1958.

49. Maisonneuve, J. "Discussion de groupe et formation de cadres," *Revue de Sociologie du Travail* 1(1960):23–28.

50. McGregor, D. *The Human Side of Enterprise*. New York: McGraw-Hill, 1960.

51. McNulty, J. E. "Organizational Change in Growing Enterprise." *Administrative Science Quarterly* 7 (1962–1963):1–11.

52. Mertens, C. *La formation à la direction des enterprises*. Paris-Louvain: Béatrice-Nauwelaerts, 1961.

53. ————. *L'influence de l'évolution culturelle sur l'équilibre psychique*. Bruxelles: Académie Royale des Sciences d'Outre-mer, 1961.

54. ————. *Psychologie et psychopathologie industrielles*. Louvain: Librairie Universitaire. 1964, p. 64.

55. ————. "La sociothérapie comme science clinique." *Revue Médicale Louvain* 10(1965):323–332; 11(1965):345–356.

56. ————. "L'intervention sur les organisations." *Revue de Psychologie et des Sciences de l'Education* 11(1966):21–44.

57. ————. "Inducing Social Change in a New Industrial Society." *Modern Government* October 1969, pp. 57–61.

58. ————. "Identification, modèles culturels et changement." *L'Evolution Psychiatrique* 1(1971):129–177.

59. Nacht, S., et al. *La psychanalyse d'aujourd'hui*. Paris: P.U.F., 1961.

60. Nuttin, J. *Tâche, réussite et échec*. Louvain: Nauwelaerts, 1955.

61. Oleron, R. "Le transfert." *Année Psychologique*. 1954.

62. Ombredane, A., and Faverge, J. M. *L'analyse du travail*. Paris: P.U.F., 1954.

63. Pages, M. "Eléments d'une sociothérapie de l'entreprise." *Hommes et Techniques* 169 (1959):158–170.

64. Pages, M. "The Sociotherapy of the Enterprise," pp. 168–185. In *The Planning of Change*, edited by W. G. Bennis, K. D. Benne, and R. Chin. New York: Holt, Rinehart and Winston, 1961.

65. Rice, A. K. *Productivity and Social Organization. The Ahmadabad Experiment*. London: Tavistock, 1958.

66. Rime, B., and Leyens, J. "Identification de l'élève au professeur: approche expérimentale." *Revue Psychologie Appliquée* 18(1968):231–240.

67. Rogers, C. R. *Counseling and Psychotherapy*. Boston: Houghton-Mifflin, 1942.

68. ————. *Client-centered Therapy: Its Current Practice Implications and Theory*. Boston: Houghton Mifflin, 1951.

69. ————. "A Research Program in Client-centered Therapy." In *Psychiatric Treatment*, edited by the Association for Research in Nervous and Mental Disease, pp. 106–113. Baltimore: Williams & Wilkins, 1953.

70. ————, and Dymond, R., eds. *Psychotherapy and Personality Change: Coordinated Research Studies in the Client-Centered Approach*. Chicago: University of Chicago Press, 1954.

71. Rosenbaum, M., and Berger, M., eds. *Group Psychotherapy and Group Function*. New York: Basic Books, 1963.

72. Salzinger, K. "An Experimental Approach to the Interview. XV. *Int. Cong. Psychol.*

73. Sargant, W. *Battle for the Mind: A Physiology of Conversion and Brainwashing*. Garden City, N.Y.: Doubleday, 1957.

74. Sayles, L. R. "The Change Process in Organizations. An Applied Anthropology Analysis." *Human Organization* 21(1962):62–67.

75. Sivadon, P. In *Vocabulaire de Psychologie*, edited by M. Pieron. Paris: P.U.F., 1963.

76. Sofer, C. *The Organization from Within*. Chicago: Quadrangle, 1961.

77. Stevens, S. S. *Handbook of Experimental Psychology*. New York: Wiley, 1951.

78. Toffler, A. *Future Shock*. New York: Random House, 1970.

79. Triandis, H. C. "Attitude Change through Training in Industry." *Human Organization* 17(1958): 27–30.

80. Van Bockstaele, J., and Van Bockstaele, M. "Note préliminaire sur la socioanalyse." *Bull. Psychol.* 12(1959):277–285.

81. Van Gehuchten, P. *Neurologie*. Paris: Masson, 1948.

82. Vansina, L. *T-groepen en leidersidentiteit. Een studie van waardewÿzigingen en onderliggende psychische processon*. Leuven: P.M.S.S.C., 1964.

83. Verplanck, W. S. "The Control of the Content of Conversation: Reinforcement of Statement of Opinion." *Journal of Abnormal Social Psychology* 51(1955):668–676.

84. Wickes, T. G. "Examiner's Influence on a Testing Situation." *Journal of Consulting Psychology* 20(1956):23–26.

85. Wolf, S. "Effects of Suggestion and Conditioning on the Action of Chemical Agents in Human Subjects—The Pharmacology of Placebo." *Journal of Clinical Investigation* 29(1950):100–109.

86. ———, and Pinsky, R. H. "Effects of Placebo Administration and Occurrence of Toxic Reactions." *Journal of the American Medical Association* 155(1954):339–341

87. Yarrow, H. R.; Campbell, J. D.; and Yarrow, L. J. "Interpersonal Change: Process and Theory." *Journal of Social Issues* 14(1958):60–63.

88. Zeigarnik, B. "Uber das Behalten von erledigten und unerledigten Handlungen." *Psychogische Forsong* 9(1927):1–85.

Editorial Note

This chapter presents drug dependence as a way of focusing on the diversity of elements that contribute to the question of human competence. In so doing, Farnsworth gives us some assessment of the variety of factors associated with drug dependence and of drug-related behavior in general. Thus, the reader is given a review of the magnitude of the drug problem, the use of drugs in different youth groups, and the variety of drugs used. (For example, Farnsworth shows our most prevalent drug to be alcohol.) But he goes far beyond the question of drugs by raising the issues of competence, coping, and identity as they occur in all of life's transition states. Competence is not just a consideration for adolescence, but for the entire life cycle sequence. In Farnsworth's scheme, if certain essential striving needs are not met in the latency period (Erikson's capacity for industry), a person may encounter difficulties later, such as, in this case, the risk of the drug-dependence syndrome.

Fundamental issues for future research are shown to relate to the effective epidemiologic assessment of drug behavior and the related socioeconomic factors associated with drug use. Farnsworth's use of drug dependence could be a prototype for the analysis of social pressures that increase the risk of dependence. These questions are posed: How did the drug-dependence behavior develop? Can the "incompetencies" that lead to drug dependence be prevented? What is the person's life history of stress and coping? What were the competence failures? How is the drug problem best treated in terms of the social system in which the person functions? How can the effect of treatment on the individual and the effects of drug behavior on society be evaluated?

B. H. K.

CHAPTER 15

Substitute for Competence: Drug Dependence and Its Amelioration

DANA L. FARNSWORTH

DRUG-INFLUENCED behavior and drug dependence are present to some degree in all cultures and societies; the form they take and the attitude toward them depend on the unique conditions of each country. In largely rural countries long tradition may have woven the use of indigenous herbs and simple concoctions into the social fiber, while industrialized urban societies evolve complex distribution systems of myriad drugs and equally complex social rituals for their acquisition and use. One culture may be able to assimilate and contain drug use so that the net result is, for the majority, a relaxation from everyday stress that makes its members more able to cope with ordinary reality. More often, use of drugs becomes misuse, with strong patterns of disintegration among those who use drugs with any regularity. Complicated importing and exporting patterns appear when one country or culture possesses the drug supply and another has the money to pay well for it.

Some countries have the reputation of being more prone to drug use than others, but in the long run probably no country is immune. Similarly, some classes of individuals are often thought to be more likely than others to abuse drugs. At certain times and in certain cultures, the young are the high-risk group; in other circumstances older people and even the aged are at greatest hazard. Moreover, each drug has its special adherents, determined by complicated interaction among its pharmacologic effects, the users' expectations, and the available supply. Drugs are a problem in all ages and societies, but the reasons vary markedly from person to person, from one community to another, and in different countries, depending on variations in customs, supply, and demand.

Addiction and Dependence

For many years the term "addiction" was applied to the condition in which a drug-using person becomes strongly desirous of continuing its use, tends to increase the dose, and develops a physical and psychological dependence upon it, with the ensuing use pattern becoming detrimental to both the individual and society. This term has outlived its usefulness for two reasons: It implies that physical and psychological dependence always accompany each other, and it has become encumbered with prejudicial overtones which interfere with optimum care of the person affected. The National Commission on Marihuana and Drug Abuse, following the lead of other professional groups, has recommended that the term "drug dependence" be used instead. This applies to all situations in which a person develops a psychological and physical dependence arising from continued use of a substance, with a strong compulsion to take it on a continuing basis in order to experience its psychic effects or to avoid the discomfort caused by its absence (pp. 126–127). [2] This definition includes both use of substances which are generally considered harmful and are distributed only through illegal channels as well as those which have a more acceptable reputation despite their danger (such as alcohol, tobacco, and improperly supervised prescription drugs).

The commission has stated it thus:

> Drug dependence should be viewed as a continuum, starting from a low degree of dependence as measured by minimal individual preoccupation with drug-using behavior and minimal disruptive effects upon interruption of the behavior, and escalating to compulsive dependence as measured by total preoccupation with drug-using behavior and serious behavioral disruption and physical discomfort attending deprivation of the drug. Drug dependence exists in innumerable patterns and in all degrees of intensity depending on the nature of the drug, the route of administration, the dose and frequency of adminis-

tration, other pharmacological variables, the personality of the user and the nature of the environment (pp. 138–139).[2]

The alternative term, drug abuse, has become synonymous with social disapproval and has lost whatever value it once had. In the commission's view, it should be deleted from official pronouncements and public policy dialogue (p. 13).[2]

Drug Use in America

Social historians are becoming more and more impressed by how intertwined the drug problem has become, in the last several decades, with a wide variety of other issues, even while it was itself changing rapidly. Realizing the dangers of opium-based products following their widespread use after the Civil War, the first major concern was centered on prevention of narcotic addiction and, due to some misunderstanding of its nature, the use of marijuana among underprivileged minority groups. Then the focus shifted to lowering the amount of alcohol used, most spectacularly by attempting to adopt a national policy of prohibition. This failed eventually because people simply refused to live without the freedom to use alcohol if they so chose. Most people of the prosperous middle and upper classes saw the drug problem as just another handicap involved in belonging to deprived social, economic, racial, or ethnic groups. Though they may have expressed concern about dependence on narcotics, marijuana, alcohol, and other sedatives and stimulants, this dependence was mainly considered to be a problem of the individual and not a vast social dilemma. Not until drug use spread from the deprived groups to the children of the middle and upper classes did people reconsider who and what was involved in the problem of drug dependence.

Then drugs began to assume a vastly increased role in the lives of everyone, as the discovery and utilization of sedatives, stimulants, antibiotics, synthetic vitamins, insulin, anticancer agents, and steroids became the subject of headlines in the papers and advertisements in all media. Many people began to think that the possibilities for human betterment through skillful use of drugs were practically unlimited. What they did not appreciate sufficiently was the fact that any chemical agent, while spectacularly satisfactory when used within appropriate limits, may be incredibly dangerous when the necessary safeguards are not observed.

To appreciate the rapid changes that have come about in most people's minds regarding the use of drugs for mind-altering purposes, it is helpful to recall that chloral hydrate was the first hypnotic drug to be introduced into medicine (1832), followed by the bromides in 1857. Barbital came into use in 1903, soon followed by phenobarbital (1912). It was not until the mid-1950s that drugs began to be widely used for the treatment of psychiatric disorders, including monoamine oxidase inhibitors such as imipramine for depression, phenothiazines, especially chlorpromazine, for psychoses, meprobamate for anxiety, and lithium salts for hypomania (p. 195).[7]

Introduction of these and many similar drugs, coming coincidentally as they did with a marked increase in interest in community mental health programs, stimulated enormous efforts to reduce the population of state mental hospitals. The subsequent reduction of hospitalized patients by more than 50 percent tended to increase the belief that drugs could be used for beneficent purposes as well as agents of control.

Those who were interested in controlling the behavior of masses of people, and those who were unalterably opposed to such manipulation, speculated with interest or trepidation on the role of drugs in such situations.

Meanwhile, Hoffmann had discovered lysergic acid (LSD), and experimenters enthusiastically (and properly) encouraged research on its role in understanding the psychoses (p. 195).[7] Other psychotropic agents, first as they occurred naturally and then in synthetic form, became the subject of laboratory study and greatly increased research. People began to speculate on how drugs might be utilized to explore areas of consciousness not usually available to an individual, with the goal of understanding better both one's self and the whole universe. In numerous instances the enthusiasm of the investigators outran their inherent caution, and the age of infatuation with such drugs was upon us.

At the same time that these drugs were becoming available, young people from the middle and upper classes in high school and college began to show increasing interest in drug experimentation. This was accompanied by wide social changes in which affluence, increased vehicles for advertising and distribution, and disillusionment with the achievements of the adult world combined to produce a youth culture which soon adopted drug experimentation as one of its criteria for membership.

The Drugs of Abuse

Although no evidence exists that use of marijuana leads to use of heroin or any other specific drug, surveys of drugs used among young people show that more multidrug users begin with marijuana than with any other drug. To become multihabituated to drugs, one must begin somewhere; the logical drug to begin with is the one most readily available, which in most instances is marijuana.

The patterns and extent of nonprescription drug use are infinitely varied, but some general principles emerge from examination of a large number of surveys. The National Commission on Marihuana and Drug Abuse made a composite compilation of 200 student surveys involving more than 900,000 individuals, and Table 15.1 gives an estimate of the drugs used and their prevalence.

TABLE 15.1
*Mean Percentage of Students Who Have Ever
Used Drugs as of 1972*

	JR. HIGH	SR. HIGH	COLLEGE
Alcohol	56%	74%	83%
Marijuana	16	40	50
Stimulants	9	19	24
Depressants	8	16	14
Hallucinogens	6	14	14
Opiates	4.75	5.2	6
Inhalants	11	9	2

Because of the complexity of such data, the pertinent sections in the report should be consulted for details (pp. 82–84).[2] The patterns of drug use were differentiated by the commission into five usage patterns arranged in order of increasing risk of danger.

1. Experimental—The short-term, nonpatterned trial of one or more drugs, either concurrently or consecutively, but no more than ten times per drug, used either singly or in combination.
2. Social or recreational—Drug use which occurs in social settings among friends and acquaintances who desire to share an experience which they regard as both acceptable and pleasurable.
3. Circumstantial—Drug use motivated by the perceived need or desire to achieve a known and anticipated effect deemed desirable to cope with a specific, sometimes recurrent, situation or condition of a personal or vocational nature.
4. Intensified—A long-term patterned use of drugs at least once daily, motivated by the individual's perceived need to achieve relief from a persistent problem or a stressful situation.
5. Compulsive—Drug use of such frequency and intensity over long periods which has produced such dependence that the individual cannot at will discontinue its use without physiological or psychological distress, practically always accompanied by gross interference with individual and social functioning.

From a public health point of view the latter two patterns are by far of the greatest concern (p. 94).[2]

We have no good evidence that extensive use of mind-altering drugs for self-realization, increased creativity, or attainment of mystical states of consciousness has been beneficial in the long run for anyone. The great hopes along these lines that were expressed a decade or two ago have not materialized. Instead, many of those who did engage in such substantial drug use are now no longer quoted seriously; their careers have been characterized by severely constricted, rather than expanded, horizons.[4]

Whenever a person uses a drug and the experience is pleasurable, he has engraved on his mind the memory that this is an effective way of reversing a bad mood or causing a good feeling. So in the future, whenever he is exposed to pain, conflict, or fatigue (as we all are), he will be more vulnerable than others because he remembers the pleasant, easily acquired solution that drug-taking afforded. The more easily available such drugs are, the more likely they are to be used without a truly objective assessment of whether their long-term complications may not be more troublesome than the original stress. We have never before had such an array of powerful psychoactive drugs, with many more being developed, so we have no specific knowledge of what would happen if they were available without restriction to all who wanted them. But all our past experience, both in this country and in others, suggests that the increased drug dependence would be striking, and the tragedy for society would be immense.

Older people usually take drugs to relieve pain, reduce misery, or bolster courage. Thus the use of strong analgesics to relieve pain, tranquilizers to blunt the edges of reality, sedatives to encourage sleep, and stimulants to give alertness and energy has become for many people a way of life. They have become dependent upon drugs—not always in the sense that they will suffer physical misery if they stop using drugs, but in the sense that they cannot cope with their lives unless they have chemical assistance. Alcohol, being a multipurpose drug from the standpoint of man's common ailments (in addition to being readily available and socially acceptable), has thus forged its way to the forefront and is far and away the most popular and most destructive of all drugs.

Since alcohol is the mind-altering drug most widely used in the United States and most other countries, a consideration of the problems it presents may serve as a paradigm for all other drugs. Strauss [9] has recently published a definitive survey of the interrelations between alcohol and society. Earlier in the same year the National Commission on Marihuana and Drug Abuse presented convincing data that alcohol presents by far the most serious drug problem in America, even though more than half the people in this country do not even consider it to be a drug.

Strauss points out that alcohol is a substance which permeates, pleases, and yet plagues most of the world. It is both functional and dysfunctional. As a medicine it has analgesic, anesthetic, antiseptic, and antianxiety properties. In social situations it relieves tension, promotes a sense of well-being, and enhances relaxation and conviviality. Excessive use, however, leads to manifestation of its disadvantages, both immediate and long-term. The most immediate problem is acute intoxication, particularly hazardous in a technological society, which leads to accidents with motor vehicles and other moving machinery, and interpersonal violence. These interact with the long-term destructive effects to produce absenteeism, family instability, suicide, crime, and ultimately poverty, mental illness, and lives of degradation. More than 24 billion dollars are expended yearly for alcoholic beverages, a sum amounting to eight to twelve times the amount spent on all other types of psychoactive drugs, both prescribed and illicit. About 100 million people in the United States use alcohol, and about 10 percent of that number use it in intensified or compulsive ways (pp. 42–43).[2]

In the United States and in many other countries alcohol and heroin are the drugs causing the most concern, while marijuana and the minor tranquilizers are less troublesome. Marijuana is not particularly dangerous unless used in large amounts over a period of time, and the minor tranquilizers, though known to produce dependence, are not seriously abused on a large scale. The amphetamines, barbiturates, nonbarbiturate sedatives such as methaqualone, hallucinogens, and cocaine fall in the intermediate group, though there are indications that the use of barbiturates and cocaine may be increasing (p. 36).[2] The use of different drugs simultaneously presents increased hazards, because many of them have synergistic effects.[1]

Adolescent Development and the Youth Culture

Since most people tend to equate the nonmedicinal use of drugs with young people (even though older people probably use more drugs of all kinds), a brief survey of current influences affecting adolescents and young adults is in order.

One student, now a physician, became so interested in the motivation for youthful drug taking that he developed his senior thesis to consider this and related problems. The answer, he said, was simple: Young people take drugs for fun (p. 15).[8] He rarely observed marijuana or LSD being taken for the compulsive satisfaction of an acute need. For most of the young people who use psychoactive drugs, the immediate stimulus is boredom. They have not been attracted to their parents' life style and have not yet developed satisfactory alternatives. He feels that most of the young people whose lives have been most disturbing to others began as alienated youths. Some reduce their feelings of emptiness by activism, others by withdrawing into the world of drug use.

A distinction should be made between two discernible groups of those who use drugs for pleasure, escape, or hope of greater awareness. The first and small group comprises those young people who have been raised under conditions of extreme hardship and deprivation, often without the support of an intact and loving family. They seek escape or diversion more than new experiences, usually in response to unpleasant conditions.

The second and by far the larger group comes from families that are comparatively affluent but in which something has gone wrong in relations between the children and their parents. This is not to say that experimentation with drugs is the fault of parents, but rather that the children appear to long for something which they are not getting, something which would cause them to feel wanted, needed, responsible, and capable of giving and receiving affection and love (pp. 181–186).[6]

What has happened during the explosion of the drug problem from the disadvantaged segments of society to the affluent or overadvantaged groups? What have we lost that will have to be regained in one form or another if we are to make sense to our young people?

Adolescence is the time when the young person starts the long task of achieving independence in place of dependence and individual identity in place of a borrowed or assigned identity. He must develop personal values, achieve meaningful social relationships outside the family, decide on his life's work, and learn how to postpone immediate gratification of desire in order to achieve long-term goals. It is natural for him to turn to peer groups for companionship, test the boundaries of authority, experiment regarding his own place in society, and desire to experience as much as possible so that he may have a clear idea of what choices are open to him in this world. Adolescents have always been impulsive, impatient, and given to risk taking. Our present group is no different from those of the past; but social, cultural and economic conditions have changed dramatically, and the young reflect these changes.

We have seen a weakening of the family structure, particularly in its functions of transmitting values and culture to the young; parents and others are even confused as to what those values and cultural components should be. The change from a rural and agrarian to an urban and technological society has progressed with great rapidity during the last half century. Accompanying the change has been an increase in mobility and a decrease in extended families, with a corresponding increase in nuclear families. Our social and political institutions have not yet learned how to support families in such a way as to foster those conditions which encourage child development.

Many children are so stimulated during the all-important developmental period between five and twelve that they do not learn to engage in an organized and sustained effort to achieve any planned goals. Called the latency period in psychoanalytic terminology, this is the time that Erikson refers to as the period when the child develops the capacity for industry, for adapting himself to a world in which attention and persevering diligence are necessary if he is to avoid feelings of inadequacy and inferiority (pp. 258–261).[3] Too many children reach adolescence unable to relate the stimuli they have absorbed from so many sources and without the capacity for fantasy. They feel stimulated rather than satisfied, and are thus ripe to be seduced into a quick solution to their tension. Ambivalence over moving from dependence leads them to accept an interim dependency, the authority of their peer group, which all too often encourages drug experimentation.

Throughout history adults have been deploring the various unsatisfactory and unacceptable ways in which young people express their feelings. The varieties of such substitutes for competence have been virtually without limit; the ones we now see most often are stealing, property damage, aggressiveness toward others, unacceptable sexual behavior, psychosomatic illness, failure in school and college, and of course drug experimentation. What many critics fail to realize is that competence is learned; it is not inborn, nor does it arise spontaneously during the years of physical maturation. It requires cultural, educational, and above all home conditions that provide the basic needs for healthy emotional development: being both wanted and needed, good role models, freedom from excessive domination, maintenance of firm but friendly discipline, encouragement for tasks well done rather than severe criticism for shortcomings, alternation between stimulation and relaxation, due regard for privacy, and absent or at least minimal prejudice. Although those who suffer from gross poverty are subject to additional risk, those whose wants are automatically furnished without effort on their part are often also seriously handicapped.

Education and the Development of Competence

Until the occurrence of widespread social upheavals fomented by those in various institutions of higher learning, most people in our colleges and universities had enormous confidence in education. They assumed that if young people could be given the facts regarding their society and its heritage, they would act in their own best interest. In drug education the expectation was that when people, young and old, became aware of the harmful as well as the beneficial uses of drugs, they would more or less automatically respond with a constructive attitude of cooperation. Instead, a steady increase in irresponsible and harmful drug use occurred as drug education programs multiplied. Whether such programs encouraged drug experimentation or merely reduced what would otherwise have been an even greater problem remains a matter of conjecture.

The notion has sprung up that drug dependence is a specific disease with a more or less standard etiology and particular forms of treatment. This idea was first promoted in regard to alcoholism, seen as an illness resulting from interaction among the pharmacological effects of the drug, the biochemistry of the user, his life situation, and his social and psychological expectations. Though alcoholism is considered somewhat different from other types of drug dependence, the concept of a dependency disease could be extended to cover other forms of drug abuse. It seems to follow logically that if such dependence is a disease, there should be a specific cure, and if it is not already known it should be discovered. There is just enough truth in these concepts to make them believable and attractive, but not enough to make them workable. Attempts to treat drug-dependent persons as if they had a specific disease usually lead to frustration on the part of therapists, since there is no known cure to be applied. Such poor results have led to understandable aversion to treating these patients; the person seeking treatment readily senses this prejudice, and what possibility of effective treatment does exist becomes less likely.

Instead of considering drug dependence as a specific disease in search of a cure, a more rational point of view is that it is a composite of social, cultural, and emotional maladaptations that may result in a wide variety of problems. Numerous life situations that have been frustrating to the individual usually coincide with or precede such disability. In most cases part, but not all, of the problems are medical ones that impair the individual's health or effectiveness and require medical treatment. Therapy therefore involves not only physicians, but many other persons whose activities relate to the patient's welfare. The multiplicity of causes and the many potentially effective therapies constitute the strongest reason for drug treatment centers to be part of total health and human service programs, rather than segregated as an exclusive specialty.

The development of extensive drug use in recent years is a result of numerous factors, including wide availability, search for new types of experience, increasing affluence with subsequent lessened responsibility on youth, loss of meaning and purpose, extended time in school and college, and weakening of family and religious influences. The commission has emphasized that simple cause-and-effect relationships are impossible to establish, but that social problems such as alienation of youth, decay of values, and decline of economic incentive are nevertheless highly important. Similarly, efforts to deal with the drug problem will have to go far beyond control of supply, punitive measures against law violators, and purely factual, didactic education; they will have to develop life styles and values that are more rewarding than methods of escape and oblivion.

A word of caution is in order concerning the treatment of those who have already become dependent on drugs, or find themselves in situations in which they feel such dependence is a predictable outcome. Drug-dependence programs should be wide-based, including "educational and informational guidance for all segments of the population; job training and career counseling; medical, psychiatric, psychological and social services; family counseling; and recreational services" (p. 366).[2] Programs staffed by volunteers and untrained personnel, such as "hot lines," are of questionable value if they are not backed up by a network of supporting consultants in the various fields in which the persons at risk need help. Treatment should be in the context of the total situation and needs, not determined by what particular drug is involved.

The primary goal of drug policy is to minimize irresponsible drug-using behavior, which can be defined as occurring when the manner or circumstances of use pose a threat to the safety of others; when the pattern of use impedes or risks the impairment of the individual's social and economic functioning; and when the pattern of use reduces the individual's options for self-fulfillment by impairing his faculties or retarding his development (pp. 205–206).[2] Establishment and implementation of such policy, to reduce the deleterious effects of drug taking by the entire population and by young people particularly, requires efforts by many persons in all areas of society. The theoretical ideal that drugs should be used only when prescribed or authorized by physicians ignores the fact that many drugs, particularly alcohol and tobacco, do not come under medical practice acts. Similarly, the reduction in availability of drugs through legal penalties for distribution and use has not been successful; in the case of cannabis preparations, it has been counterproductive. Many have considered education to be the essential component in any program of prevention, yet experience strongly suggests that many drug-education programs stimulate rather than discourage experimentation.

Nevertheless, each of these procedures (inadequate when applied exclusively or inappropriately) has constructive elements. To the greatest extent possible, competent persons who are aware of the dangers should supervise use of any potent drug. Nonprescription drugs which are harmful when used excessively should be limited in their distribution by whatever consensus can be achieved in each community, state, or nation. The use of drugs known to have no medical value can be lessened by legal sanctions against distribution, provided these sanctions are established so that they avoid doing more harm than good. Knowledge is still preferable to ignorance, hence drug education is necessary, but it must be in a form that constitutes an effective deterrent. Factual information should be available not just in classroom programs, but in school and public libraries for all to explore when they need it, and in a form that is not so technical as to be confusing and self-defeating. Such information should be directed toward development of constructive attitudes about drug use fully as much as toward transmitting technical knowledge. Probably most important of all, we need to study the social influences that encourage indiscriminate drug taking, clarify their effects, and develop counterinfluences that will create alternatives to drug use which are more satisfying than diversion and escape.

Among the persons and groups who are most concerned, physicians must exercise greater restraint in prescribing psychoactive drugs. Patients should be made aware of the limitations and hazards of drug use. Law-enforcement officials need to concentrate their efforts on large-scale drug traffickers rather than individual users, while suppliers of legitimate drugs need to limit production and reduce diversion to illegal channels. For those who have misused drugs, restraint or deprivation of liberty should be reduced to the minimum amount consistent with the optimum application of therapeutic procedures. Religious groups have a major responsibility for the elaboration of philosophical, moral, ethical, and spiritual questions. They have a basic role in dealing with the many issues of private moral choice which are outside the realm of social policy (pp. 15–22).[5]

The most important change must be a shift from overreliance on government restrictions to a reactivation of informal, nonlegal controls on drug-using behavior. School, church, family, business, community organization, and service organization, each working from its own perspective and values, will have to encourage self-discipline with regard to drug use. The primary aim should be to guide the individual to other satisfactions and other coping mechanisms instead of resorting to drugs. In fact, there are good reasons why preventive programs should emphasize total personality, social, and educational development without emphasizing drugs at all.

Educational programs should involve all members of the community (local, state, and national), and not be confined to the schools. Furthermore, they should be low-keyed, objective rather than moralistic, and without exaggeration—the facts are sufficiently impressive when clearly and accurately stated. In whatever ways are possible, information should be freely available to parents, young people themselves, teachers, and others in the community whose aid is enlisted when specific problems arise. Attitudes encouraging responsible use of drugs are most effective when mediated through families (especially when relations between parents and children are good) and peer-group members.

In our educational efforts so far, we have been so concerned with keeping people, especially young ones, out of trouble that we have not sufficiently encouraged efforts to help them learn to do this themselves. Because of the great variety of drugs available, and the fact that new ones are constantly being developed, there is little possibility of controlling their use through external restraint, legal or otherwise. The only truly effective controls will be learned by the young people (and older people as well) in the form of self-control. Attention to the sources of supply, whether by regulation of manufacture or restrictions on distribution, can only be partially effective, even though it is desirable and necessary (pp. 234–238).[5]

15 / Drug Dependence and Its Amelioration

Our main hope lies in working with the young people from the time they enter the educational system, before they have come under the tyranny of peer-group influences based on a combination of errors and unfulfilled emotional needs. Alternatives to drug use must be developed and made attractive. This should not be too difficult if we set our minds to the task, because those alternatives form the basis of any civilization that is both satisfying and enduring. They are integral parts of the personality that has learned to cope with the problems and enjoy the rewards of both intrapsychic and interpersonal competence.

REFERENCES

1. Davis, J. M.; Sekerke, H. J.; and Janowsky, M.D. "Drug Interactions Involving the Drugs of Abuse." *Drug Use in America: Problem in Perspective.* 2nd Report of the National Commission on Marihuana and Drug Abuse, app. 1, pp. 181–208. Washington, D.C.: U.S. Government Printing Office, 1973.

2. *Drug Use in America: Problem in Perspective.* 2nd Report of the National Commission on Marihuana and Drug Abuse. Washington, D.C.: U.S. Government Printing Office, 1973.

3. Erikson, E. H. *Childhood and Society.* 2nd ed. New York: W. W. Norton, 1963.

4. Farnsworth, D. L. "Drugs—Do They Produce Open or Closed Minds?" *Medical Insight* 2(July 1970):34–44; 2(August 1970):22–31.

5. *Final Report of the Commission of Inquiry into the Non-medical Use of Drugs.* Ottawa: Government of Canada, 1973.

6. Gerzon, M. *The Whole World's Watching.* New York: Viking, 1969.

7. Goodman, L. S., and Gilman, A., eds. *The Pharmacological Basis of Therapeutics.* 4th ed. New York: Macmillan, 1970.

8. Pope, H., Jr. *Voices From the Drug Culture.* Cambridge, Mass.: The Sanctuary, 1971.

9. Strauss, R. "Alcohol and Society." *Psychiatric Annals,* 3(1973):9–103.

Part IV

Research and Evaluation

ALTHOUGH estimates vary, it is safe to conclude that psychiatric disorder is one of the most common chronic diseases. Therefore, we need to have a better assessment of social and mental functioning. Furthermore, can we improve the evaluation of the treatments we use? Can we secure a more accurate picture of the large variety of "sick" behavior patterns? These are the important questions of this section of the book.

Altering harmful social conditions is a message at least as old as Isaiah. Evaluation research—whether the evaluation of social risk factors or of the efficacy of programs—is the current term for an old conern, that is, improving the human condition through directed change.

How much "health" is possible? Committed as we are to reducing social sources of emotional illness and to improving therapy, is there a limit to how much "health" is possible? Are we caught, with inevitable contradictions, conflicting traits, suffering over acceptance and rejection, over life itself?

Editorial Note

This chapter sets out to develop a system for assessing the level of health in populations by measuring morbidity, subjective feelings of well-being, and social participation. The authors provide a conceptualization of health as a process which is best assessed in terms of level of functioning rather than only by absence of illness. Second, they emphasize that health has to be considered in its social context; and third, they present a model for representing the functioning of people in natural settings.

This chapter is an illustration of a major effort to measure health and adaptation. It is economical conceptually in providing a profile of people who should be high risks on a social measure of health. Obviously, the framework of this book, that of integration-disintegration, is strikingly illustrated in this attempt to give weight to and operationalize measures of social effectiveness.

Durkheim would have been pleased to read this chapter; he set out to examine the level of social functioning in his classic work, Suicide. His four etiologic conditions for precipitating suicide—the egoistic, the altruistic, the anomic and the fatalistic—all relate to the level of social functioning in terms of the relationship of the individual to the group, to optimizing real affiliations, and to the nature of effective social functioning.

What are the implications of this approach? It raises questions about indicators of a healthy social system in the spirit of Durkheim. Could we develop scales on egoistic, altruistic, and anomic social arrangements? It also suggests consideration of the need for better criteria for assessing social effectiveness in the areas of family competence, work satisfaction, leisure, religion, and socialization.

B. H. K.

CHAPTER 16

The Measurement of
Health in Populations*

ROBERT C. BENFARI

MORTON BEISER

ALEXANDER H. LEIGHTON

JANE M. MURPHY

THIS CHAPTER is concerned with presenting a conceptual model whereby the measurement of health in populations can be accomplished. The point of departure is the desire for a method by which the health of individuals can be estimated and, on this basis, frequency distributions obtained of different health levels in a population.

It is probably unnecessary to elaborate on the importance of this kind of measurement, but it may be worthwhile to note that it implicates two main kinds of use: (1) estimating the health needs of populations; and (2) monitoring whatever changes occur as a result of introducing health programs. This second point is to be distinguished from the kind of evaluation that analyzes the functioning of

* This work, conducted as part of the Harvard Program in Social Psychiatry, was supported in part by Public Health Service Grant MH-12892 from the National Institute of Mental Health and also by Public Health Service Contract HSM 110-71-240 from the Health Services and Mental Health Administration.

a hospital or agency in terms of number of patients seen, treatment given, percent cured, and so on, but which does not assess the actual impact on the health of the total population of the area served. The screening of populations with mobile x-ray units illustrates the notion we have in mind, although the emphasis there is on illness and on surveying everyone. Our concern is with health and with making estimates by means of samples.

From the foregoing it is evident that our theory visualizes health in both biological and psychological terms. In Chapters 9 and 10 it is pointed out that adequate and even excellent functioning can occur in the presence of pathology. This suggests that measures of *functioning* may be as important in health assessment as tabulations of morbidity. If one takes decline in morbidity as a sole criterion of the effectiveness of a health service, the curve of apparent health improvement in the population may flatten after a time, while the actual curve of (functional) improvement continues to rise. That is to say, morbidity studies alone may fail to show adequately what has been accomplished because they do not sufficiently take into account the totality of the individual.

As suggested in Chapter 10, one approach to the assessment of functioning is the individual's participation in the social group of which he is a part. This can be visualized in terms of work, family, and community participation, and of scales which would reflect degree of contribution to group needs versus degree of dependency. Thus a person with permanent damage from polio can be toward either of two poles: contributive in matters of work, family, and community, or dependent.

In putting these several considerations together, we have arrived at a tripartite conceptualization of health. The components are: (1) morbidity (biological and psychological); (2) subjective feelings of well-being; and (3) social participation. The total process is conceived as taking place in a sociocultural context.

The Model for Analysis

The ideas just sketched make evident the need to develop analytic procedures that are capable of handling data in the form of multiple, interrelated variables. In such a situation it is the common practice to devise a conceptual model as a guide.

Models are common among the sciences. The double helix, for instance, is a well-known model employed as an aide in understanding and investigating the nature of chromosomes. An illustration from medicine is to be found in the representation of the cardiovascular system as a pump circulating fluid through a network of pipes. While such a model is an oversimplification, it nevertheless helps conceptualize such variables as stroke volume and frequency; amount of fluid in the system, its specific gravity and viscosity; peripheral resistance; and pressure in the system.

In the social and behavioral sciences the models tend to be more abstract. The ideal model is one that can be stated entirely as a mathematical formula (an equation of functions). In practice, however, it is frequently more feasible to start with models consisting in geometric representations of systems of variables. As with the pump illustration, they serve to highlight interrelationships of the system and provide a basis for developing a research strategy.

Everyone recognizes, of course, that models do not accurately represent reality, and their application must always be conducted with this in mind. On the other hand, the oversimplification characteristic of models does serve to help separate major considerations from minor. As the work goes along and the results of first analytic treatment of data come to hand, the model can be refined and errors corrected, moving through successive approximations closer and closer to nature. Thus, a model is developed through its use.

A first step in constructing our model was the utilization of prior findings and current theory to select a preliminary set of major variables. We assumed that we are always dealing with an open system (e.g., a community) that has components. One of the components, obviously, consists in the individual organism, or person, which can vary in frequency in different parts of the total system. In other words, a major category of inquiry is to answer questions of the general form: *How many individuals* in this or that part of the system have variable X?

This leads to conceptualization of variable X as a next step. One possibility consists in the various types of behavior patterns which persons display. We take these as a second major category in the model; it is concerned with questions in the general form: *What are the frequencies of behavior patterns* $X_1 X_2 X_3 \ldots X_n$ among various groups of individuals?

It may seem a little curious to posit behavior patterns as independent of persons when there can be no behavior without persons. While this is true, it remains that any given behavior may vary in frequency from 0 to 100 percent in a population of persons, and this seems sufficient justification for treating the phenomenon as conceptually independent.

Next we may note that the particular categories of behavior we have in mind are, of course, those which pertain to illness, sense of well-being, and social participation.

The final major category is that of societal systems implied by the word "groups" toward the end of the paragraph above concerned with the frequency of behavior patterns. What is meant here can be illustrated by family, socioeconomic class, ethnic membership, and so on. It pertains to questions in the general form: What classes of human groups are there which display variables X and person-frequencies Y?

Our model, then, in gross outline, has three major categories, each considered able to vary more or less independently from the others. Because of this, it points up possibilities for investigating relationships. This can be illustrated by a geometric device invented by Cattel [1] for showing potential systematic relationships among three sets of variables. (See Figure 16.1.)

The covariation diagram might equally well be called a correlation cube, and it shows the possible systematic interrelationships of three types of statistical procedures. These involve the major categories already described: (1) the reference point or person; (2) the terms in which the observation is made, namely behavior variables; and (3) the societal subsystems or setting in which the observa-

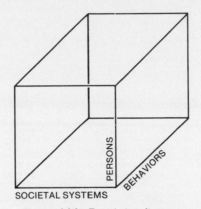

FIGURE 16.1. Covariation diagram.

tions take place. The cube has six facets, each of which involves correlations of two variables while holding the third constant. Our focus will be on the three facets most relevant to the goals of our project, and will not attempt an exhaustive investigation of all the logical possibilities.

Facet I is shown in Figure 16.2 and is called "V-analysis" for variable analysis. It has to do with the correlation of persons and behaviors while holding societal systems constant. Derivable from this are dimensions of behaviors which are "reliable" in the sense that they are shown to occur commonly among people. In other words, this analysis reveals those variables (behavior patterns) which do show up with a sufficient frequency as to make them worthy of attention.

Facet II is shown in Figure 16.3 and is called "O-analysis" for object analysis: This refers to the category of persons as the objects. It also has to do with the correlation of persons and behaviors, but from a different perspective. Having found through V-analysis that certain dimensions of behavior occur with suf-

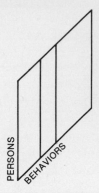

FIGURE 16.2 Facet I—V-analysis.

ficient frequency to be of interest, the question now is: How do these dimensions group together in individuals? Are there characteristic combinations or profiles of behavior dimensions which go together so as to constitute personality types? In short, O-analysis reveals types of people who show up with sufficient frequency to make them worthy of attention.

Facet III is shown in Figure 16.4 and is called "S-analysis" for situation (societal) analysis. This refers to correlations of societal systems and behavioral dimensions while holding persons constant. Derivable from this are empirical classifications of societal systems in terms of the behaviors characteristic of the people in them.

From this overview of the model we must proceed to some more detailed specifications before it can be applied to actual data. Thus each of the three major categories have to be considered in terms of subcategories before they can be employed in analysis. These subcategories, furthermore, must be in the form of dimensions—that is to say, they must be measurable properties. Inasmuch as it is impossible to investigate every conceivable dimension within a major cate-

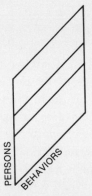

FIGURE 16.3. Facet II—O-analysis.

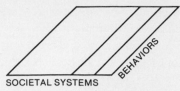

SOCIETAL SYSTEMS

FIGURE 16.4. Facet III—S-analysis.

gory, selection has to be made. This choice, in our case, has been carried out in terms of the goals and theory of health outlined earlier.

I. Category of persons.
    Dimensions:
        a. Age
        b. Sex
II. Category of behavior.
    Dimensions:
        a. Illness
            1. Organic symptoms
            2. Psychological symptoms
            3. Impairment (negative part of social participation related to above symptoms)
        b. Health
            1. Sense of well-being
            2. Social participation
III. Category of societal systems.
    Dimensions:
        a. Socioeconomic status
        b. Ethnic membership
        c. Urban setting versus rural setting
        d. Social integration (degree of social cohesiveness of a group)

The dimensions listed above are themselves susceptible to being broken down into numerous subdimensions, e.g., there are many types of organic symptoms, and further choices among large numbers of possibilities will have to be made.

It is apparent that in the selection of dimensions, especially under II, many aspects of behavior have been omitted that may turn out to be important, such as IQ and unconscious motives. We think it important to keep in mind that the model we are constructing does have these omissions and that at some point it may be necessary to reconsider them.

Of the three major categories, the last, societal systems, is perhaps the most in need of taxonomic development. This is a growing field. Krause [2] has proposed that there are seven subclasses of social "settings," and other authors approach the problem in terms of other dimensions. The emphasis on "social integration" has grown out of our own work and is being further explored with regard to quantifiable indicators. The topic is taken up in Part V of this book.

A look at the dimensions, as we have laid them out, makes it apparent that those within a single major category may have relationships to each other parallel to the relationships among the categories. For example, organic symptoms and the sense of well-being may, as noted earlier, vary more or less independently of each other. This, however, brings us to the limits of the model in purely geometric terms. More than three simultaneous variables cannot be represented in real space. They can, however, be handled through matrix algebra and multivariate techniques and this is the extension of the model developed for the analysis of dimensions and their interrelationships. More specifically, the model encompasses factor analysis and cluster analysis.

Trying Out the Model

Previous work has given considerable information with regard to illness behaviors, but much less regarding health. We have focused therefore on searching for dimensions indicative of the sense of well-being and of social participation.

The analysis to be described is related to two different data banks—questionnaire responses from a sample of adults living in New York City, and from adults in Stirling County. In accordance with the model, the first step will be concerned with V-analysis and the next with O-analysis.

I. DESCRIPTION OF SAMPLES

a. *Urban Sample.*   Seven census tracts in New York, six in Brooklyn, and one in Queens were selected as survey areas for the urban study. Tracts were chosen to represent a range of socioeconomic status, on the basis of the 1960 public record data.

Blocks were defined within each tract, and a representative selection of the blocks was made. Next, a quota was established of the number of dwelling units for a subsequent random draw of households; then one adult was chosen from any single dwelling unit drawn for the sample. There was an attempt to alternate males and females in the draw.

An initial sample of 640 was drawn to insure at least 500 respondents; 530 completed interviews were obtained.

Table 16.1 gives the age and sex distribution of the sample. It shows that there is a more or less equal distribution of males and females in the age categories under 30, 50–59, 60–69, and 70 +, and that there is an overrepresentation of females in 30–39 and 40–49 ranges (155 females to 104 males).

TABLE 16.1

Urban Sample Age and Sex Distribution

	UNDER 30	30–39	40–49	50–59	60–69	70 +	N
Male	51	56	48	41	26	14	237
Female	52	75	80	45	22	21	294
	103	131	128	86	48	35	531

b. *Rural Panel:* Stirling County, a small town and rural county with some 20,000 inhabitants, forms the backdrop for this group. A sample of 404 adults living in thirteen villages, ranging in size from 100 to 400 inhabitants, was interviewed with a structured questionnaire designed to elicit information about psychiatric and other symptoms.

From this sample, a subsample of 123 individuals was drawn to approximate the following controls:

1. Equal representation by sex.
2. Equal representation of three age categories (young, middle, and old).
3. Equal numbers of ill and asymptomatic individuals. (See Table 16.2.)

TABLE 16.2

Composition of the Rural Panel

		PSYCHIATRICALLY ILL		ASYMPTOMATIC	
		M	F	M	F
Age					
Young	(18–35)	5	12	10	11
Middle-aged	(36–54)	13	16	6	7
Old	(55 +)	10	8	14	11
Sex		28	36	30	29
Health ratings		64		59	

The rural panel was seen annually for a total of five years by a team of psychiatrists. During the last year of interviewing a questionnaire schedule was administered.

These two data banks may be viewed as different but complementary in a variety of ways:

1. Urban versus rural.
2. Extensive data on a large group in one case, intensive data on a small group in the second instance.
3. As will be detailed later, somewhat different, although overlapping, information was obtained for each group.

II. SELECTED FINDINGS—V-ANALYSIS

The first goal was the development of the behavioral dimensions of illness and health in accordance witn the V-analysis outlined earlier. In essence this consisted of factor analysis of questionnaire responses across people. From this we were able to show empirical groupings of responses in order to form behavioral dimensions of health and sickness. Once a set of dimensions had been identified, we proceeded next to the O-analysis to see how these clustered in people. By this means person types are identified.

These two procedures, V-analysis (dimensional analysis) and O-analysis (person analysis), were sequentially carried out in the two samples—Urban Sample and Rural Panel. It is necessary to keep in mind that each sample had different levels of behavior assessment. In the Urban Sample there was an emphasis on psychological and physical symptomatolology plus impairment, with a lesser emphasis upon signs of positive health. Yet these signs of positive health were still present and used in the analysis. The Rural Panel, on the other hand, focused more heavily on the behaviors of health and had lesser emphasis on sickness behavior.

The aim in analyzing these data banks, it will be recalled, is to provide the empirical evidence necessary for the construction of an index of health that encompasses the range of health and illness behavior and will have maximum predictability for general population use.

a. *Urban Sample.* The following dimensions were isolated in the V-analysis of some 150 questionnaire items.

Health behaviors:

1. Self-esteem (a subclass of the sense of well-being).
2. Good neighbor behavior (a subclass of social participation).
3. Sociability with others (another subclass of social participation).

Illness behaviors:

1. Psychological
   a. Anxiety
   b. Topical depression
   c. Physiological process disturbance
   d. Nonspecific neurotic complaints
2. Physical
   a. Sensory problems
   b. GI problems
   c. Musculoskeletal problems
   d. Female problems
   e. Skin problems
   f. Allergy problems
   g. Respiratory problems

    h. Cardiovascular problems
    i. General health problems
3. Impairment
    a. Role impairment (family, social, and work)
    b. Sickness behavior (staying in bed, visiting MD, stay in hospital, and
        sense of feeling ill)

   b. *Rural Panel.** The V-analysis of a twenty-six item questionnaire
(measuring health) yielded the following dimensions.
   Health behaviors:

1. Negative affect
2. Positive sense of involvement
3. Long-term sense of satisfaction
4. Self-esteem

III. O-ANALYSIS
    a. *Urban Sample.* After the preliminary V-analysis had been conducted
on the sample of 530 respondents, it will be remembered that we used the fifteen
psychological and physical illness dimensions as a basis for typing people. This
was done to derive stable types of symptom-based classifications. The types
formed a baseline upon which to project the dimensions of "health." In addition
to the dimension of health, we used demographic characteristics such as age,
sex, and educational level as control variables.
    Seven clearly defined types of people emerged from the O-analysis of the fif-
teen dimensions and the 530 respondents. A subset of 100 unique profiles also
emerged, which in a sample size of 530 and fifteen dimensions is not uncommon. The 100 uniques represent individuals who have very high scores on one
or two dimensions but do not fit the profiles of the seven stable types. In order to
merge the unique individuals into other types, more subjects would be needed in
the study. The score patterns of the seven types on the fifteen dimensions are presented in Table 16.3. The characterizations of the types are presented in
Table 16.4.
    One of the interesting findings from the study is the complex relationship
between the dimension of self-esteem and the various types. High self-esteem is
positively related to the basically symptom-free type (TI), but also positively
related to a group who presented general health problems. Low self-esteem is associated with Type V (female problems) and Type VI (psychological disturbance). It is thus apparent that self-esteem is an independent dimension across
the sample, and has differential relationships with subgroups in the population.

* The actual items and the loadings, domain validities, and reliabilities of the dimensions in
both the urban and rural we hope to present in future publications dealing with the specific method-
ologies and results. For the overview purposes of this chapter, only procedures and highlights of the
results will be given.

TABLE 16.3

O-Types in the Urban Sample

	SCORE PATTERNS OF PERSON TYPES							
DIMENSIONS	I	II	III	IV	V	VI	VII	UNIQUE N
1. Anxiety	low-low	average	low	low	high	high-high	low	high-high
2. Cognitive depression	low-low	average	low	low-low	low	high-high	high	high-high
3. Physiological depression	low-low	average	low	average	average	high-high	average	high-high
4. Anxiety/depression	low-low	average	average	low	average	high-high	high	high-high
5. Self-esteem	high	average	average	high	low	low	average	low-low
6. Nonspecific neurotic	low-low	high	low-low	low	average	high-high	average	high-high
7. General health index	low-low	high	low	high-high	average	average	low	high-high
8. Sensory problems	low-low	average	average	high-high	low	average	low	high-high
9. GI problems	low-low	low	average	average	low	average	average	high-high
10. MS problems	low	average	low	high-high	average	low	low-low	high-high
11. Female problems	low	low	low	low	high-high	low	low	high-high
12. Skin problems	average	low	low	average	low	average	average	high-high
13. Allergy	low	low	high-high	low	low	high	low	high-high
14. Respiratory problems	low-low	average	average	average	low	average	average	high-high
15. CV problems	low	high-high	low	low	average	low	low-low	high-high

low-low = scores on a dimension well below the group mean
low = scores on a dimension significantly below group mean
average = scores equal to the group mean
high = scores significantly greater than the group mean
high-high = scores highly significantly greater than the group mean

TABLE 16.4

Characteristics of the O-Types in the Sample

Type	I	characterized by lowest scores on symptom dimensions and highest score on self-esteem
Type	II	moderately high score on nonspecific neurotic complaints
		high score on general health complaints
		highest score on cardiovascular problems
Type	III	generally low scores or average scores on psychological and physical health dimensions but a high score on allergy problems
Type	IV	high self-esteem
		high score on general health problems
		high score on sensory problems
		high score on musculoskeletal problems
		low allergy score
		low cardiovascular score
Type	V	moderately high anxiety score
		low cognitive depression score
		low self-esteem
		moderately high score on sensory problems
		moderately high score on gastrointestinal problems
		high score on female problems
		low allergy score
		low skin problems
Type	VI	highest scores on all psychological dimensions
		lowest score on self-esteem
		moderately high score on allergy
		low score on cardiovascular problems
		low score on musculoskeletal problems
		low score on female problems
Type	VII	moderately high score on cognitive depression

Use of self-esteem as an indicator of health by itself obscures some important factors. When self-esteem and impairment are both used as variables of health, the relationship of health to illness types become clearer.

For example, the pattern of scores on the three dimensions of self-esteem, role impairment, and sickness behavior are depicted below for the seven types and the unique group:

TYPE	SELF-ESTEEM	ROLE IMPAIRMENT	SICKNESS BEHAVIOR
TI	high	low	low
TII	medium	medium	high
TIII	medium	low	medium
TIV	high	low	medium
TV	low	medium	high
TVI	low	high	medium
TVII	medium	medium	low
Unique	low	high	high

If one indicator is used, the following groups are identified as healthy or ill:

Types Falling Into Ill-Well Classification
By Univariate Indicator

INDICATOR—DIMENSION	ILL	WELL
Self-esteem	TV, TVI, and unique	TI, TIV
Role impairment	TVI and unique	TI, TIII, TIV
Sickness behavior	TII, TV, and unique	TI, TVII

It can be seen from the above that if one indicator is used, one or more groups are left out of the categories of ill and healthy. Type I is consistently seen as healthy and the uniques are seen as in ill health, but Type IV would be missed if sickness behavior is used as an indicator without scales measuring self-esteem and role impairment. This type is an older group who have some complaints of illness associated with old age, but function quite well on the inner level and in roles.

b. Rural Panel. While there are fewer subjects in this sample than in the urban study, several variables are available for use in classifying people who are more clearly on the "health" side. Furthermore, the fact that those individuals were given repeated clinical assessment provides a point of triangulation which is unique.

The panel study began with people classified into two major groupings—ill and well. During the ensuing five years, considerable change occurred in the clinical status of these people—some who were ill recovered, some who were well developed psychiatric symptoms, while others were consistent in their health behaviors over the five years.

One hundred and twelve of the original 123 panel members were seen annually and, on the basis of the wealth of data obtained, they may be classified according to the clinical picture they presented over the five-year period. Those groupings are shown in Table 16.5

It is interesting and instructive to compare these clinical assessments with a classification of the same individuals based on health behaviors.

The four dimensions which emerged in the V-analysis—negative affect, positive sense of involvement, long-term sense of satisfaction, and self-esteem—were used to construct typologies. The result was eight discrete types and one residual category.

In Table 16.6 these types are described based on scores obtained on the four health dimensions. They are compared with the clinical ratings already presented.

TABLE 16.5
Clinical Ratings Over a Five-Year Period

A group which remained consistently ill	30
"Vulnerable" (ratings were inconsistent, but in a symptomatic direction; many of them represent "latent" cases or people "vulnerable" to development of frank psychiatric disorder)	17
Improved (lost symptoms)	23
Worse (developed new symptoms)	3
Consistently well	39
	112

First the types are listed, with summarizing names. These names are based on the score profiles for the four dimensions. Next comes the number of people classified as belonging to each of the types. The pattern of scores achieved by the individuals in each cluster is then listed; these patterns suggested the summarizing names for the groups. $\bar{H}$ is a statistic which reflects the homogeneity of the groups with respect to their scores on the defining dimensions. The closer $\bar{H}$ is to unity, the more homogeneous the type. Most of the groups reveal a fairly "tight" pattern. Type 9 is an obvious exception and is therefore classified as "Residual."

Finally, the clinical ratings are presented. The percentage figures here have as their referent the rating categories. For example, 29 percent of the vulnerable group fall within the Stolid Solid type, 12 percent within the Reactor type, 6 percent in Neurotic Type A, and so on.

The whole numbers have the types as their referent. Thus five of the seventeen Stolid Solids are "vulnerable," three of them improved, and nine are in the consistently well group.

One striking feature in this table is that practically all of the consistently well group fall into three different types: 85 percent in Types 1, 2, and 3. In other words, somewhere between one-half and two-thirds of each of these types are people who have been well over the entire period of the study.

Type 7, the Reactors, which on inspection of its profile might also seem to be a "healthy" pattern, has no clear-cut relationship with any of the clinically rated groupings.

Types 4, 5, and 6 seem to be fairly clear groupings primarily of ill or illness-prone individuals, constituting 46 percent of the ill group among them. Each type also contains a high proportion of ill people.

The empirically derived types have also been examined with respect to a number of different sociodemographic, psychological, and other variables. Of particular interest is the relationship of the types to one measure of social effectiveness—participation in community organizations. In Table 16.7 each type is compared to the group as a whole with respect to mean score on a scale of social participation.

TABLE 16.6
Empirical Types and Clinical Classifications

					TYPES					
	1 STOLID SOLIDS	2 INVOLVED SOLIDS	3 MR. AVERAGE	4 NEUROTIC TYPE A	5 NEUROTIC TYPE B	6 PSYCHIATRIC ILLNESS	7 REACTORS	8 DISSAT-SATISFIEDS	9 RESIDUAL	TOTAL
Profile Levels and Homogeneities										
Negative affect	low	low	low	high	high-high	high-high	high	average	average	
Pleasurable involvement	low	high-high	average	low	average	low-low	high	average	low	
Satisfaction	high	high	average	low-low	high	low-low	high	low-low	average	
Self-esteem	high	high	average	low	low	average	high	average	low-low	
H̄	.92	.92	.91	.64	.83	.45	.92	.75	.23	
Clinical Ratings Comparison										
Ill	0%(0)	13%(4)	7%(2)	23%(7)	10%(3)	13%(4)	10%(3)	7%(2)	17%(5)	100%(30)
Vulnerable	29 (5)	0 (0)	18 (3)	6 (1)	12 (2)	0 (0)	12 (2)	6 (1)	18 (3)	101 (17)
Improved	13 (3)	13 (3)	13 (3)	13 (3)	0 (0)	4 (1)	17 (4)	22 (5)	4 (1)	99 (23)
Worse	0 (0)	0 (0)	0 (0)	0 (0)	0 (0)	0 (0)	100 (3)	0 (0)	0 (0)	100 (3)
Well	23 (9)	36 (14)	26 (10)	3 (1)	0 (0)	0 (0)	3 (1)	5 (2)	5 (2)	101 (39)
	17	21	18	12	5	5	13	10	11	112

low-low = mean score 1 or more standard deviation below the mean
low   = mean score ½ to 1 standard deviation below the mean
average = signifies an average value
high   = mean score ½ to 1 standard deviation above the mean
high-high = mean score 1 or more standard deviation above the mean

TABLE 16.7
Empirical Groups and Social Interaction Variables

| | ORGANIZATIONS | | HOBBIES | |
TYPES	LEVEL	H̄	LEVEL	H̄
1. Stolid Solids	average	.418	average	(−)
2. Involved Solids	high	(−)	average	.520
3. Mr. Average	average	.46	average	.62
4. Neurotic Type A	average	.62	high	.33
5. Neurotic Type B	average	.71	average	.73
6. Psychiatric Illness	low	.87	high	(−)
7. Reactors	high	(−)	high	(−)
8. Dissatisfieds	very low	(−)	average	(0)
9. Residual	low	.86	low	.77

The Involved Solids and the Reactors contain in their midst some people who are very active in the community. However, there is evidence of considerable heterogeneity in each group with regard to this variable. Thus some members probably participate very little and others are certainly average.

The Psychiatric Illness group and the Residuals participate very little, whereas the other groups are very comparable in this dimension.

The implications of these findings are consistent with those from the urban analysis. No one measure by itself is satisfactory at the current level of development for measuring health and illness. Thus there are individuals who express negative affect, but who are apparently also capable of feelings of pleasure and satisfaction. The sense of pleasurable involvement does show a relationship to social participation, consistent with other studies utilizing this dimension. The sense of long-term satisfaction, however, which is surely an important aspect of psychological well-being, varies independently of negative affect, pleasurable involvement, or participation in community organizations.

It is clear that one could construct a series of "hit-miss" tables for illness and wellness similar to that described in the section on the urban sample, if any one dimension were used as *the* measure of health. For example, scores on long-term satisfaction would lump together people who are definitely well (Stolid Solids and Involved Solids) with people who have definite indications of illness (Neurotic Type A), and some people among the Reactors. Furthermore, the Mr. Average group would be left out of a wellness rating, even though they do exhibit a pattern of consistent, if low-keyed, positive adaption.

In conclusion, it can be said that this analysis of the questionnaire data banks enhances the range of our concepts and develops the analytic model with empirical data. The tripartite concept of health is given specific content and some indication is achieved of the actual distribution of health patterns in populations. One can see, therefore, the beginning of indices that will take into account the way different properties relating to health interact with each other to produce a total effect.

REFERENCES

1. Cattel, R. B. *Factor Analysis*. New York: Harper and Brothers, 1952.

2. Krause, M. S. "Use of Social Situations for Research Purposes." *American Psychologist* 25(1970):748–753.

Editorial Note

The advent of a more rational, deliberate posture toward the solution of social problems is aptly symbolized by the concentrated attention currently being devoted to evaluative research. Our time is becoming, as Edgerton claims in Chapter 18, preëminently the "age of accountability." If social change is increasingly planned change, so the implementation of the plans is ever more closely monitored. One meaning of evaluation is to heighten our awareness of change processes and their outcomes. Doing evaluative research forces more careful and sustained thinking about why we are performing certain operations in social action programs, how we are doing them, and what we hope to accomplish.

Rieker and Suchman underline the character of evaluation as part of an ongoing process. Research on the effectiveness of social psychiatric programs is only occasionally a one-time, sharp judgment about assets and deficits; most often it is an integral element of those programs, a durable exercise in self-surveillance. Thus the authors aver that "the purpose of evaluation is not to 'pass' or 'fail' these activities, but instead to feed back information for their more effective operation."

A significant feature of this chapter is the impressive variety of evaluative modes it describes. The analysis is rather general and abstract, applicable to a wide range of social change efforts, and outlining multiple strategies and tactics of evaluation. It is distinguished by a catholicity of approach in which research is not locked into a single model or design (such as the classic experiment). Instead, the authors are generous toward the whole armamentarium of investigatory methods, including the often-maligned case study and the modest descriptive history. Such hospitality to evaluative alternatives is important, especially since we so frequently encounter an all-or-nothing attitude in assessing programs, in which helpful observations and measurements are mistakenly foregone in the belief that an elegant experimental proof is the only worthwhile research model.

The surveillance of staff behaviors that is intrinsic to program evaluation offers at once a hazard and an advantage. An enhanced self-awareness among the members of a treatment team, for instance, may contribute to the "Hawthorne Effect" *in which their work is improved by the sheer fact of its being observed. In such a case we are hard put to identify specifically altered behaviors and to attribute specified outcomes to the techniques employed. On the other hand, one can argue that the Hawthorne Effect may have very efficacious practical consequences: if the stimulation derived from the very process of scrutiny contributes significantly to the program, then we may choose to forsake scientific rigor (or make it more problematic) in favor of policy benefits.

R. N. W.

* Roethlisberger, F. J., and Dickson, W. J. *Management and the Worker.* Cambridge: Harvard University Press, 1939.

CHAPTER 17

Prescriptions for Evaluation

PATRICIA PERRI RIEKER
EDWARD A. SUCHMAN *

Purpose of Evaluation

EVALUATIVE STUDY is an essential and expanding area of social research intended to contribute to our conceptual knowledge of planned social change, as
well as provide information with which administrators and practitioners can
choose alternative courses of action with some idea of the positive and negative
consequences associated with that choice. Generally, such studies are aimed as
much at understanding the factors influencing the desired change as they are at
understanding whether or not the desired change was achieved. In this chapter
we want to suggest that evaluation has a twofold contribution: The first is to assist
in the administrative aspects of mental health programs; the second is to further
the conceptual development of new modes of thought and practice, such as community or social psychiatry. This twofold contribution is only possible when the
evaluator can attribute the success or failure of a specific program either to the
principles or assumptions guiding the program, or to the operation or implementation of the program.

* This chapter is based in part upon an unpublished speech given by the late Edward A. Suchman in 1968. Dr. Rieker is responsible for reorganizing, writing, and elaborating on certain of Dr.
Suchman's seminal concepts, in addition to her own observations.

From our point of view, evaluation studies are research studies and as such they have to conform, as much as any piece of applied research can, to the basic tenets of the scientific method. The difference between evaluative research and nonevaluative research is a difference in purpose and not a difference in methodology. So the question becomes: What is it that we are trying to do in evaluative research which differs from what we are trying to do in nonevaluative research?

At the most general level, evaluation refers to the process of determining worth or value. The process may range from a subjective assessment based on personal experience to a highly controlled experiment based on the scientific method. In theory, the object of evaluation may be as broad as federal policy on community mental health centers or as narrow as some individual patient's diagnosis. In most cases, however, the purpose of such evaluation is to direct future actions or decisions. Thus evaluation is closely related to decision making, whether the decision involves some personal act or major social policy.

Given the wide range of application, it is easy to understand why so much confusion and debate exists today about what constitutes the most appropriate method of evaluation. Our position in this debate is that different purposes and contexts will require different evaluation designs. The issue is not a question of methodology per se, but rather how to determine the object of evaluation (what exactly is to be evaluated) and, after completion of the study, how the findings can be translated into action. Thus evaluative research is a problem enterprise with a clear-cut relationship to some decision-making function.

However, in addition to practical considerations, it is essential to stress the potential theoretical importance of evaluative research, not because such an emphasis is fashionable, but because it is necessary if serious scholars are to enter the field. More importantly, it is our conviction that evaluative research aimed at testing the underlying principles of social psychiatry or any social intervention program will have greater utility in the long run than evaluation limited to specific program operations.

Innovative mental health programs, as well as professional practice in any field, should be based upon the best available scientific knowledge and theory of that field. From this standpoint, evaluations of the degree to which a program achieved its desired goals (when they are known at all) are ultimately tied to the confirmation or rejection of the underlying assumptions. However, it is common knowledge that specific activities as well as entire programs are carried out largely on the basis of tradition, without sufficient attention to the rationale for believing that they are capable of producing the desired results. On the other hand, "academic" disciplines continue to develop basic theories which fail to tie into professional practice. Evaluation studies which can distinguish between a "technical" versus a "theoretical" failure could aid the development of theoretical models which can link professional models to desired social outcomes.

Evaluation–An Experimental Methodology

One way of formulating some elementary but fundamental conditions for an evaluative study would be to ask about the *kind* of change desired, the *means* by which this change is to be brought about, and the *measures* according to which such change can be recognized. Unless one can visualize an *objective* involving change from some less desirable to some more desirable state of affairs, an *activity* or *program* designed to produce this change, and *criteria* by which one can judge that change has taken or is taking place, one cannot conduct an evaluation study.

Our perspective is to regard evaluation as an experimental methodology applied to the study of human behavior, as moving the experiment out of the laboratory and into some natural setting. We would argue that when you move out into the community with any type of mental health program, basically you are trying to set up an experimental-type situation within an administrative framework which serves as a test of basic hypotheses concerning the way in which services have to be organized to achieve what are considered desirable objectives.

There are several key elements or requirements necessary to this formulation. The first involves the setting up of some administrative programmatic activity (such as a satellite office) that can serve as the *independent* variable or our so-called manipulated stimulus in a field experiment. What is necessary (though not sufficient) in evaluative research, just as in any social experiment, is a clear-cut understanding of what is extraneous to what you are isolating or attempting to manipulate. One needs to ask what are the "causative" factors affecting achievement of the desired outcomes. What is it that you are hypothesizing will produce certain effects?

A second element has to do with the desired effect or objective of the particular experiment. In ordinary applied research this objective is largely one that has to do with the administration of program. In evaluative research it takes on an additional aspect of applying professional practices. The word "evaluative" has real meaning here; namely, there is *value* attached to the objective. People care what happens.

It is not that you are doing an experiment such as applying some drug or a different therapeutic approach in order to see what happens. To fulfill the requirements of our suggested experimental approach you have to specify the value or the desired objective that you wish to achieve with the program or activity. You cannot simply conceive of some series of activities, such as a way of operating a community mental health center, a way of developing some psychotherapeutic regimen, or some drug therapy, just to see what happens. To us that is an inadequate statement, insufficient for evaluation. It is inadequate in the sense of not satisfying one of the basic requirements of methodology: specification of the dependent variable. In the field of evaluative research it becomes extremely important to formulate your desired objectives as dependent variables which have values attached to them, so that if you get one kind of result you can judge it as fair, and if you get another kind of result you can say it is good. *Evaluative* research *cannot* be based upon a nonevaluative hypothesis such as "If I heat iron it will expand" without indicating that you care whether it expands or not. It must be stressed that in evaluative research you care about your objectives, and the hypotheses have to be formulated in that sense. Quite often evaluative research is defined in terms of knowing of what the program consists, but not being at all clear about what effect, outcome, output, or results someone wanted to achieve with the program.

The third requirement that should be considered in conceiving of evaluation as an experimental methodology has to do with the process that joins the independent (planned programs or intervention) to the dependent variable (the desired objective). That intervening process becomes extremely important for social and/or community psychiatry. The intervening process is what we mean by theory and what we are referring to when we talk of trying to aid the conceptual development of social and community psychiatry. What gives us any right to believe that a certain program will achieve the kind of objectives that people want it to achieve? The only thing that can give us such a right is basic theory—an understanding of what it is exactly about our experimental program, about our actions or interventions, that will produce the desired outcome. This means that you have to have some knowledge of what can be seen as interfering with or promoting your desired objectives. You have to have some knowledge of what it is about your program that can intervene in the underlying process.

In a very real sense, then, the intervening variables, as we use the term in social research, become the intervention, as we use the term in social change or experimental research. If a program fails, therefore, you have at least two elements to look at that are more important in evaluative research than in nonevaluative research. In nonevaluative research you are basically testing some hypothesis such as: if "a," then "b." What you attempt to demonstrate is that a change in "a" will produce a change in "b," and then you introduce a series of control variables which will test the validity of the relationship: Is "a" truly related to "b," or is the correlation we observed due to some spurious factor that both "a" and "b" have in common? Then the association between "a" and "b" is simply because they possess this factor in common and not because there is a real causal relationship.

In nonevaluative research a spurious intervening variable can in a sense be traced to a theoretical mistake which somebody else can easily catch and reformulate. An undetected intervening process in evaluative research can lead you to mount an entirely wrong community program which has only a spurious relationship to the real objective. And then you find yourself manipulating an independent experimental variable that has no real association.

The nonevaluative hypothesis, "the more 'a,' the more 'b,' " becomes the evaluative hypothesis: By changing "a" through a planned program, I will increase the possibility of "b," which I judge to be desirable. The evaluative hypothesis concerning the relationship of activity "a" to objective "b" requires critical examination according to control factors which test whether it was really activity "a" that achieved objective "b," and which elaborate upon how and why the activity was able to achieve the objective. *This is the heart of evaluative research.*

To state it another way, the input, the experimental program, may lead to some output which in evaluative research represents the desired objective. Then we anticipate a relationship between programs we implement and outputs or objectives judged to be desirable. It is important to stress here that the inputs in evaluative research have a limitation which they do not have in nonevaluative research. *They have to be socially approved and publicly financed and funded inputs.* They are not simply ideas that you test out in a laboratory, but must be supported by society.

You cannot simply test any interesting hypothesis. You have to get the funds to finance the program in which you have some interest. Those *inputs* become *in a way socially legitimated inputs* rather than *just experimentally justified inputs,* and the outputs *become objectives* that have values attached, as we have indicated earlier. The fact that values are attached to inputs, and more especially to outputs, contributes to the politicization of the conduct and use of evaluation research.

The connection between these inputs and outputs that is most important for social psychiatrists is an understanding of the process whereby a particular input will lead to a particular objective, or, to be concrete, whereby any form of community mental health activity will lead to a lower incidence of nonfunctioning individuals. Another example might involve how certain community mental health activities reduce bed occupancy in mental institutions. Exactly what it is about community mental health programs that leads one to believe that such an objective might be achieved can only be answered by an understanding of the process that creates nonfunctioning people, and which leads your program to change this process and its undesirable outcome. You have to start with a basic theory of the underlying elements that affect the outputs you wish to change. If your program, your input, fails to produce the desired outcome, you can locate the "problem" in either the underlying theory or the operation of the program. Then the evaluative question becomes: Did the community mental health center activities fail to produce the desired results because they technically—in reality—

never got started, or because the theory behind them was inadequate or wrong? So you have a sticky interchange between "causes" of the failure—that is, whether you failed on a technical level because you never really got started, or whether you failed on a theoretical level because you started a good program, but your theory was inadequate.

Take the following example of the definition of mental illness. Can we study the effectiveness of community mental health programs if we don't know exactly what mental health or mental illness are, and we want to promote the former and prevent the latter? We can't, except by convention; we arbitrarily decide that although we do not know exactly what mental health is, we do know that it is good for some people to be with their families and not locked up in institutions. So whether that is mental health or not, one can *define* it as a socially desirable objective and try to attain it. Our concern is that you can get caught up in the disease model of physical medicine, in which you accept the notion that until you define mental illness as a disease whose incidence you can show you've reduced, you can never justify your existence. And we would suggest that a definition of the problem in those terms is very limiting.

Obviously, you must study people who have the effects you're interested in to detect what factors are present in their background in order for you to come up with a diagnosis and some kind of ameliorative action. But it must be recognized, as any medical practitioner or psychotherapist realizes, that this diagnosis and prescription are not derived from conducting an experiment on the person; instead they are derived from the practitioner's familarity with all the theoretical knowledge of the field. But that process still involves an evaluative statement, in the sense that a diagnosis is an evaluative statement about cause, and prescription is an evaluative statement about treatment.

Evaluation—Nonexperimental Methods

Not all scientific activities, especially evaluations, can approximate the experimental model. And so we would argue that case studies, clinical studies, community studies, studies of single mental health centers, and observational descriptive studies of particular programs, all have a legitimate place in the field of evaluation. However, you must remember that what you are doing is diagnosing and prescribing in terms of a single, particular case. You are not *testing* in the sense of *proving* that your prescription and diagnosis is correct, but are applying theoretical knowledge that has been built up through more systematic testing. Which points up one of the purposes of systematic research—to enable practitioners to do case-study evaluation. But the case study is just one level of evaluation.

A second level involves expanding the number of case studies so that you have a collection of them to make up a survey. At this level you can survey a large population of patients, a cross-section of a community, a sample of the clients at a clinic, patients in a hospital, or divisions in a community health clinic. The survey expands upon a case study because it includes a random sample representative of some meaningful population in which you not only have cases of the disease or problem area, but also cases without the disease or problem. This is what we broadly mean by "epidemiology."

The strength of the whole field of epidemiology, the basis on which we get so much of our knowledge of the chronic diseases, has to do with comparison within a population of the characteristics which we distinguish as related to the presence or absence of a disease. So epidemiology is evaluative research in the sense that it compares two groups, as opposed to the case-study method, which deals with only one group.

A third level involves expanding the survey method to what the social scientists call the "panel study," or what in epidemiology or community research has been called the "prospective" or "longitudinal" study. At this level we get four measures by starting with a population which at time one does not have lung cancer; we know a lot of their characteristics, but none of them have the disease. At time two some of them have developed the disease, or the effect in which we are interested; the others have not. We can now go back and examine the differences between the two groups at a time when neither had developed the disease. The effect of this is that it examines the population which doesn't have lung cancer and compares them with those who developed lung cancer to see if they were the ones who started to smoke. This kind of prospective design allows you to make predictions, set up risk factors, develop risk quotients, and develop probabilities for the development of the disease, but it does *not* permit you, in the experimental sense, to really go out and, in a controlled way, divide the population at random and force some people to smoke and make others refrain from smoking. However, it is as close as one can get.

So our argument is that the case-study level is extremely important for clinical diagnosis and prescription, for an understanding within a single case of the dynamics that relate your independent to your dependent variables, and for the development of hypotheses. You do not have case-study methods in the physical sciences because all you can see when you heat iron is that it expands; you cannot really study the iron as you would a case study of an individual *developing* anger as a result of being heated, ignored, or some other social action.

Therefore the case-study method, far from being weak, is a strength of those sciences which deal with individual growth, because it is through the case-study method that you understand what happens in the developmental process of health or illness. Evaluation on this level can be extremely useful and informative. The prospective study, however, starts with a disease-free population or a community as a whole, and over time looks for the development of certain effects, at the same time that it keeps track of *process*, so that *process* can then be related to effect. To us this is the most meaningful design for evaluation and the closest approximation to the experimental model.

Unfortunately, there is a tendency to view program evaluations in terms of the classical experimental design, so people are inclined to think of ongoing mental health programs as if they were new drugs being introduced into therapy, and the model used to *evaluate* them is the traditional "one-shot" evaluation. This model is not appropriate for most mental health programs because they are an ongoing activity. An ongoing organization like a hospital, a community mental health center, or a community program of any sort are not the same as a one-shot program. The one-shot program is the reference for most discussions of evaluation because it fits the traditional (medical) approach more closely; namely, one thinks of a new "cure" and then proceeds to test the effectiveness of this "cure." And if you evaluate in terms of the experimental model, you think of a one-shot test.

Theoretically that is a sound way to proceed, but in reality the situation is somewhat different. In everyday practice we move into an ongoing situation which already has built into it a lot of current activities, and the purpose of evaluation is not to "pass" or "fail" these activities, but instead to feed back information for their more effective operation. (We are becoming more convinced that the real contribution of evaluation in the area of chronic disease—that is, in an area where you don't have a single cause of a disease, where you cannot hope to develop a single antitoxin or something similar for elimination of that disease, but where you have an ongoing process like mental illness or heart disease, a degenerative kind of process, where there is not hope for a cure in the sense of multiple causes—is to provide feedback into a continuous regimen of care, an ongoing operation, a method of treatment, as opposed to an experimental cure.)

Evaluation—an Incremental Approach

In light of the above, we would propose an operational model of evaluation as perhaps more relevant than the experimental model of evaluation, under certain conditions. It is an operational model which builds on administrative terms like

315

pilot or demonstration project, model program, and prototype, but which can have logical differences when viewed from our suggested perspective.

For illustrative purposes, let's begin with the pilot project. In a pilot project we are concerned with trying to test specific approaches to a particular problem and evaluate these varied activities in an experimental sense on a one-shot basis. The point is, either they work or they do not work; if they work we maintain them, and if not, change them. A pilot project should be under constant revision, should change approaches in midstream, and should be flexible enough to revise its procedures as it goes along. The design of this pilot project should contain provisions for "quick" evaluation information that could be used to revise the original idea by changing elements, such as introducing a public health nurse, or removing a psychiatrist, or putting them together as a team. In other words just move back and forth on a true empirical basis, that is, proceed by trial and error. Thus the pilot project would not be evaluated as if it were an ongoing, institutionalized activity, but strictly as a demonstration type of activity.

Emerging from the flexible, trial-and-error, revised pilot project is what we may now call a model program. The model program requires a more experimental type of evaluation because, on the basis of pilot studies, we have now set up what we consider an ideal type of program; in this sense the model program is an ideal. What we want to do is test the evaluative hypothesis that, given the right conditions, the proposed activities (model program) will achieve the desired objectives. At this stage we are not asking how realistic the conditions or inputs are, but rather stating that if *these* conditions are obtained, then we will solve the problem to some degree of satisfaction. To test that hypothesis we need the traditional experimental design (one-shot evaluation), and the model program has to be set up in a way that satisfies all the requirements for this classical design.

If the evaluation indicates that the model program achieves its objectives, then we develop a prototype which embodies and puts into operation as much of the model program as possible. If the evaluation indicates that the model program does not achieve its objectives, then we cannot set up a prototype; instead we should go back to the pilot project level and begin to revise on a trial-and-error basis until a new model program is ready to be tested. In true experimental fashion we move between pilot and model programs until we develop a model program that works, and then see to what extent the model program can be translated into a prototype for an ongoing operational program within given resources.

In order to evaluate the prototype program we need an operational or systems model. The question for an operational system does not involve judging success or failure. What you have at this level is mainly a feedback, recycling, revision type of system which permits you, as you evaluate your program operations, continuous feedback of information for self-evaluation. This then becomes a form of monitoring, a form of quality control, a form of built-in evaluation. The pilot and model program evaluations are important for the development of knowledge, and the operational system is important for the application of knowledge.

All of the foregoing suggestions assume that you can state clear-cut program objectives. Is evaluation research possible without clear-cut program objectives? The starting point for evaluative research is a statement of objectives. To us, the statement of objectives requires that we ask of ourselves such questions as: What do we want action for? Why do we want to reduce mental illness? Why do we want community mental health centers? Why do we want to eliminate social pathology?

The statement of objectives becomes an important problem that has to be resolved in terms of social values. Objectives are set by the value system. Before an evaluation can be carried out, you have to determine the objectives in terms of the value premises. Then these objectives have to be stated in some kind of meaningful framework. Because never-achieved ultimate objectives are unrealistic, you have to break down an intervention program into a series of immediate and intermediate steps moving toward the unattainable ultimate objective, with the ultimate being refined as you make progress with your intermediate objectives. If you accept this notion of incrementalism—moving toward ultimate objectives only in terms of always moving toward the next immediate objective— then a very interesting process occurs. In terms of the means and ends schema, the immediate objective becomes the means to the intermediate objective, and that in turn becomes the means to the next objective. So as you move step by step your objective always is to develop the means to attain a new objective. The independent variable which achieves a dependent variable changes that dependent variable into an independent variable for achieving a new dependent, and so on ad infinitum.

Along with this ongoing, stepwise notion of measurement of objectives, it is useful to think of four major groupings of criteria. The first of these we call *effort*, which refers to your ability to implement the program. This is measured in terms of resources, personnel, time developed, cases seen, cases found, admissions—a whole network of immediate effort. Second you move to a measure of *performance*, which refers to the results of the effort. Here you try to get at achievement, namely, what has been accomplished as a result of that effort. When you get an answer to performance, you raise the third question of *adequacy*. Given this degree of performance, how adequate is it to a reasonable or meaningful solution of the problem? No matter how much effort I put in, and no matter how good that performance, if I still find that it reaches only 2 percent of the people who need treatment, then the fourth criterion, *efficiency*, must be applied. This criterion can be applied only when you have a series of alternately adequate ways to solve a problem, and then you choose in terms of cost-benefit analysis (or some such value) which alternative is the most efficient. This then becomes another way of addressing the question of objectives.

Evaluation Model Related to Purpose

The primary goal of evaluative research is usually to aid the decision-making process concerning some social problem or policy. In the conduct of evaluation studies, administrative considerations will often have precedence over scientific ones. It seems unproductive to continue arguments over whether the classical experimental design is the only model for evaluation research. We have suggested that in the early stages of evaluating a new program, it would probably be more fruitful to utilize a rather fluid, clinical case-study, "anthropological" type of design. Increased understanding of the problem and more detailed specification of the type of activity to be carried out could then be followed by a survey evaluation design which would provide preliminary evidence as to the effectiveness of one's program on an ex post facto or longitudinal basis. Finally, when the stage is reached for a definitive test of some particular program, it would be possible to proceed to a more rigorous experimental design.

It does not make sense to argue in the abstract about which "approach" is "correct." In this chapter we found it useful to distinguish between pilot projects, in which the main objective is to try out different program elements and in which a flexible, case-study approach provides the greatest amount of information, and model projects, in which the emphasis is upon testing a program under ideal conditions and a more rigorous experimental design is indicated. Prototype projects call for an operations research design whose main emphasis is upon the feedback of information for program improvement.

Finally, we have argued that these practical considerations do not rule out the need to view evaluation research within a broader theoretical or methodological perspective. We found it most fruitful to link the evaluative research models to that of the independent-intervening-dependent variable sequence of multicausal analysis. In terms of this logic, the program activity becomes the independent variable which is to be manipulated or changed. The intervening process represents the causal factors which promote or inhibit development of the valued goal. The dependent variable then becomes the desired objectives or changed conditions. The model we propose inherently requires a close linkage between professional practice and academic theory, thus permitting the evaluator to distinguish between what we might call a "technical" versus a "theoretical" failure. Without this distinction, evaluation research will not contribute to either decision making or theoretical knowledge.

BIBLIOGRAPHY

Ackoff, R. G. "The Development of Operations Research as a Science." *Operations Research* 4 (1956):265–295.

Borgatta, E. "Research: Pure and Applied." *Group Psychotherapy* 8 (1955):263–277.

———. "Research Problems in Evaluation of Health Service Demonstrations." *Milbank Memorial Fund Quarterly* 44 (1966):182–199.

Brooks, M. "The Community Action Program as a Setting for Applied Research." *Journal of Social Issues* 21 (1965):29–40.

Campbell, D. T. "Validity of Experiments in Social Settings." *Psychological Bulletin* 54 (1957):297–312.

———. "Administrative Experimentation, Institutional Records, and Nonreactive Measures." In *Improving Experimental Design and Statistical Analysis*, edited by J. C. Stanley. Chicago: Rand McNally, 1967.

———. "Reforms as Experiments." *American Psychologist* 24 (1969):409–429.

———. "Considering the Case Against Experimental Evaluations of Social Innovations." *Administrative Science Quarterly* 15 (1970):110–113.

———, and Stanley, J. C. *Experimental and Quasi-Experimental Design for Research*. Chicago: Rand McNally, 1966.

Caro, F. G., ed. *Readings in Evaluation Research*. New York: Russell Sage Foundation, 1971.

Chapin F. S. *Experimental Designs in Sociological Research*. New York: Harper and Brothers, 1947.

Coleman, J. S. *The Evaluation of Equality of Educational Opportunity*. Baltimore, Md.: Center for the Study of Social Organization of Schools, Johns Hopkins University, 1968.

———. *Policy Research in the Social Sciences*. New Jersey: General Learning Corporation, 1972.

Cottrell, L. S., Jr., and Sheldon, E. B. "Problems of Collaboration Between Social Scientists and the Practicing Professions." *Annals of the American Academy of Political and Social Science*. 346, March 1963.

Doby, J. T. *An Introduction to Social Research*. New York: Appleton-Century-Crofts, 1957.

Elinson, J. "Effectiveness of Social Action Programs in Health and Welfare." In *Assessing the Effectiveness of Child Health Services*. Report of 56th Ross Conference on Pediatric Research. Columbia: Ross Laboratories, 1967.

Evans, J. W. "Evaluating Social Action Programs." *Social Science Quarterly* 50 (1969):568–581.

Freeman, H. E., and Sherwood, C. C. "Research in Large Scale Intervention Programs." *Journal of Social Issues* 21 (1965):11–20.

French, J. "Experiments in Field Settings." In *Research Methods in Behavioral Sciences*, edited by L. Festinger and D. Katz. New York: Holt, Rhinehart, 1953.

Glock, C., ed. *Survey Research in the Social Sciences*. New York: Russell Sage Foundation, 1967.

Greenburg, B. G., and Mattison, B. F. "The Whys and Wherefores of Program Evaluation." *Canadian Journal of Public Health* 46 (1955):293–299.

Gruenburg, E. M. ed. "Evaluating the Effectiveness of Mental Health Services." *Milbank Memorial Fund Quarterly* 44 (1966): pt. 2.

Herzog, E. *Some Guidelines for Evaluative Research*. Washington, D.C.: U.S. Government Printing Office, 1959.

Hyman, H. *Survey Design and Analysis: Principles, Cases and Procedures*. New York: Free Press, 1955.

————, and Wright, C. R. "Evaluating Social Action Programs." In *The Uses of Sociology*, edited by P. F. Lazarsfeld, W. H. Sewell, and H. L. Wilensky. New York: Basic Books, 1967.

————; and Hopkins, T. K. *Applications of Methods of Evaluation: Four Studies of the Encampment for Citizenship*. Los Angeles, Calif.: University of California Press, 1962.

Klineberg, O. "The Problem of Evaluation Research." *International Social Science Bulletin* 7 (1955):347–351.

Lynd, R. S. *Knowledge for What?* Princeton, N.J.: Princeton University Press, 1969.

Merton, R. K., and Devereaux, E. C., Jr. "Practical Problems and the Uses of Social Science." *Transaction* 1 (1964):18–21.

Pelz, D., and Andrews, F. M. "Detecting Causal Priorities in Panel Study Data." *American Sociological Review* 28 (1964):836–848.

Reicken, H. W. *The Volunteer Work Camp: A Psychological Evaluation*. Cambridge, Mass.: Addison-Wesley, 1952.

Rieker, P. P. "Reflections on Evaluative Research." Mimeographed. Pittsburgh, Penna.: Department of Sociology, University of Pittsburgh, 1971.

————. "Utilization of Evaluation Studies." Paper presented at American Sociological Association in New Orleans, La., 1972.

————. "The Utilization of Evaluation Research: The Social Organization of an Intellectual Activity." Ph.D. dissertation, University of Pittsburgh, 1974.

Rosenthal, R. *Experimental Effects in Behavioral Research*. New York: Appleton-Century-Crofts, 1966.

————, and Weiss, R. "Problems of Organizational Feedback." In *Social Indicators*, edited by R. Bauer. Cambridge, Mass.: MIT Press, 1966.

Rossi, P. H. "Boobytraps and Pitfalls in the Evaluation of Social Action Programs." *Proceedings* of the Social Statistics Section, American Statistical Association, 1966, pp. 127–132.

————. "Evaluating Social Action Programs." *Transaction* 4 (1967):51–53.

Schulberg, H. C., and Baker, F. "Program Evaluation Models and the Implementation of Research Findings." *American Journal of Public Health* 58 (1968):1284–1255.

Suchman, E. A. "Principles and Practices of Evaluative Research." In *An Introduction to Social Research*, edited by John Doby. New York: Appleton-Century-Crofts, 1957.

————. "A Model for Research and Evaluation on Rehabilitation." In *Sociology and Rehabilitation*, edited by Marvin Sussman. Washington, D.C.: American Sociological Association, 1966.

————. *Evaluative Research*. New York: Russell Sage Foundation, 1967.

————. "Evaluating Educational Programs." *Urban Review* 3 (1969):15–17.

————. "The Role of Evaluative Research." *Proceedings* of the 1969 Invitational Conference on Testing Problems, pp. 93–103.

Weiss, C. H. "The Politicization of Evaluation Research." *Journal of Social Issues* 26 (1970) 57–68.

————, ed. *Evaluating Action Programs: Readings in Social Action and Education*. Boston: Allyn & Bacon, 1972.

————. *Evaluation Research*. Englewood Cliffs, N.J.: Prentice-Hall, 1972.

Weiss, R. S., and Rein, M. "The Evaluation of Broad Aim Programs: A Cautionary Case and a Moral." *Annals of the American Academy of Political and Social Science* 385 (1969):133–142.

————. "The Evaluation of Broad Aim Programs: Difficulties in Experimental Design and an Alternative." *Administrative Science Quarterly* 15 (1970):97–109.

Wright, C. R., and Hyman, H. H. "The Evaluators." In *Sociologists at Work: Essays on the Craft of Social Research*, edited by Phillip E. Hammond. New York: Basic Books, 1964.

Editorial Note

In the following selection Edgerton underlines Rieker and Suchman's concern (Chapter 17) with evaluative research as an integral part of mental health programing. He stresses the effect of research on ongoing program operations, seeing in it a cybernetic, self-steering function: "The growing necessity for solving social problems through planned action requires a self-correcting system for the conservation of resources and the detection of unexpected and undesirable consequences." More and more clearly, what Max Weber in The Theory of Social and Economic Organization, foresaw as "the rationalization of life, the disenchantment of the world" entails evaluation as an imperative, routine accompaniment of action itself.

The editorial discussions of Chapters 3 and 4 (pp. 29–45, 46–73) point to problems besetting the community mental health movement today. In one sense the array of assessments reviewed by Edgerton form a response to some of the most telling criticism of the centers' operations. Edgerton is low-keyed and shrewd in his analysis of the history of community centers, the overexpectations aroused by early enthusiasm for this scheme, and the energetic attempts to come to grips with the measurement of effectiveness. He makes the revealing observation that the long-standing state mental hospital system, which the centers were designed to complement or even supplant, has itself never been subjected to full evaluation. The discussion includes encouraging reports on techniques for measuring the bedrock criterion of efficacy: the changing health states of treated populations.

Finally, Edgerton stresses that the measurement enterprise is value-laden. He notes, for instance, that there is a continuing problem of divergency among the views of staff, patients, and others in the community on the choice of treatment goals and the estimates of relative success in reaching them. In this he supports Rieker and Suchman's contention that evaluative research must begin precisely here, with values per se. One of its chief merits is that such research demands that our values be examined and articulated in a much more thoroughgoing fashion than has usually been the case.

R. N. W.

CHAPTER 18

The Measurement of Mental Health Center Program Effects

J. WILBERT EDGERTON

THE IMPACT of mental health center programs on the recipients of service, on the mental health services delivery system, and on the structure of community services in general, has been a matter of controversy. Opinions differ as to the validity of judgments brought so soon in the life of the mental health center movement, either on the side of the efficacy of centers or on their not having lived up to their promise.

There is no reliable basis for disagreement on the long-range impact of mental health center programs, for the era of the comprehensive mental health center has been in existence for only a relatively brief period. Federal legislation authorizing construction monies [23] was enacted in October 1963, and authorization of staff support [25] two years later. The first center received approval for construction in 1965, and the first federal grant for staffing was not awarded until 1966. Following that and through Fiscal Year 1973, when the Nixon administration halted support for new staffing or construction proposals, it was expected that 515 mental health centers would be funded. Of these, 152 would be supported for construction only, 128 for staffing only, and 235 for both construction and staffing. They would serve 76 million people, or 36 percent of the population of fifty states, Puerto Rico, and Guam. It was estimated that approximately 324,000 children (aged zero to nineteen) and 700,000 adults would receive direct services from the operating mental health centers in Fiscal Year 1973. The federal dollar investment in the 515 centers was approximately $625 million.[27]

As of December 1972, only 340 of the federally funded centers were operational. Minimally, these operating centers were furnishing the five essential services, as defined in federal regulations,[24] of inpatient, outpatient, partial hospital, emergency, and consultation and education services.

Other activities included rehabilitation services, training, research and evaluation, and special services for children and adolescents, the retarded, the geriatric, alcoholics, and drug abusers. These operational centers covered 182 of the 502 catchment areas defined as poverty areas in the country.

Positive Effects of Mental Health Centers

In phasing out federal support for the mental health centers program, the office of the secretary of the Department of Health, Education, and Welfare declared that the program was a significant one which had proven itself. Indeed, the secretary could cite a number of indications that mental health centers have made an impact on the mental health delivery system, particularly the state mental hospitals. Where community mental health centers had been in operation three years or more, persons from those catchment areas had a 30 percent lower chance of being a resident in a state mental hospital than as true for the country as a whole. Residents of catchment areas where mental health centers had been in operation for as long as one and one-half years had a 17 percent lower chance of being a resident in a mental hospital than for the country as a whole. Admission rates of residents of catchment areas where mental health centers had operated for three or more years were 22 percent lower than for the country as a whole.[27]

A specific study of the effect on state hospitalization of a community mental health center is that by Wolford and associates.[39] They matched as closely as possible census tracts from their center's catchment area with census tracts from a catchment area without a center on the demographic variables of age, race, education, and income. Both areas were served by the same state hospital. They compared admission rates of the two areas over a two-and-one-half-year period following the opening of the center. Rates of admission from the center catchment area declined 5 percent, as compared with 1.9 percent for the matched noncenter catchment area. The unmatched tracts from the center catchment area showed an even greater decline in rate of admissions: 8.1 percent, with people being older, more educated, and affluent. Hospitalization for more than one year showed significant differences in declines as between the center's catchment area tracts and their matched noncenter counterparts after the center went into operation. The center catchment area tracts showed 18 percent decline in patients hospitalized for more than a year, while the noncenter tracts showed only a 3 percent decline. The lowest income areas showed the greatest decrease in rates of admission to the state hospital, and a study of referrals from emergency service to the mental health center showed high rates of patients who previously would have been sent to the state hospital. Nationwide, 16 percent of patients being seen at mental health centers had been previously hospitalized in state hospitals. [11]

Criticism of Mental Health Centers

Perhaps the most focused critique, and most critical review of the mental health center program to date, is one conducted by Ralph Nader's Center for the Study of Responsive Law. [22] Presuming to speak from the consumer point of view, this review takes the National Institute of Mental Health, the federal body responsible for administering the centers' programs, to task for not assuring that the program fulfilled the anticipated effects proclaimed at its initiation. It accuses National Institute of Mental Health officials of misrepresentating the effects of centers and programs, of not enforcing its own operating regulations, of designing a program that extends the medical model to the alleviation of social ills, and perhaps with the most vehemence of all, of not having eliminated state mental hospitals or even truly reducing their patient loads. Other criticisms were imposition of catchment areas by population size rather than by ecological grouping, specification of primarily clinical services as "essential" services, omission of rehabilitative services as "essential," and nonspecificity of the definitions of "reasonable volume of services" to those unable to pay, of continuity of care, of coordination with other agencies, and of adequate community involvement. Furthermore, there was criticism of the lack of earlier evaluation of the mental health centers program by the National Institute of Mental Health.

This is not the place for the resolution of any differences in viewpoints on the impacts of centers. It does seem obvious that state mental hospitals and the systems that support them are alive and well, and the most telling criticism of the mental health centers program is that generally it is a parallel system of care and hardly the keystone of the whole network of mental health services that was envisioned. The main reason for this is finances. Mental health centers usually are not well-enough supported by federal, state, or local funding to enable them to provide long-range care for but a small percentage of those unable to pay. State budgets for mental health still go overwhelmingly to state hospitals, commonly in the 80–90 percent range, and the powerful bureaucracies built up over the years in and for mental hospitals are relatively unyielding as regards unitary financing of institutional and community-based care. Tradition and the legal statutes uphold this point of view. Political and economic factors also play a large part in the resistance to change in mental health agencies toward the decentralization of resources necessary for a viable unitary community-based system of mental health care. Closing or reducing substantially an established mental hospital is perceived as working a hardship on the economy of the immediate community, and results in citizen protests and legislative arousal.

With only about one-third of the country's catchment areas covered by mental health centers (515 of 1,498), and just over one-third of the people (36 percent), the locus of power is clearly on the side of perpetuating state hospital systems for some time to come. To have expected the mental health centers program to turn this state of affairs around in the time it has had, and with the political odds against it, is to have expected the impossible. There is clear evidence that centers do make a difference in rates of admission and chances for being a resident in state mental institutions where they exist, but it is probably expecting too much for such a difference to be reflected in national statistics, in view of the relatively small coverage.

The Problem of Evaluation

Whatever the current status of valid evaluation data on mental health center programs, the times emphatically require evaluation operations to be carried out. It is no accident that valid and reliable methods have been relatively slow in development. For one thing, the press of treatment service needs for the time of mental health services personnel has essentially precluded their involvement with formal program evaluation practices. For another, service personnel as a group, while interested in treatment outcomes, are not usually disposed personally to formalize the criteria for particular outcomes. In general, they have not had the requisite skills and knowledge for effective functioning in this complex area. Mental health center administrators, as a rule, have felt their budgets could not accommodate the salaries of qualified program evaluation staff. There are exceptions to this, of course, and some state mental health agencies have designated program evaluation staffs, with requisite budgets to support them. A few states have statutes requiring program evaluation or utilization review. But it is probably safe to say that no state is carrying out systematic evaluation of mental health center program effects throughout its community program. Legislators have been more interested in responding to the service demands of their constituent citizens.

This press for services has also led to emphasis on program efforts rather than on program effectiveness. Mental health agencies, national, state, and local, in order to justify program budgets, have demonstrated the number of programs launched, the number of patients seen, the estimated size of the problem, and the number of personnel needed compared with those employed. In short, statements have been made on the efforts expended with the resources provided, in comparison with the estimated size of the problem. The population has generally been pleased to know that something was being done for its mentally ill, but without any real knowledge of the effectiveness of such measures. It is striking that in the period of more than a century in which state mental hospitals were the primary mental health program in this country, never has there been a really concerted effort to determine program effectiveness. There were individual efforts to determine some particular clinical treatment outcomes, but no systematic built-in program evaluation activities in this multibillion-dollar public program expenditure.

Another factor in the absence of effective and working program evaluation designs is the complexity of the variables involved. For example, the quality at issue, mental health, exists not in discrete categories, but as a continuous variable. It exists in degrees of more or less, not as present or absent.[13] Furthermore, the relationship between mental health and the product of the impairment of mental health, mental disorder, has not been specified. It has not been established whether mental health and mental disorder vary inversely, or indeed whether they exist on the same continuum. These qualities do not exist in observable absolute quantities because an end point of zero, at which they are nonexistent, from which to measure or establish units of direct measure, has not been specified. So we can only describe changes in mental health or mental disorder.

Describing such changes or assessing the mental health or mental disorder of an individual means making judgments as to the degree of its existence in comparison with some implicit or explicit standard, some criterion. These judgments are really inferences based on observable behaviors defined as indicative of health or disorder. Changes in the behaviors imply changes in mental health or mental disorder. The task in evaluation is to define the criterion in explicit terms and then to determine the amount or nature of change attributable to the specified intervention. A central problem has been the complexity of the criterion behaviors, depending as much as they do on the accuracy of self-reporting of psychic states. The intervention techniques have also been difficult to specify, and the necessity of being certain that they are causal of behavior change only adds to the methodological difficulties in evaluating treatment outcomes or program effectiveness.

If the variables are complex in evaluating treatment procedures, they are even more problematical for program-level or community-level interventions and effects. Controls in design, as practiced in the experimental laboratory, are rarely, if ever, possible with mental health center programs. Matching treated with untreated groups raises ethical questions. Matching one population group with another may introduce gross imprecision. Since the mental health of the population group served by a mental health center is a function of the social, economic, and political environmental systems, and since these three systems are admittedly highly interdependent, measuring the mental health impact of interventions at the community level on any one of them requires very sophisticated conceptual models, perhaps beyond anything so far perfected.

It is also no accident that there is an awakening consciousness of the need for accomplishing mental health center program evaluation. Some impetus for this has come from the realization by the taxpayers, by mental health professionals themselves, and by government administrators that a program so potentially costly as the mental health center program should demonstrate its effectiveness if it is to be continued. Furthermore, evaluation data are a necessity for program modification. So in order to assure program change to meet changing conditions in social systems or populations to be served, evaluation procedures must be present.

We have also entered an era which stipulates that health care, including mental health care, is a right, not just a privilege. Implementation of that ideal includes the concepts of comprehensiveness of program, coordination of services, and continuity of care. It also includes the concept of financial, geographical, and psychological accessibility of services to all people. Evaluation activities are the means for rational choices of services, for information on coordination of mental health services in the community, including and extending beyond the mental health center, for proof of continuity of care throughout the network, and for assurances that services are accessible to all ethnic and socioeconomic groups, near and far.

The needs in the mental health field have been so acute and broad in scope that it has been the custom to accept new programs on faith. But we can no longer afford the luxury, either morally or financially, of developing just any mental health program on the premise that it will be a contribution. The growing necessity for solving social problems through planned action requires a self-correcting system for the conservation of resources and the detection of unexpected and undesirable consequences. This will be particularly true as we attempt preventive interventions for whole population segments. The mental health center has a mandated preventive program along with its services of remediation and rehabilitation. The measurement of program effects follows necessarily, given this set of forces in action.

There is a growing trend toward appraising health programs through cost-benefit or cost-effectiveness analysis. The perfection of this analysis enables the program manager to decide whether the expected benefit warrants the expenditure of the resources that would be necessary to achieve it, or even to know if he has sufficient resources available. Or the manager may be enabled to see that he has achieved a certain benefit at a certain cost, but the expected increments of benefit beyond that will consume disproportionate amounts of resources. With this information he may decide that the additional costs would not be well expended. Cost-benefit or cost-effectiveness analysis can help to answer the growing number of legislators and program managers who want knowledge of the return rate on program appropriations.

Perhaps the most important index of the awakening consciousness of the need for effective mental health center program evaluation is the federal legislation stipulating that up to 1 percent of congressional appropriations for mental health programs be available to the secretary of the Department of Health, Education, and Welfare for program evaluation.[28] Monies totaling several millions of dollars have thus been available for program evaluation, whereas before the time of the legislation none had been available specifically for that purpose. No more tangible evidence of the arrival of the "age of accountability" could be adduced. Some of this was brought about as a result of the extensiveness of the programs of the early and middle 1960s which were designed to eliminate social, economic, educational, health, and mental health deficits and deprivation. The magnitude of expenditures for these programs essentially forced some accounting of effectiveness.

Early Mental Health Center Evaluation Strategy

The press for accountability led to the use of the available funds in a number of ways. Known as the "1 percent monies," they were divided three ways: .25 percent to the office of the secretary, .25 percent to the Public Health Service's Health Services and Mental Health Administration, and the other .50 percent to its operating agencies. These monies first became available to the National Institute of Mental Health (NIMH) for community mental health center program evaluation in the latter part of Fiscal Year 1969. In that year and the successive two years, the sums for all three echelons were respectively $793, $838, an $900 thousand.[38] Total NIMH money for mental health program evaluation ii Fiscal Year 1973 was $6.1 million, with the largest portion going for evaluatioi of mental health centers (p. 19).[4]

At the time of the availability of the first evaluation monies, given the un certainties and exigencies of the timing of the federal appropriations, NIMH hac neither the full-time staff nor the schedule through which to develop a gradual step-by-step program. Consequently, most early efforts went to develop method: with which to do evaluation, and others focused on the degree and circum stances under which "process" objectives were met. For example, for the objec tive of responsiveness of services to community needs, contracts were let for the development of methods of catchment area analysis and for procedures foi utilization review and for evaluating citizen participation processes. For the ob jective of availability of services, contracts were let to study the financial, psy chological, geographical, and temporal factors related to accessibility.

Contracts were also let to study factors in equity of services to different so cioeconomic classes, to study models of children's services, and to look at the im pact of centers on availability and quality of services in four specific counties. A methods study related to the objective of availability of services attempted to de velop the criteria for program consultation to schools (p. 4).[38]

Examples of contract studies related to the objective of organization of ser vices for continuity of care and efficiency of operation are: (1) the development of methods to measure continuity of care; (2) methods of cost finding in centers; (3) comparing day care with inpatient care; (4) studies of the integration of mental health care with other health services delivery and other care-giving agencies; (5) a study of administrative functions in relation to improved services; and (6) a study on the application of systems technology to the mental health center pro gram (p. 4).[38]

Other objectives or principles of center programs to which funded studies have been directed include shifting the locus of care to the community, which necessitates studying the impact of centers on state mental hospital utilization as well as the relationships between the two facilities, and increasing community support, which requires studying available sources of funding (p. 4).[38]

The Evaluation of Effort

The yield from these studies has not been definitive evaluations of center pro grams, but more of a description of program effort, and in some cases the devel opment of workable methods for evaluating some process aspect of center programing.

Program effort describes the application of resources in manpower, facilities, or funding, and is often reflected in service indices of numbers and categories of consumers served, hours devoted to a given program activity, or numbers of agency contacts or liaisons developed. An example of a study of program effort is one directed at the possible differential factors in the growth of mental health resources in two counties with federally funded mental health centers, as compared with two comparable counties without centers.[26] Although all four counties progressed substantially in the development of mental health resources in the period of 1958–1970, the two counties with federally funded centers progressed much more substantially than did the two without the centers. Federal funding enabled the two programs to include significantly more preventive elements, such as education, and to have more impact on other allied programs, such as vocational rehabilitation and corrections. Having mental health services available in the local communities was also an important factor in the reduction in use of the state hospitals. It was also shown that the existence of significant local mental health programs is a function of funding, leadership, and community organization skills from state and national levels. This was a study in quantity of services, or effort, as opposed to quality of services, or program outcomes.

Another example of a study of program effort was a contract attempt to determine child services in selected mental health centers, and to describe models for the delivery of services to children.[35] Through a mail survey of 206 centers, it was shown that although all responding centers provided some services to children or youth, there were significant gaps in services. Of the five "essential services" for federal funding, partial hospitalization and inpatient services for children are the most deficient. Of responding centers, only 63 percent provided all the five "essential services" for children, and only 79 percent did so for adolescents. While these findings could not be generalized for the country, the early results impelled NIMH to implement a policy that all five essential services should be provided to children. (The five services, as stated earlier, are inpatient, outpatient, partial hospitalization, emergency services, and consultation and education.)

There are many other contract studies of program effort, or for information on center programs, which could serve as the basis for national policy or consulting activity changes, but which do not represent quality of program or a measure of effectiveness of services. Some of these include such subjects as community involvement in program planning and policy decisions, in obtaining political, financial, and psychological support, and the delivery of services; the hours of the availability of emergency care, partial hospitalization, and outpatient care in mental health centers; sources of center funding; and studies of the impact of mental health centers on state hospital systems. In Colorado, as a case in point, it was determined that regions served by centers experienced a greater rate of reduction in state hospital resident population over the same time period than those not served by centers (p. 9).[32] In addition, the admission rates for regions served by centers declined significantly from 1966 to 1970, whereas the admission rates for regions not served by centers increased significantly over the same period (p. 13).[32]

Additional findings of the Colorado studies established that state hospitals and mental health centers served essentially different populations.[33] Hospitals served an older population, a less-educated population, and a higher proportion of widowed and divorced persons than did centers. Mental health centers did not serve the aged and the very young, nor persons with junior high school education and less, as represented proportionally in the population base of catchment areas. Centers served a higher proportion of widowed and divorced persons than their representation in the population base warranted. Coincident with these differences, and correlated, since income and education correlate very highly, is the fact that hospitals served a lower-income population than did centers. However, centers served a lower-income group proportionately than their representation in the population warranted, suggesting that groups with higher income seek private care, or have fewer mental health service needs.

The Colorado study showed for 1969–1970, that different clinical populations were served by state hospitals and mental health centers. Centers treated higher percentages of diagnosed neurotics, child adjustment disorders, psychophysiological disorders, personality disorders, social maladjustment, and transient situational disorders than did state hospitals. Hospitals treated higher percentages of the psychotic, alcoholic, and brain-disordered patients than did centers, essentially serving those requiring intensive and perhaps long-term residential care (p. 61).[31]

The Development of Methods

Several contract studies produced methods for later use in program evaluation of mental health centers. An important early study aimed at developing a method for cost finding and rate setting in centers, to result in establishing fees for services and negotiating with third-party payers, and state and federal funding sources.[34] Four methods were developed, including a pencil-and-paper approach and a sophisticated computer-based cost-finding method derived from a Bayesian theory of analysis. The methods were tested for three months in a mental health center, and led to widespread interest in the field and a demand for training.

Another methods study involved the development of a system for measuring continuity of care in a mental health center.[1] The product was the Continuity of Care Inventory, tested in a single-facility center but designed for use in multiunit centers as well. The Inventory is adaptable to small centers, and to a center's capacity for evaluation. It requires no elaborate data-collecting equipment and is not burdensome to therapists. The data provide a picture of continuity in all the direct services, and can serve as a basis for program description which may lead to program improvement. These are data relative to admission and movement of patients within the center and out, to stability of patient-caretaker relationships, to communication among caretakers relative to a patient, and to the retrieval of patients who miss appointments or who are on unauthorized leave. The Inventory's usefulness lies in monitoring the processes of continuity of care in a mental health center.

A third study was devoted to the development of methods and instruments for evaluating school mental health consultation programs.[29] Models for three types of program consultation were put forward, each in stages and with suggested measures for evaluation. The three types of consultation are agency-centered staff development, client-centered staff development, and project development. The instruments facilitate the statement of explicit expectations by both consultant and consultee, and evaluation of consultation outcomes. Film presentations on children with problems are included, along with instructions for their use in assessing consultation results. It is not known how greatly employed or how effective these methods are for assessing school consultation program outcomes.

A fourth study in method concerned itself with developing, testing, and implementing a program-monitoring system in eleven alcoholism treatment centers.[36] Aimed at determining the extent to which the alcoholism treatment centers were meeting the objectives of the National Institute of Alcohol Abuse and Alcoholism, the contracter developed a procedural manual for data collection and conducted a two-month operational test of the monitoring system. Beginning with the explicit goals of the alcoholism treatment centers in providing direct services and indirect services, taking into account the administrative and management means to deliver services, and also specifying appropriate assessment measures for progress toward the goals, all together comprised the necessary strategy for measuring program outcomes. The information at hand shows the system devised produced client and population profiles within catchment areas, information on community and interagency relationships, and some information on effort expended on indirect services.

As to treatment outcomes, the assessment of direct services effectiveness, three indices of the severity of alcoholism were derived. They are the criterion measures of client improvement as a result of treatment. By name they are the

Quantity-Frequency Index for alcohol intake, the Impairment Index for the individual due to alcoholism, and the Self-Perception Index, or the individual's perception of his ability to cope with the alcoholism problem. Early data show these indices changing with treatment and follow-up of clients at 30-day, 90-day, and 180-day intervals. Facilitating this data yield was an automatic data processing system with appropriate forms to provide individual client and statistical output reports, which could in turn be used for program monitoring and to support decisions for program improvement. Other data collected were those required to satisfy the information requirements for administration and management, cost accounting and budget, program planning, and research. The total effort in this project seemed to produce a very useful tool for program evaluation, and one that can be expanded and adapted as needs specify. However, the data were not available as of the 1972 report for assessing the effectiveness of treatment procedures for alcoholics in the eleven alcoholic treatment centers.

Impact on Community Structure

In prescribing continuity of care and comprehensiveness of services, the conceptualizers of the comprehensive mental health center at the NIMH visualized linkages of mental health services with existing care-giving agencies. This would mean a network of services providing for the mental health needs of clients, but also for their vocational, physical health, subsistence, and other needs as well. From this point of view, it is important to know the impact of the advent of the mental health center on the community's network of services and upon the structure.

To this end, a number of studies have been focused on interagency relationships and citizen participation. Two will be reviewed here. In one of these, six mental health centers in four states, all serving some poverty area populations, became the basis for case studies.[8] Extensive interviewing was conducted in each community, including key administrative and lower-level staff, directors of other care-giving agencies, and representatives of citizen groups.

Three relatively middle-class patterns of citizen participation were identified: elitist governing board, narrowly advisory, and mixed. In all three of these, the interests of the professionals and community leaders are dominant, practically to the exclusion of the interests of other consumers. This state of affairs is likely to be accompanied by fairly traditional treatment programs and the feeling by poverty-area residents that the center program is not responsive or accountable to community needs. Three other patterns of citizen participation were identified as activist-adversary advisory boards, consumer control, and participation through staff.

Patterns of interagency relations that emerged from this study were categorized as isolationist-independent, informally interdependent, or totally interdependent. The first may produce conflicts among agencies that seriously hamper continuity of care, and removes the center from accountability to the residents it serves. The informal interdependent pattern relies on the mutual interests of cooperating agencies and is thus easily terminated. An integrated network of services which avoids duplication of effort is the expected product of the totally interdependent pattern of interagency relationships, and this is, of course, the ideal.

The study concluded that the responsible involvement of consumer representatives in planning, administration, control, and evaluation is desirable. This is an important factor in solving the problem of having mental health centers responsive and accountable to the poverty-area citizens they serve. A second conclusion was that more responsive services can be provided through the utilization of new-career persons in responsible staff roles. But there must be opportunities for advancement and remuneration commensurate with their responsibilities. Finally, it was concluded that alternative solutions to the problems of citizen participation and interagency relationships must be recognized by professionals and lay persons in the community. Some possibilities would be through the use of newsletters, workshops, consultants, and technical advisors.

In a second study of the impact of the mental health center on the community's network of services, a stratified sample of nine centers was chosen on the basis of having been in operation for at least two years, on median income, on percent nonwhite in the catchment area, and on number of inpatient facilities.[30] The relationships among these centers and the other care-giving agencies in the community (schools, law enforcement, welfare, public health, social agencies, other mental health agencies) were examined, focusing on staff members and boards of centers, and the staffs of other agencies. Respondents were asked to describe, through mail questionnaires and structured interviews, the nature and extent of the relationships among the mental health centers and other agencies, and to explain how the relationships affected accessibility, continuity, and comprehensiveness of care.

Through ranking mental health centers on four variables, an Interagency Network measure was derived. The variables were: (1) proportion of staff time devoted to consultation and education; (2) proportion of consultation and education staff time directed to care-giving agencies; (3) proportion of referrals of new clients to the center from other care-giving agencies; (4) proportion of clients referred to other agencies at the termination of treatment. The data from which these variables were developed were contained in the Annual Inventory Reports prepared by the centers for NIMH.

The measures for accessibility, continuity of care, and comprehensiveness came from ratings of satisfaction of the centers' staffs and staff members of other agencies with the interaction of center staff and other agency staff, and the referral of clients between centers and other agencies. A five-point scale of satisfaction was used.

The proportion of staff time in the nine centers devoted to consultation and education varied from 5 percent to 30 percent. There was no relationship between the proportion of staff time given to consultation and education and the proportion of referrals received by the centers from other care-giving agencies. This being true, it is not surprising that no correlation was found between accessibility and interagency network measures. Negative correlations were found between the interagency network measure and continuity and comprehensiveness. In the nine centers continuity and comprehensiveness were moderately and positively correlated, but accessibility was negatively correlated with continuity and comprehensiveness. Decentralization seemed to have more relationship with accessibility than did the index of interagency network.

This study suffers from lack of definitive criterion measures of accessibility, continuity, and comprehensiveness. It also lacks sufficient information on referral practices on which the interagency network index was based. These weaknesses preclude any definitive conclusions. However, the case studies revealed a wide range of strategies for initiating, developing, and maintaining program interaction with other care-giving agencies. The strongest conclusions from the study were that decentralization of services is related to accessibility, and that sharing of staff also promotes accessibility of services.

Methods of Measuring Treatment Outcomes

While the measurement of the impact of mental health center programs on the recipients of service cannot feasibly be done independently of the processes through which services are delivered, clearly the measurement of services' effects is at the heart of the efforts to determine if the center is reaching its goals. A center exists primarily to deliver its direct treatment services and its services of consultation and education for the ultimate benefit of individuals and the whole community. All other aspects of its program exist in order to facilitate delivery of those services. So it is understandable that most evaluation efforts have been expended in developing workable techniques, valid and reliable, for determining the impact of treatment services on recipients. The principles by which the indirect services of consultation and education are evaluated are, of course, exactly the same, but the variables and logistics are considerably more complex.

Over the past decade several major efforts have been directed at the construction of methods of treatment evaluation which focused on outcomes for individual patients. Referred to as "individualized goal attainment measures" (p. 23),[9] the methods embody a statement of behavioral goals for each patient in relation to a course of treatment for a stated period of time. Because the goals are stated in terms of observable overt behaviors—for example, "works x-days weekly," "sleeps x-hours nightly," "attends class regularly," "uses hallucinogens less than once a month"—concrete outcomes are more easily noted than in the use of more generalized adjustment or well-being scales, which depend so much on the subjective judgment of patients, therapists, and family members. The chief disadvantage for some of the methods is found in the individuality itself. When behavioral goals are set for and with the patient in terms of his presenting behaviors, and he is later appraised against only his own baseline, information is not usually provided which compares him with other patients on a given characteristic. Measurement against outside and independent criteria, such as would be effected through the use of standard nosological descriptions of disorders, or even through the highly fallible judgment of treatment effectiveness by the lay society, is not in this manner effected.

In spite of the lack of the benefit of generalization, or the criterion of normativeness, there are important dividends in the use of individualized goal attainment measures (p. 23).[9] In the first place, the patient benefits directly. Improvement in service delivery should follow this method of focusing on specific, individual, patient progress. Patients cannot help but benefit from the efforts they and the staff, family, and other persons expend in fulfilling the explicit goals that are established. Second, staff can be provided important new incentives. Such concrete client change provides timely feedback for effectiveness of effort and treatment method employed. The relationship between effort and reward will be much more clearly understood and can lead to appropriate and more immediate differential treatment approaches.

Third, these methods seem to be adaptable to a broad range of management procedures and research efforts. Whenever management goals can be specified in outcome behavioral terms, goal attainment can be ascertained. The methods can be used with individual staff, supervisor, or administrator behaviors. Even promotional and monetary rewards can be tied to the behavioral outcomes. They are an essential part of comprehensive evaluation programs, and lead to the increasingly important procedures of cost-benefit and cost-effectiveness determination.

Brief descriptions of four individualized goal attainment methods developed for treatment evaluation will be presented here:

GOAL ATTAINMENT SCALING

Goal Attainment Scaling, as developed by Thomas J. Kiresuk at the Hennepin County Mental Health Center in Minneapolis, is probably the best-known of the methods of individualized goal attainment.[18,19,20] The methods have had wide dissemination through presentations to numerous agencies and conferences, consultation with potential users, a widely circulated newsletter, and published manuals, brochures, journal articles, and government reports.

Although Goal Attainment Scaling was devised to measure treatment outcomes for individual patients, it may be applied to program services, administrative activities, or any other set of activities for which outcomes may be set and operations set in motion to achieve them. Through its use, the relative effectiveness of various modes of therapy may be determined, and as a program evaluation instrument it delivers a numerical value as a measure of program effectiveness. The attainment of one goal may be compared with that of another, even though the criteria of attainment of the two goals are different. Another important advantage of the method is that the scales allow for the attainment of success levels beyond those expected, facilitating the possibility of providing special rewards for those achieving the success.

In using the model, three operations must be performed. An objective statement must be made as to what a patient or program will accomplish on a given task at a particular point in time. Then, following treatment or program operations, the state of affairs with regard to that stated goal is determined by measurement or observation. Following this observation a standard score is calculated, which permits comparison of one score with another as to their distance from what would be an "average" or predicted score. The scores can be interpreted in relation to attainment of more or less than was predicted, and with what probability.

Technically, five procedures are required: (1) a set of tasks for the patient or program to accomplish is delineated; (2) weights are assigned to each task according to its adjudged importance; (3) for each task two degrees of attainment above and below the expected outcome are described (with expected outcome scored at zero, and two degrees above or below at respectively $+1$, $+2$, -1, -2, a five-point scale is constructed which allows attainment at more than expected success and at less than expected success; each point on the scale is given meaning in terms of descriptive behaviors appropriate to the attainment of that level of success); (4) follow-up scoring on the set of tasks is done; and (5) a score is calculated which summarizes the outcome scores of all tasks in the original set.

In implementation the scaled and weighted tasks are arrayed horizontally in

337

a grid, the vertical dimension being the five-point scale attainment levels. This grid constitutes the goal attainment follow-up guide, and in use is marked as to where the patient is in relation to expected level of treatment outcome at the time of intake, and again at the predetermined time subsequently. The overall score at follow-up can be compared with the score at intake for an indication of change during the treatment. In the case of program administration or management processes, the grid-arranged follow-up guide would be utilized in exactly the same way. A sample grid appears in Figure 18.1.

Extensive studies have been carried out with the measures derived from the method of Goal Attainment Scaling. Among these are comparisons of methods of treatment, comparisons between professional disciplines, comparisons of particular medications with placebo, studies of selected population and problem groups, and studies of the accuracy of clinician's indicators of progress in therapy. Other studies done by the Program Evaluation Project at the Hennepin County Mental Health Center have been of direct utility to management processes. These include a study of the relationship between treatment outcome and method of patient intake, and a study of the effect of feedback to therapists on subsequent outcome scores. Methods of relating scale content and outcome to management goals and related cost estimates are being developed.

Statistically the Goal Attainment Score is practically symmetrical in its distribution; it has a mean of 50, a standard deviation of 10, and ranges from 20 to 80. Outcome scores on two different follow-up guides for the same client, constructed independently by different staff at different times, correlate .70 (Pearson r).* Agreement between the scores of follow-up workers scoring the same guides at different times is approximately .75 (Pearson r). A correlation of .88 is obtained between separate content analyses done on follow-up guides constructed for the same client by different staff members. In an effort to develop standard scales it has been found that twenty scale headings might be necessary for most clinical settings, and that these would include most of the needed content. For the therapists and clientele of a place such as the Hennepin County Mental Health Center, the scale headings include aggression, alcohol/drug abuse, anxiety/depression, education, family/marital, interpersonal relationships and social activities, legal/financial, living arrangements, physical complaints, psychopathological symptoms, sexuality, suicide, treatment, and work. Others may be added that are special to a given client or setting.[12]

Goal Attainment Scaling has been applied in numerous situations and with various population, ranging from disturbed children to delinquent youths and adults, adult outpatients, geriatric patients, and graduate students. These population groups can assist in constructing and scoring the follow-up guides themselves.

* r = Pearson product moment coefficient of correlation.

FIGURE 18.1

Sample Clinical Guide: Crisis Intervention Center. Program Evaluation Project. Goal Attainment Follow-Up Guide

Check whether or not the scale has been mutually negotiated between patient and CIC interviewer.

SCALE ATTAINMENT LEVELS	SCALE HEADINGS AND SCALE WEIGHTS				
	SCALE 1: EDUCATION ($w_1 = 20$) YES __ NO X	SCALE 2: SUICIDE ($w_2 = 30$) YES __ NO X	SCALE 3: MANIPULATION ($w_3 = 25$) YES __ NO X	SCALE 4: DRUG ABUSE ($w_4 = 30$) YES X NO __	SCALE 5: DEPENDENCY ON CIC ($w_5 = 10$) YES X NO __
a. most unfavorable treatment outcome thought likely (−2)	Patient has made no attempt to enroll in high school. ✓	Patient has committed suicide.	Patient makes rounds of community service agencies demanding medication, and refuses other forms of treatment. ✓	Patient reports addiction to "hard narcotics" (heroin, morphine).	Patient has contacted CIC by telephone or in person at least seven times since his first visit.
b. less than expected success with treatment (−1)	Patient has enrolled in high school, but at time of follow-up has dropped out.	Patient has acted on at least one suicidal impulse since her first contact with the CIC, but has not succeeded. ✓	Patient no longer visits CIC with demands for medication but continues with other community agencies and still refuses other forms of treatment. ✓	Patient has used "hard narcotics," but is not addicted, and/or uses hallucinogens (LSD, Pot) more than four times a month. ✓	Patient has contacted CIC 5–6 times since intake.
c. expected level of treatment success (0)	Patient has enrolled, and is in school at follow-up, but is attending class sporadically (misses an average of more than a third of her classes during a week).	Patient reports she has had at least four suicidal impulses since her first contact with the CIC but has not acted on any of them.	Patient no longer attempts to manipulate for drugs at community service agencies, but will not accept another form of treatment. ☆	Patient has not used "hard narcotics" during follow-up period, and uses hallucinogens between 1–4 times a month. ☆	Patient has contacted CIC 3–4 times since intake.
d. more than expected success with treatment (+1)	Patient has enrolled, is in school at follow-up, and is attending classes consistently, but has no vocational goals. ☆		Patient accepts non-medication treatment at some community agency. ☆	Patient uses hallucinogens less than once a month.	
e. best anticipated success with treatment (+2)	Patient has enrolled, is in school at follow-up, is attending classes consistently, and has some vocational goals.	Patient reports she has had no suicidal impulses since her first contact with the CIC.	Patient accepts non-medication treatment, and by own report shows signs of improvement.	At time of follow-up, patient is not using any illegal drug.	Patient has not contacted CIC since intake. ☆

Source: T. J. Kiresuk, "Goal Attainment Scaling at a County Mental Health Service," Evaluation 1, special monograph, 1973.

Level at Intake: ✓
Level at Follow-up: ☆
Level at Intake: 29.4
Goal Attainment Score (Level at Follow-up): 62.2
Goal Attainment Change Score +32.8

GOAL-ORIENTED AUTOMATED PROGRESS NOTE

Researchers and staff at Fort Logan Mental Health Center have developed the Goal-Oriented Progress Note, which serves both as a communication instrument, facilitating information exchange of treatment plans and outcomes for individual patients among staff, patients, and family/community others, and as a program evaluation tool, providing information for clinical and management decision making. [10,37] Treatment programs may be revised or abolished, methods of therapy compared, or the effectiveness of a therapist, a therapeutic team, or a hospital division determined.

The researchers set out to develop an individualized goal attainment measure which could be weighted differentially on more important goals in calculating outcomes, could lend itself to input from the patient himself and from relatives or friends involved with the treatment process, and would be comparable across patients and at different times. Additional requirements were that the treatment methods for each goal should be stated clearly and their helpfulness toward individual goals determined; feedback on outcomes should be available quickly and in a meaningful form so as to contribute effectively to planning for treatment in process; clinical staff should not be burdened with additional paperwork, and even existing record keeping should be replaced; finally, data processing should be used in order to reduce error and facilitate rapid feedback, and maintaining the system in operation should be relatively inexpensive.

The instrument consists of 703 goal statements developed in collaboration with clinical staff, and is felt to include 99 percent of patient treatment goals at Fort Logan Mental Health Center. These statements are grouped in seven categories: (1) medical; (2) symptom alleviation; (3) self-concept; (4) patient-initiated interactions with others; (5) other-initiated interactions with the patient; (6) community environment; and (7) disposition plan. They are printed for automated optical scanning, thus eliminating the need for coding and keypunching. An average time of only three minutes is required for staff to use the form for recording both the previously determined treatment goals and the methods of treatment for each patient. By means of interview, goal statements are secured from patients and family or other relevant community members, and recorded on the same forms as used by staff, thus producing the "tri-informant" goal listings.

The computer then produces a record of goals and methods in narrative form. Following this, the computer printout shows each goal printed above two scales, one permitting a rating of the importance of the goal for the patient on a five-point scale from "Least" (important) to "Very" (important), and the other for recording patient goal attainment on a six-point scale. The six-point scale is constructed as follows:

(1)	(2)	(3)	(4)	(5)	(6)
Much Further From	Further From	No Change	Somewhat Closer	Much Closer	Sufficient Attainment

A five-point scale is also used by the staff on which to rate the helpfulness of the methods of treatment selected. The data from the three scales are keypunched and summarized for each goal in the third computer printout. The first progress note made available to clinicians and others is comprised of the original goal-method selection form and the summary of the ratings of the first goals and methods.

Staff, patient, and community others rate progress on their initial goals after one month and again at patient discharge. In addition, staff members rate patients' progress toward staff goals, and the helpfulness of methods, each week of the first month of treatment in order to revise goal-method selections if indicated.

These ratings figure in a success score which is a comparison of actual attainment with maximum possible attainment, including importance ratings as factors. The possible range is 0.00 to 1.00, with a score of 0.40 equal to No Change, and all smaller scores interpreted as failure. This formula for success allows for comparisons among patients, treatment methods, staff teams, demographic groups, and patient aggregates.

The Goal-Oriented Progress Note was tested over an eleven-month period by three adult psychiatric teams at Fort Logan Mental Health Center in a sample of sixty-seven patients for whom the staff had enumerated goals. It was possible to record 79 percent of patient goals and 84 percent of community-other goals. Interview data were available to staff within one week. Reliability between interviewers for goal setting was .94. Over a three-month interval, interview-reinterview reliabilities were .93 and .96 for two interviewers. The coefficient of agreement among fourteen staff members coding goals for the same seven patients was .92. Divergence among staff, patient, and community others on goal choices and success scores continues to be a problem, unless these various perspectives are indeed valid.

The measure is compatible with use of other data on patients available in the center, such as the usual demographic, historical, medical, psychiatric, and length-of-stay data. It also forms a necessary part of the data required to relate treatment effectiveness to costs of a particular program for management decisions. Data on treatment success are reported to various managers at various levels for teams, services, or the center as a whole. It is a central measure for relating costs to benefits, a concept of increasing importance in the mental health field.

CONCRETE GOAL-SETTING

This individualized goal attainment measure was developed by Theodor Bonstedt in the day hospital at Rollman Psychiatric Institute in Cincinnati, Ohio.[3] Similar in principle to Goal Attainment Scaling and the Goal-Oriented Progress Note, Concrete Goal-Setting is somewhat simpler in operation and ease of communication. It came into being in a small patient population in a day hospital and is thus practically applicable to small services. It could be extended to larger populations and the multiservices of the mental health center, but would probably require more systematic methods, and even the use of computer facilities.

Concrete Goal-Setting was a response to a range of factors prevailing in the day hospital that made objective measurement of patient progress in treatment a frustrating experience. Staff was composed of many disciplines with a variety of treatment orientations. Patients came from a variety of sources and were in the day hospital from one to five days weekly. The goals of referring personnel would be broad and different from the rather more concrete goals of an activities-oriented day hospital staff. Evaluation of patient progress would proceed from many frames of reference and thus be difficult to specify or quantify in terms acceptable to the variety of evaluators.

In order to facilitate the stating of treatment goals in concrete terms and to enable an appraisal of progress at any point, brief information is recorded on a five-by-eight-inch card for each patient. Besides name, age, and date of admission, five columns respectively record date of review, treatment goals set prior to the review, method of treatment to be used, persons taking major treatment responsibility, and date of the next review.

Goals are set in behavioral terms, specifying the changes expected quantitatively, such as "sleeping eight hours a night without medication," or "spending one hour daily in conversation with another person." The selected method depends on the interest and skills of the therapist, knowledge of what methods usually are effective for the kind of problem faced by the patient, and the goal to be achieved. Therapist choice depends on the skill of the therapist with respect to the kind of problem. The date of the next review is set as the time at which, with the given goals and methods of treatment, minimum change, positive or negative, will have occurred. At review the goals, methods, and staff persons responsible can be changed, and the date set for next review or termination or transfer.

After experience of a year and a half at the Rollman Institute, it was shown that stating goals in behavioral terms facilitated agreement among staff on progress of patients and gave a focus for determining change in status. Patients could be discharged because behavior change could be specified. New goals could ensue with achievement of earlier and less complicated clinical goals.

There were some problems with staff resistance to a "behaviorist approach," but no particular method of treatment was imposed.

Concrete Goal-Setting as used here would seem to be applicable to all the services of the mental health center and lends itself to comparison of methods of therapy, particularly for the instruction of mental health personnel in training. It also bids fair to improve patient care, in that systematic review reveals inefficiency of some methods and facilitates change to treatment methods that might be more effective.

CLIENT-THERAPIST CONTINGENCY CONTRACT TREATMENT GOAL SETTING

This approach to an individual goal attainment measure is an application of behavior modification techniques to the treatment contract between the therapist and the client. In the Huntsville-Madison County Mental Health Center where this is taking place, the methods are also being applied to the program components, both direct and indirect services, and to the performance of the individual staff persons within the center. [14,15] In the treatment situation the therapist and the client establish a contract which specifies explicitly what is expected of each. The goals of treatment are established in specific behavioral terms, for example, "to increase social contacts to ten or more a week" or "to increase school attendance to 90 percent of school days or more." Goals are assigned priorities of importance and records are kept on the frequency of occurrence of the particular behaviors or modifications. The type of therapy is specified, as, for example, assertive training and role-playing, or relaxation training. Initially the client may be sent to a group in order to help him or her work out the measurable goals that will constitute the contract. This also helps the client define explicitly his reasons for being at the center.

Baseline rates are established on three targets of behavior, and these three are those for which the therapist is held accountable, although many more items may be listed as goals for the client. For each goal, the percentage of success is determined at the time of the termination of the contract. At termination the treatment could have been successful with no further intervention necessary. Alternatively, treatment could be successful but further intervention needed in another service within the center or with some other community resource. Termination may also take place with referral of the client to another center service or some other community resource following unsuccessful treatment. Unsuccessful treatment may also be followed by a refusal of the client to attend further sessions, and thus be terminated. In evaluation, treatment success may be correlated with such variables as duration of problem behavior, type of treatment, number of therapy sessions, and score on the Client Evaluation of Therapy questionnaire. Evaluation also includes follow-up of clients at six- and twelve-month intervals. This includes those who received treatment and were terminated and those who were not in need of treatment and terminated. Those clients who were referred to other agencies instead of receiving treatment at the mental health center are followed up immediately.

In a manner similar to that developed for client intervention, specified behavioral goals are set for all of the service elements of the mental health center's program. The facilities to be used are indicated, the amount of staff time and specific staff persons designated, and the exact procedures for providing this service spelled out. The criteria for evaluating the success of the program are also specified, and at the end of a given period of time it can be determined if the program goals have been reached. Such procedures are outlined for inpatient services, outpatient services, day-treatment services, the aftercare service, the crisis service, and the alcoholism services. All specifiable tasks of the center are developed in this format, including such items as research and evaluation, training, and the satellite operations service. Consultation and education services are also carried out through contract arrangements within the mental health center and with those agencies for whom services are provided. For evaluation, those data are collected which enable the determination of whether the goals have been reached.

Such a program requires a philosophical commitment to these procedures as well as some special staff to manage the overall application of behavior modification principles. Considerable paperwork is involved, but completing this in a specified time is made part of the performance goals of each person so involved. Personnel performance tasks are delineated and a contract made with each staff person for carrying them out. Criteria are explicitly specified and both the staff person and his supervisor can easily determine the degree to which performance goals are met. Salary raises may be tied differentially to these degrees of attainment, with larger raises accruing to those who far exceed the goals set down. A particular advantage of these concrete program results is that data are available from which to calculate costs for individual patients, for a service, or for the overhead of the mental health center. From this it is a relatively small step to calculating cost-effectiveness of various services or of intervention modes. Management decisions can then be made as to the best use of available resources.

A criticism of the contingency contract method of goal setting is sometimes aimed at the fact of internal consistency without external criteria. What is to prevent the therapist from setting goals that are easily fulfilled, and thus always accomplished? The truth is that such a state of affairs cannot exist for very long in the community. For one thing, referral agencies will know about the outcomes of treatment and consultations, and data from such agencies are always included in the valuation criteria of a mental health center that is serious about its program outcomes. For another, satisfaction of clients is an important force. Here again, follow-up data on client outcomes as well as client satisfaction with the services he receives are crucial. Even setting the treatment contract with the client provides a hedge against the therapist setting too-easily-achieved goals. Other remedies for this criticism could include having the goals set by the intake worker who is not the therapist, developing goals for similar patients, and having a review by a qualified reviewer from outside the program of goals set as against outcomes achieved. A quality control or utilization review group within the mental health center itself can also be an important control procedure. In the last analysis, clients of direct services and indirect services will speak for themselves in one way or another. Hopefully, it will be through valid mechanisms built into the planning and evaluation procedures of the center program. Contingency Contract Treatment Goal Setting seems to offer many advantages.

Systems Approaches to Evaluation

A program evaluation which focuses on treatment outcomes for cohorts of patients rather than upon individualized goal attainment measures has been developed by James A. Ciarlo and associates at the Community Mental Health Center at the Denver General Hospital.[6,7] This approach focuses on the change in program outcome levels over time, comparing one cohort of patients with another as to level of treatment outcomes. These outcome measures are applicable across all treatment modalities and across all kinds of patients. Inpatient programs, daycare services, emergency care, and outpatient services can be compared with these measures, as can alcoholics, drug addicts, chronic psychotics, and patients of other classifications. Various kinds of therapy may also be compared in this system which focuses only upon outcomes.

Since the mental health center exists primarily to assess and remediate mental and emotional ills of the population, the heart of program evaluation is the determination of the impact of treatment on those persons admitted for services. Evaluation also takes into account the impact of the program on other care-giving agencies, but assessing this becomes a formidable enterprise, except as other agencies are able to apply appropriate evaluation techniques to the outcomes of their mental health center-supported interventions. Because the evaluation data must be available to mental health boards and community funding structures as well as to mental health center staff members and clients, it seemed appropriate to the Denver investigators to choose goals and outcome measures easily understood by all. This meant selecting concrete behavioral terms in which to state the goals and outcome measures developed. Obviously, outcome measures should be related to the program goals and should assess behaviors that are indicative of the patient problems presented.

Seven usable outcome scales were developed, as follows: (1) psychological distress, which means feelings of discomfort or malaise, which are experienced as unpleasant or negative; (2) interpersonal isolation, which refers to lack of involvement with family and friends; (3) nonproductivity, which means failure to pursue constructive, socially valued, vocational, volunteer, or educational activities; (4) substance abuse, which implies frequency of use of drugs or alcohol and the troublesome consequences of such abuse in work, family relationships, or self-satisfaction; (5) trouble with the law, which has to do with arrests or other involvement with police for various criminal acts; (6) dependency on public systems, which has to do with maintenance of the patient through public resources as to his health, welfare, and social functioning; and (7) client satisfaction, which relates to the feelings the client has about the program services provided to him in the mental health center.

These scales are sufficiently reliable to be useful, and their validity is very promising. Beside the face validity of the items, correlations between the report of the client and judgment of the follow-up interviewer are very high. These scales allow for the weighting of particular dimensions which most appropriately measure the objectives set for patients, and data have already been amassed as to which dimensions of the scale are most applicable to particular kinds of patients. So far the instrument is applicable to adults between the ages of eighteen and sixty-five, but it is expected that similar forms with appropriate items may be fashioned for children and for persons over sixty-five years of age. Because of its generality with respect to treatment careers, it is especially well-suited to the program of a comprehensive community mental health center which offers a large variety of services to any client for which they are appropriate. Furthermore, the data collected on individual clients lend themselves very well to measuring accessibility of services, continuity of care, and the extent to which the community service minimizes the referral of patients to long-term care in distant state hospitals.

A further advantage of this continous monitoring system is that it lends itself nicely to procedures for measuring cost-benefit ratios. Program managers can determine the cost of resources consumed in order to achieve a particular outcome measure for a particular set of patients. From this measure it is possible to determine what additional resources are needed to produce a better outcome level. Programs may then be changed or modified in accordance with the particular value placed on a particular outcome. The program manager may wish to settle for a smaller outcome level in favor of a greater number of clients in need of treatment. Or he may modify the treatment regimen itself in favor of the one that proves to be most effective for a smaller number of clients. The political realities of the situation may very well dictate the strategic choice.

Another important advantage to this method is that the outcome measure on a group of clients may be compared with the measure on a random sample from the community. This can serve as an outside criterion of effectiveness of center program interventions. Incidentally, the outcome measure developed in this scheme is taken at ninety days after intake, regardless of where the client is. The system can be utilized with two staff members, one to supervise data collection and analysis procedure and the other to locate clients in the community for the purpose of conducting the standard follow-up interview. A reliable record-keeping system is also imperative, but those centers that maintain good clinical records will have the minimum requirements for evaluation as well. Some punch card system is probably necessary for small mental health centers, but computer service is essential in those centers having 5,000 or more patient contacts each year.

Another systems approach is one called Key Factor Analysis, developed by Irwin M. Jarett at Southern Illinois University.[21] It is basically an information system designed to enable the organization to determine the extent to which goals are realized through specified indicators. Goals are expressed in population aggregate terms and are time-limited. For example, "by x year, y percentage of the teenage population will have access to routine screening for emotional health." Programs for accomplishing the goals can then be mounted, with explicit specifications as to facilities, staff, and budget. Provision is made for collecting indicator information as to the degree of success in reaching the goal. This is a logical system applicable to a catchment area population or to a state mental health system. So far, however, the methods for installing Key Factor Analysis are complex and time consuming, and seem to generate tremendous resistance in mental health staff. The system seems to need intermediate payoffs for its participants, because the ultimate rewards seem to follow only long development periods. In successful operation, it should provide managers with the information they need at the time for making crucial decisions as to allocation of resources or program activity. The results can be linked with program costs for enabling decision as to the greatest benefit per unit of cost.

A specific application of general systems theory to the evaluation of service delivery systems is that of network analysis.[5] Network analysis, as focused on client flow through the system of mental health delivery facilities, is process-oriented. Treatment outcomes must be inferred. By looking at client pathways in the system it is possible to determine the length of time and number of admissions or readmissions to a given element of the various program services. From this it can be determined which pathways are followed by longest stays in the community or independent living, and which have services to which given clients go repeatedly. Inferences may then be made as to the adequacy or effectiveness of given services, as, for example, the inpatient service, the outpatient service, or aftercare service. Nonproductive or ineffective services may be located and modified. Gaps in services may appear from such an analysis, or it may be shown that appropriate interventions are not available for a particular disorder, client age group, or group with a special history, such as hospitalization in a state hospital. Network analysis permits the computation of costs of client careers in the various segments of the network of services. In order to utilize the information from network analysis maximally, outcome evaluation criteria for various elements of service must be developed.

Outcome Value per Unit Cost

The ultimate utility of outcome measures of program effectiveness is to enable the program manager to make decisions on the allocation of his resources of time, money, facilities, and staff for the maximum benefit of the clients served. The question has to do with the return on optimal resource investment in terms of benefits to clients and to society. A method for determining output value per unit cost has been developed at the Fort Logan Mental Health Center.[2,17] This scheme involves the level of impairment in clients admitted to the mental health center and the intensity and extensity of the therapeutic process in which they participate. The results are measured by the Output Value Index. Impairment is measured by a score for predicting the amount of resources the patient will use in the course of his treatment. Units of resources are the days in each kind of treatment, such as inpatient or outpatient, weighted by the cost of each treatment status. Prediction of the resources used is based on the demographic items from the admissions form and items from the mental status examination. The more impaired a patient is, the more resources it is expected that he will use. Program characteristics are measured by the actual percent of time in formal therapy for different program elements. The number of days in each treatment modality weighted by the percent of time in formal therapy constitute the extensity of therapeutic involvement. The intensity of therapeutic involvement is computed by dividing the sum of the weighted days by the number of days actually in treatment.

The results of treatment were defined in terms of the value of the discharged patient for the community. This value was based on two factors, his estimated economic productivity (what will he actually earn) and the estimated economic value of his response to treatment. The Output Value Index is the number representing the amount of value returned on the investment of resources. As would be expected, patients of low impairment would require the least amount of resources and would show the highest return for the program dollar. All of this relates to a judgment that the client is of the most value when he is functioning in the community. The Output Value Index has the advantage of being useful in determining the critical point at which further investment of resources is not economically feasible in terms of improvement value in the client. It is at such a point that the program manager may decide to use a minimum of inpatient services, for example, because of the intensity and extensity of resources required. But this has to be weighed against such factors as the community's value of optimal assistance to the most people versus maximum assistance to a relatively few, and the prevailing sentiment for supporting services. All too frequently the community values treatment of those in need of services more highly than it does the financing of measures of prevention which might prove to be more economical in the long run.

Prospective

The final verdict on the effectiveness of mental health centers is not yet in. Studies do show less likelihood of being admitted to or becoming a resident in a state mental hospital from the catchment areas of functional mental health centers. Services available in the community are utilized in preference to the inpatient facility of the state hospital which is geographically farther away, all other things being equal. All other things are not equal enough for mental health centers to have replaced state hospitals, although the character of hospitals is changing. Unfortunately, we have come too close to developing two parallel systems of mental health care, though the hospital system continues to command a much higher proportion of the resources. Perhaps two systems is the only viable route to a unitary system in which more and more of mental and emotional ills are attended to in local communities, with attendant gradual shift in resources. This certainly seems likely as the pool of chronic long-term patients diminishes, long-term hospitalization becomes less and less necessary, and more and more of treatment needs are met in community mental health centers.

The efficacy of mental health centers, both financially and in effects of services on recipients, is yet to be established. But the climate for accountability for the resources expended is developing to the point that funding may soon be conditional upon the effectiveness of programs and services. Appropriation bodies and taxpayers are demanding information on outcomes of services financed.

Pressures for effectiveness data which can be translated into unit costs have resulted in widespread efforts to develop means and methods of evaluating mental health center programs. Since the most salient of services is clinical services,

349

most of the efforts have gone into the evaluation of direct treatment services. Several workable individualized goal attainment models have emerged from these efforts. Systems models of program evaluation also have an important place, in that they call attention to the processes involved in mental health center operations. Measures of comprehensiveness of care, continuity of care, and accessibility of services are essential in the assessment of these process outcomes envisioned by the progenitors of mental health centers.

In the final analysis, some form of goal attainment for individuals and then cohorts or patient aggregates is necessary in determining treatment effects. Of the models developed, none has yet been widely adopted, although Goal Attainment Scaling is probably best known. There is the problem of costs, and managers of mental health centers generally have not yet seen fully the possible payoffs. What is required is a system simple enough in concept as well as in operation that produces the needed data without the necessity of adding very much evaluation staff or of preempting significantly the time of all existing staff persons. Another problem is linking evaluation outcomes with administrative decision, but this should diminish as evaluators answer questions in practical terminology and administrators are required to justify program support. There is every reason to believe that managers and administrators will come to see that the costs of evaluation efforts will be more than repaid through the benefits of specified, measurable goals. There are satisfactions in achieving treatment contracts with individuals and in reaching program performance goals. Practical evaluation efforts will simplify and facilitate the financial support processes and enhance net financial inputs.

A climate that is pressing for outcome evaluations, and successes in developing workable models and procedures, bode well for integrating evaluation with the regular fabric of mental health center operations. It will be wise, however, to continue to include a spirit of experimentation or empiricism with attitudes favorable to evaluation. Self-correcting schemes are mandatory, or the feedback loop must be short and yield results of practical utility.

Of models in use for all the services of a mental health center, the contingency contract approach for treatment, personnel performance, and costing of services may be the most easily utilized. It does require a philosophy that is accepting of a behavioral approach, and there are some resistances to the amount of paper work necessary. But the positive reinforcements for specified goal attainment are powerful!

From the various approaches to outcomes measurement have come scale dimensions that are quite similar in describing client behavior. From this commonality it is not too much to expect that a system can be devised which may be applied, with some modification, to the operations of almost any mental health center. Successful adoption would depend upon the leadership, appropriate incentives, and techniques for integrating the model with ongoing operations.

The prospect of the development of some form of national health insurance in the United States serves to underline the necessity for quality control of services. Already there are program-monitoring schemes and services utilization review methods in development and use. These methods begin with the goals of services and programs and represent a mode of evaluation. The next step is outcomes criteria. As mental health centers become units of supra-agencies incorporating the primary human services, or as they unite with health maintenance organizations to promote mental and emotional health, the advantages of efforts to measure program effects will be even more apparent. Efforts to assess the impact of the mental health center upon the structure of community services and upon the total mental health problem, both given relatively little attention so far, will be of increasing importance.

As we look to the future, we must anticipate that new models will emerge in the service of measuring mental health center program effects. We have understandably been bound to the classic experimental model for deriving valid data, conscious all the while of the fact that community and field conditions rarely approximate those of the laboratory. We have constantly qualified our findings and made the most cautious of inferences. Applying quasi-experimental designs and using unobtrusive measure when possible have helped.

Although we shall continue to try to perfect and apply our experimental models, we shall also look to methods that incorporate contextual interaction. It is not enough to adopt a model for which data of any kind are suitable. Guttentag [16] has pointed to some alternative methods in evaluation which include context effects. In one method the units of measurement include social and situational effects, and have been called "eco-behavioral units." They are units of persons in time-space boundaries, and say that a person's behavior is related to the ecology of his setting. In another method, called "social area analysis," the total social context in which programs occur is included. Data from multiple sources, such as census, courts, health, welfare, and schools, are subjected to multivariate analysis. Through this, trends for a given geographical area may be established in such domains as disrupted families, substandard housing, and ethnic population densities, in relation to social agency data. Establishing a program may change trends, and the change is the measure of the program effect. This approach allows comparisons of social area profiles from one area to another, as well as before-and-after measures on the same area.

We can expect further refinement of these methods, but whether they will prove to be feasible for application through the resources of the average mental health center is yet to be determined.

REFERENCES

1. Bass, R. D. A *Method for Measuring Continuity of Care in a Community Mental Health Center*. Rockville, Md.: National Institute of Mental Health, Office of Program Planning and Evaluation, 1971.

2. Binner, P. R.; Halpern, J.; and Potter, A. "Patients, Programs, and Results in a Comprehensive Mental Health Center." *Journal of Clinical and Consulting Psychology* 41 (1973):148–156.

3. Bonstedt, T. "Concrete Goal-Setting for Patients in a Day Hospital." *Evaluation* 1, special monograph (1973):3–5.

4. Buchanan, G. N., and Whaley, J. S. "Federal Level Evaluation." *Evaluation* 1 (1972):17–22.

5. Burgess, J.; Nelson, R. H.; and Wallhaus, R. "Network Analysis as a Method for the Evaluation of Service Delivery Systems." *Community Mental Health Journal* 10 (1974):337–344.

6. Ciarlo, J. A. "A Performance-Monitoring Approach to Mental Health Programs." *Evaluation*. Paper presented at American Orthopsychiatric Association Convention, 1972, Detroit, Michigan.

7. ———; Lin, S.; Bigelow, D.; and Biggerstaff, M. "A Multi-Dimensional Outcome Measure for Evaluating Community Mental Health Programs." Paper presented at American Psychological Association Convention, September 1972, Honolulu, Hawaii.

8. *Citizen Participation in Community Mental Health Centers: Issues and Program Implications for Community Mental Health Centers*. Boston, Mass.: Tufts University School of Medicine, Contract with NIMH, 1971.

9. Davis, H. R. "Four Ways to Goal Attainment: An Overview." *Evaluation* 1, special monograph (1973):23–28.

10. Ellis, R. H., and Wilson, N. C. "Evaluating Treatment Effectiveness Using a Goal-Oriented Automated Progress Note." *Evaluation* 1, special monograph (1973):6–11.

11. Feldman, S. "Ideas and Issues in Community Mental Health." *Hospital and Community Psychiatry* 22(1971):325–329.

12. Garwick, G., and Lampman, S. "Typical Problems Bringing Patients to a Community Mental Health Center." *Community Mental Health Journal* 8(1972):271–280.

13. Glidewell, J., and Domke, H. "Health Department Research in Community Mental Health." Paper presented at American Public Health Association Convention, Cleveland, Ohio, 1957.

14. Goodson, W. H., Jr. *An Empirically Based Community Mental Health Center*. Huntsville, Ala.: Huntsville-Madison Mental Health Center, 1973.

15. ———, and Turner, J. *Behavior Modification Applied to a Mental Health Center*. Huntsville, Ala.: Huntsville-Madison Mental Health Center, 1971.

16. Guttentag, M. "Models and Methods in Evaluation Research." *Journal of the Theory of Social Behavior* 1(1971):75–95.

17. Halpern, J., and Binner, P. R. "A Model for an Output Value Analysis of Mental Health Programs." *Administration in Mental Health*, National Institute of Mental Health, Winter 1972:40–51.

18. Kiresuk, T. J. "Goal Attainment Scaling at a County Mental Health Service." *Evaluation* 1, special monograph (1973):12–18.

19. ———. *Progress Summary*. Minneapolis, Minn.: Mental Health Program Evaluation Project, Hennepin County Mental Health Center, 1973.

20. ———, and Sherman, R. E. "Goal Attainment Scaling: A General Method for Evaluating Comprehensive Community Mental Health Programs." *Community Mental Health Journal* 4(1968):443–453.

21. Longhurst, P., Jr. "Key Factor Analysis: A General Systems Approach to Program Evalua-

tion in Mental Health." In *Systems Approach to Program Evaluation in Mental Health*. Boulder, Colo.: Western Interstate Commission for Higher Education, 1970, pp. 23–47.

22. *Mental Health Complex. Part I: Community Mental Health Centers*. Washington, D.C.: Center for the Study of Responsive Law, 1972.

23. Mental Retardation Facilities and Community Mental Health Centers Construction Act of 1963. Public Law 88–164, 88th Congress. Washington, D.C.: U.S. Government Printing Office, 1963.

24. "Mental Retardation Facilities and Community Mental Health Centers Act of 1963: Regulations." Public Law 88–164. *Federal Register*, May 6, 1964.

25. Mental Retardation Facilities and Community Mental Health Centers Construction Act Amendment of 1965. Public Law 89–105, 89th Congress. Washington, D.C.: U.S. Government Printing Office, 1967.

26. Moore, J. H. *The Development of Mental Health Resources in Two Pairs of Counties Between 1958 and 1970*. New York: National Study Services, Contract with NIMH, 1972.

27. National Institute of Mental Health, U.S. Public Health Service, Department of Health, Education, and Welfare, Rockville, Md.

28. Partnership for Health Amendments of 1967. Public Law 90–174, 90th Congress. Washington, D.C.: U.S. Government Printing Office, 1967.

29. *Procedures for Evaluating Mental Health Indirect Service Programs in Schools*. Alexandria, Va.: Human Resources Research Organization, Contract with NIMH, 1971.

30. *Relationships Between Community Mental Health Centers and Other Care-Giving Organizations*. Chicago, Ill.: National Opinion Research Center, Contract with NIMH, 1971.

31. Rittenhouse, J. D. "The Diagnostic Spectrum of Center Treated Patients." In *The Impact of the Community Mental Health Center's Program on the State of Colorado*, pt. 3. Contract with NIMH, 1970, pp. 52–68.

32. ———. "The Impact on the State Hospital System." In *The Impact of the Community Mental Health Center's Program on the State of Colorado*, pt. 1. Contract with NIMH, 1970, pp. 1–20.

33. ———. "Representativeness of Center Client Populations." In *The Impact of the Community Mental Health Center's Program on the State of Colorado*, pt. 2. Contract with NIMH, 1970, pp. 21–51.

34. Sorensen, J. E. *Cost-Finding and Rate-Setting for Community Mental Health Centers*. Rockville, Md.: National Institute of Mental Health, Office of Program Planning and Evaluation, 1972.

35. *A Study of Mental Health Services for Children in Community Mental Health Centers*. Joint Information Service of the American Psychiatric Association and the National Association for Mental Health, Contract with NIMH, 1971.

36. Towle, L. H. *Alcoholism Program Monitoring System Development*. Menlo Park, Calif.: Stanford Research Institute, Contract with NIMH, 1972.

37. Wilson, N. C. "The Tri-Informant Goal-Oriented Progress Note." Research Report PN 17, American Psychological Association Convention, September 1972, Honolulu, Hawaii.

38. Windle, C. "National Institute of Mental Health's Evaluation of the Community Mental Health Center Program: An Interim Appraisal of the Evaluation." Paper presented to the Program Evaluation Forum, October 1971, Brainerd, Minn.

39. Wolford, J. A.; Hitchcock, J.; Ellison, D. L.; Sows, A. C.; and Smith, F. "The Effect on State Hospitalization of a Community Mental Health/Mental Retardation Center." *American Journal of Psychiatry* 129(1972):202–206.

Editorial Note

How does one gather valid data on behaviors of psychiatric interest? How can our data systems for measuring the dependent variables—these behaviors of psychiatric relevance—be better developed and, in this case, computerized? These are the dominating questions for this chapter by Robert C. Benfari and Alexander H. Leighton. These are also the critical considerations for developing a more effective system of discovering who has how much of what behaviors of psychiatric interest, and why.

In setting a direction for more valid behavioral assessments, this chapter also rigorously systematizes a variety of behaviors of psychiatric epidemiological interest, such as stress and cardiovascular symptoms, allergic responses, worry, tension, anxiety (psychological), restlessness, and low mood. In addition, the universe of relevant symptoms is factorially analyzed into six factors: (1) anxiety-depression; (2) allergic; (3) psychosomatic; (4) aggressive-tense; (5) social deviancy-psychotic indicator; and (6) activity-intellect.

The authors demonstrate how their approach to the analysis of symptom categories can be used to develop a psychiatric symptom dictionary for content analysis of field epidemiological surveys.

B. H. K.

CHAPTER 19

The Uses of the Computer in Psychiatric Behavioral Epidemiology[*]

ROBERT C. BENFARI

ALEXANDER H. LEIGHTON

IN THE FIELD of psychiatric epidemiology there is the perpetual task of making standardized assessments and evaluations from field surveys concerned with mental health. Much of the data is collected from respondents by means of structured questionnaires. Additional data on respondents can be gathered from unstructured interviews, hospital records, and physicians' comments. Each of these sources represents impressions by or about the respondent that, when taken together, form an assessment of the mental health of the individual.

The Stirling County assessment procedure is an attempt to triangulate on the phenomena of mental health and illness, using as many data sources as are feasible in large-scale epidemiological surveys: questionnaires, psychiatric interviews, collateral information from family doctors, key informants, and so on.[8]

* This report is based on work conducted as part of the Harvard Program in Social Psychiatry and supported by Mental Health Grant P. H.-43-68-1045 from the National Institute of Mental Health.

Information on a respondent which may be missed in one phase of data collection will often be acquired through another source. For example, a respondent may give reliable complaints of certain psychiatric phenomena such as anxiety, depression, tension, and phobia, but poor information regarding his own social behavior.

Analysis of questionnaire data offers few problems. Questionnaire items are easily coded and prepared for computer processing. Since the items are close-ended, the inputs for each respondent are standardized. A computer program with the logic necessary to simulate the human judgment process of these same inputs has been devised.[2]

On the other hand, less structured verbal data in the form of open-ended interviews demands a different approach. An example of this in the Stirling County study was a survey in which psychiatrists conducted open interviews and rated them based on the evaluation system in the Stirling County assessment procedure.

Starting from common clinical psychiatric practices of classification and appraisal, the method was developed step by step to fit the needs of the epidemiological work, to provide consistent standards and procedures so that reliability of judgment among raters could be achieved, to establish descriptive qualitative and quantitative units which could be used to compare groups within the same cultural setting, and, finally, to compare groups in different cultures. It is distinct from the usual clinical diagnosis or diagnostic formulation, for it consists in an objective scrutiny of the evidence rather than a diagnosis with inherent etiologic and prognostic implications. The evolved categories are essentially phenomenal.

Nevertheless, despite all of this, some of the content, when rated by the psychiatrist, is still clinical judgment: the rater makes assessments based on his impression of a protocol as it compares with others in his experience. Clinical judgment is at times idiosyncratic to the assessor and raises questions of reliability. This problem, coupled with the time and expense involved when professionals hand-rate the interviews of a large survey, led us to consider the construction of a computer program designed to analyze verbal reports.

These reports are accounts of the verbatim interview material of the respondents. They are not the exact verbalizations of the interviewee. They are both descriptions of his behavior and impressions of the psychiatrist about the respondent.

Computer models for the evaluation of standardized questionnaires and objective tests, such as the Stirling County Psychiatric Evaluation and the MMPI, have been developed. However, these instruments are structurally defined and in no way exhaust the raw data on any one respondent. In order to further the purposes of both descriptive and analytic epidemiology, personal interviews, verbal reports, therapy notes, and other text documents should be assessed to evaluate the dependent and independent variables under study. We attempted to go one step beyond these models and to make the evaluation process more comprehensive in scope by including other materials for assessment and by increasing the number of variables under consideration.

We decided that a computer could serve as a reliable aid to the awareness of human intuition and handle the mechanics of formal analyses. Research on this level is not considered by us to be a one-step processing operation, but can be used to encourage repeated, cumulative interactions between the processing by the machine and the thinking of the investigator. This is close to the process of construct validation.[6] A program that analyzes interview, key informant, and respondent verbal reports could be integrated with other data bases of the individual. The goal was to get an accurate picture of the whole person which we may call his "personality sphere." Currently, we have concentrated on behaviors of psychiatric interest and are hoping to include other aspects of the personality at another stage.

The focal point of our research project was the development and application of a psychiatric dictionary for field epidemiology. Our main areas of concern in the development of the instrument were:

1. The construction of categories for the psychiatric dictionary.
2. The cross-validation of the dictionary using an external criterion as the standard.
3. Application of the dictionary in a research situation.

A content analysis dictionary is similar to any dictionary in that it gives descriptions or meanings of words. A specific content dictionary is a concrete representation of the investigator's theory as it relates to verbal data about the person. The words, phrases, and sentences are linked by theory to a collection of content analysis categories. The language-relevant variables are clearly specified in terms of content categories. Most of the categories in our present system were devised for use with the epidemiological surveys of psychiatric disorder in the Stirling County study. In psychiatric epidemiology a common frame of reference is necessary in order to permit comparable judgments of the data. That is to say, since we are dealing with mental health constructs that pertain to the psychiatric and psychological status of the individual, a theoretical frame of reference must be built.[7]

Although over the past years a number of researchers have evolved dictionaries for use with the General Inquirer system,[13] the present study is unique because the categories were constructed so that they could be compared with an outside criterion measure—the psychiatrist's evaluation—to test the degree of concurrent validity. The problem of validity in our study took into account this discriminate level of measurement plus an attempt to see if the categories fit into a theoretical network (construct validity).

The dictionary that was devised for the study is called CASE, which stands for Computer Assigned Symptom Evaluations. Since we were working in an epidemiological frame of reference, our concern is with the manifestation or prevalence of symptoms.

Sample and Data Base

From a 1962–1964 field survey of a sample of 405 adults in a rural area, a subsample of 123 was selected from those having or not having symptoms currently, so that about half were at the A (ill) end of the ABCD or "caseness" rating, and most of the remainder at the D (well) end. [10]

This subsample was also selected in such a way as to secure representation of both sexes and of people from a range of different ages and socioeconomic circumstances.

Five psychiatrists participated in the study and each interviewed between fourteen and thirty-two sample members. The 123 individuals made up what is referred to as the Rural Panel. The sample in the present study was 120, since three were dropped due to processing difficulties.

It is appropriate to discuss in detail the purposes and intent of the Rural Panel study and the methods of data collection. The overall plan was to reassess annually the Rural Panel for five years. Thus each individual was contacted five times by a psychiatrist, and one of the primary goals of the study was the validation and clarification of psychiatric constructs. At the end of this time there would be a resurvey, with questionnaires in addition to the psychiatric interviews. One important operation was to refine constructs so that they would be, as far as possible, mutually exclusive.

In terms of operations, it was decided to leave the clinical interviewers as free as possible to conduct an open-ended interview. A questionnaire would probably have resulted in discomfort for both interviewer and interviewee. On the other hand, it was necessary to obtain as much information as possible in a systematic fashion; otherwise meaningful analysis would have been precluded.

The clinical interviewers were presented with three major tasks: (1) to review all relevant case materials for each respondent and to summarize this in as standard a fashion as possible; (2) to interview the respondents using a checklist to insure as full coverage of topic as possible; and (3) to make a series of ratings, based upon the information from (1) and (2), which would enable us to answer some of the questions with which we are concerned. For all the respondents in the rural panel the clinical folders contain the following information: (1) abstracted information from the 1962–1963 questionnaire interview; (2) comments by interviewers who conducted the questionnaire interviews; (3) comments secured from the panel's family doctors; and (4) open interview conducted by a psychiatrist.

Research Design

The design for this analytic project is broken down into four separate but interlinked stages: Stage I, Category Construction; Stage II, Dictionary Construction; Stage III, Dictionary Validation; and Stage IV, Application of Case to selected research problems. Stage I, Category Construction, is the basic link between the theory underlying the evaluation model and the empirical operations of assessment. The categories used in our study were conceptualized and operationally defined. Table 19.1 lists the CASE categories (tags) * used in the present study. Recently we have expanded CASE to 167 categories, of which some tags cover positive mental categories plus other relevant behavioral and social variables. The focus of the present chapter, however, will be on CASE I, containing ninety-seven tags or categories.

Stage II, Dictionary Construction, was considered the keystone phase of the preliminary stages of the project, during which the empirical derivation of the language signs were inferentially linked to the various categories.

It is not possible, due to space limitations, to recapitulate all of our category definitions and tagging examples. In the following paragraphs seventeen selected categories are presented with the operational definition and examples of the language signs in order to give the reader a flavor of the process of dictionary construction. Each category has multiple entries for defining the concept. Some of the tags contain 100 or more language signs. In the interest of brevity we have selected only two language signs for the tags presented. We have not described the intricacies of the tagging procedure.†

Selected Tags and Language Signs

TAG 06 RESPIRATORY SYMPTOM

Minor respiratory symptoms which are not of sufficient severity to be entered in Tag 05 are found here, described as: trouble breathing, tightness in chest, short-winded.

---

* Tags and categories will be used interchangeably in the chapter.
† The reader interested in the technical aspects of computer content analysis should refer to the two volumes of the *General Inquirer*.[12,13]

TABLE 19.1
Tag Names and Numbers: CASE Dictionary

TAG NO.	TAG NAME	TAG NO.	TAG NAME
01	Skin	50	Confusion
02	Marker Tag	51	Phobic Reaction
03	Musculoskeletal Disorder	52	Cyclothymic Label
04	Musculoskeletal Symptom	53	Conversion Reaction & Trance
05	Respiratory Disorder	54	Apathy
06	Respiratory Sympton	55	Obessive Label
07	Gastrointestinal Disorder	56	Paranoid Label
08	Gastrointestinal Symptom	57	Jealousy
09	Cardiovascular Disorder	58	Aggressiveness
10	Cardiovascular Symptom	59	Anger
11	Genitourinary	60	Suspiciousness
12	Hemic Disorder	61	Dissociation Label
13	Hemic Symptom	62	Depersonalization
14	Endocrine	63	Judgment
15	Headache Ordinary	64	Poor Work Role
16	Headache Sick	65	Passive Attitude
17	Allergy	66	Histrionic Label
18	Subjective Body Sensations	67	Mental Deficiency
19	Overweight	68	Subnormal Intelligence
20	Underweight	69	Trouble School
21	Sense	70	Antisocial
22	Marker Tag	71	Dyssocial
23	Negation *	72	Alcohol
24	Nervousness	73	Drug Addiction
25	Worry	74	Sexual Deviation
26	Tense	75	Psychotic Indicators
27	Anxiety, General	76	Schizophrenia Label
28	Anxiety, Physical	77	Affective Psychosis Label
29	Marker Tag	78	Acute Brain Syndrome
30	Restlessness	79	Chronic Brain Syndrome
31	Depressive Label	80	General Motor Disturbance
32	Low Mood	81	Special Symptom Reaction
33	Concentration Difficulties	82	Untrustworthy
34	Low Energy	83	Eccentric
35	Marker Tag	84	Grief Reaction
36	Hypochondriasis	85	Insecure
37	Trouble Appetite	86	Drug Tag
38	Trouble Sleeping	87	Exhibition
39	Compulsive Label	88	Inadequate
40	Rigid	89	Guilty
41	High General Activity	90	Suicidal Label
42	Perfectionist	91	Blocked Affect
43	Compulsive Habits	92	Detached
44	Emotionally Unstable	93	Marker Tag
45	Social Activity	94	Defensive Label
46	Social Isolation	95	Self-disparagement
47	Euphoria Label	96	Rumination
48	Undifferentiated Reaction	97	Once *
49	Projected Disparagement		

* Descriptions of Tag 23 (Negation) and Tag 97 (Once) are not included in the body of this chapter. They are used to avoid mistaggings. Most entries in the dictionary check for proximity to these tag numbers. If found, the entry word will be ignored. Marker Tags serve similar functions.

Examples:

(a) Respiratory, admits to shortness of breath, a smothering feeling which has recurred at night on several occasions generally during the last year.
(b) He does have shortness of breath, paroxysmal nocturnal dyspnea, and a feeling of strangulation, nausea.

TAG 07 GASTROINTESTINAL DISORDER

Entered here are gastrointestinal ailments which are chronic or frequent— diarrhea, constipation, gastritis.

Examples:

(a) Indigestion and gastritis often after eating, accompanied by severe pain.
(b) Constipation has been a continual problem for most of his life.

TAG 08 GASTROINTESTINAL SYMPTOM

Complaints of the GI tract which are not severe or chronic are classified here. Stomach cramps, epigastric pain, gastric upset are listed. We are keying on words indicating GI trouble which is not clearly incapacitating or frequent but which should not be overlooked.

Examples:

(a) The respondent admits to occasional gas pains from things she would eat.
(b) Constipation occasionally when cheese binds her.

TAG 09 CARDIOVASCULAR DISORDER

Serious cardiovascular illnesses which are likely to be long-lasting and impairing are tagged, including heart attack, stroke, high blood pressure, angina.

Examples:

(a) He went to Doctor L. for further examination and Doctor L. again commented on his high blood pressure and gave him some more pills for hypertension.
(b) The respondent attributed her CVA to continual worry.

TAG 10 CARDIOVASCULAR SYMPTOM

This tag includes CV complaints which are probably less severe than those found in Tag 09, such as rapid heartbeat, trouble with circulation.

Examples:

(a) He has an occasional chest pain in the left and right when he raises his hands, and he can hear his heart beat fast when he lies with his ear on the pillow.
(b) He said he has had palpitations for many years, but this has caused him no disability.

TAG 17 ALLERGY

This tag classifies the allergic conditions:

1. Used in addition to respiratory when asthma or hay fever are mentioned.
2. Used in addition to skin when eczema or other probably allergic skin conditions are mentioned.
3. Used on their own merits when unspecified allergies are mentioned by respondent or M.D., etc.

Some entries are asthma, allergy, eczema, hay fever.
Examples:

(a) She suffered from eczema in her infancy which disappeared in her puberty.
(b) Allergy: She is allergic to sulfa drugs.

TAG 18 SUBJECTIVE BODY SENSATIONS

We introduced this symptom pattern in order to have a place to register the rather common complaints of feeling worms, heat, creeping sensations in the skin, body, or head, pressure in the head, and expanded head and gooseflesh. In addition, key words include tingling feelings, choked-up feelings, body quivers, internal shakiness.
Examples:

(a) She has some weakness and light-headedness just before her period and feels shaky, but she never goes to bed or stops working.
(b) She recounts that from time to time she feels that she is looking out of one eye only and that even that eye is blurred and at the same time she has a headache and the fingers of one hand go numb.

TAG 25 WORRY

Too small an indicator to be tagged "anxiety," words expressing "worry" were kept separate under this tag.
Examples:

(a) His wife remarked that the respondent worries much more than he lets on and that he really worries for no good reason.
(b) He says he is very much of a worrywart.

TAG 26 TENSE

This tag includes words explicitly indicating a tense feeling: tenseness, tension, stiffen up.
Examples:

(a) In the past, she states she was frequently so tense that she felt she would explode.
(b) Some thirteen years ago she had an episode characterized by tension and anxiety, during which she put on a good deal of weight and she overate a good deal.

TAG 27 ANXIETY, GENERAL
TAG 28 ANXIETY, PHYSIOLOGICAL

Anxiety in the present system of evaluation is a diffuse reaction of an organism that cannot cope with the demands of its environment. In our assessment of anxiety we rely heavily on its neurophysiological concomitants; these processes are seen as one phase of the hierarchy of organization of the organism. Anxiety in this sense is a reaction that is so pervasive and fundamental that it cannot be related to a specific neurophysiological base, and we depend on such symptoms as palpitations and hands sweating.

In describing anxiety we have chosen to separate the physiological concomitants from the feeling state. The latter is tagged *Anxiety, General* and describes feelings of agitation, anxious states, bad dreams, and nightmares. On the other hand, *Anxiety, Physiological* describes sensations related to diffuse feelings of apprehension; i.e., jumpy, hard heartbeat, profuse sweating, tightness in the throat, violent shaking.

Examples, Tag 27:

(a) The patient has suffered considerably for most of her adult life from marked psychoneurotic disorders, most notably chronic, incapacitating fatigue, depression, and anxiety.
(b) An intelligent, responsible, and likable woman with significant impairment growing out of physical and psychological symptoms, particularly anxiety.

Examples, Tag 28:

(a) She felt as though she had a lump in her throat and she felt run down.
(b) Sometimes while in bed his heart will beat just as fast as it can beat and he will feel frightened.

TAG 30 RESTLESSNESS

Used in combination with Tag 26, *Tense*, to assess a tension state, this category includes expressions such as can't sit down, always jumping about, never still, cannot wait.
Examples:

(a) She was restless and unable to sleep.
(b) He stated that he can't sit down for a minute, must always be moving and active or else he gets nervous.

TAG 31 DEPRESSIVE LABEL

TAG 32 LOW MOOD

Depression in our system is a phenomenal characteristic of the organism in which feelings of low mood, dejection, loss of appetite, lowered initiative, and gloomy thoughts predominate. Guilt and object loss are not necessary components of our operational definition and they are excluded on the grounds of etiological bias. Tag 31, *Depressive Label*, is really a high-order label in which the assessment of depression is made in a global fashion rather than by describing the feeling state or behaviors of the individual; i.e., depressed, depression, melancholia. Tag 32, *Low Mood*, defines the behavioral components of depression as: (1) feelings of dejection; and (2) disrupted body functions.

Examples, Tag 31:

(a) R is a thirty-five-year-old woman with an important psychophysiologic illness (peptic ulcer) associated with mild amounts of depression and anxiety.

(b) Depression when in the city, sitting home at night he feels miserable.

Examples, Tag 32:

(a) She does get quite nervous and sad and discouraged because the arthritis prevents her from getting at her work.

(b) She said she couldn't really understand why she was low in spirits.

TAG 45 SOCIAL ACTIVITY *

Entries in this category record statements referring to an active involvement in social (community/religious) events: active in church, hard worker in social activities.

Examples:

(a) The respondent said she is a steady member of her church, active in its social functions.

(b) He often participates actively in sports events with his church group.

TAG 46 SOCIAL ISOLATION

This category tags indications of subjective isolation from friends and community. Some entries are: stays to himself, doesn't like to mix, distant from people, recluse.

Examples:

(a) He prides himself in having no friends, not particularly wishing to establish close relationships.

* This tag was added to differentiate between a very active person (Tag 41, *High General Activity*) and a person active in social organizations.

(b) She belongs to no organizations because she doesn't like to mix with the people around.

TAG 65 PASSIVE ATTITUDE

Entries key on expressions indicating passivity and dependency. Helplessness, cling to other, stubbornness, and dependent are among them. It is used with Tag 58, *Aggressiveness*, and/or Tag 59, *Anger*, to assess a passive-aggressive profile.

Examples:

(a) She seemed rather dependent upon her children and certainly was a rather anxious woman with quite a few fears. She said that usually she was in a bad temper when she first woke up in the morning.
(b) He seems to have the feeling that the community should support him and owes him a living. He is rather chronically angry that he can't get anybody to satisfy his dependent needs and support him.

Stage III, Dictionary Validation, was the logical offshoot of Stage II. It was the cross-validation, on a second subsample, of the results obtained in the previous stage. Stage III represented an advance in dictionary construction in that a concurrent criterion (psychiatric evaluation on the category level) was used as a comparative yardstick for the computer dictionary. The procedures and results of the cross-validation study are described in detail in our 1972 CASE publication.[3] It can be noted that our level of agreement for our overall validation test was 91 percent (Kappa coefficient of agreement $= .67$, significant at less than the .01 level). The remainder of this chapter will deal with the application of CASE to research in psychiatric epidemiology and further implications for development.

Application to Research Problems

One of the persistently difficult and unresolved problems of psychology and psychiatry is the classification of behavior in meaningful, operational units. Human knowledge about personality and abnormal behavior is still at a rudimentary level of sophistication. As Cattel points out,[4] the systematizing of human knowledge about personality has fallen into three historical phases:

1. Literary and philosophical phase, a game of personal insight and conventional beliefs extending from the first thoughtful caveman to the most recent novelist and playwright.

2. The stage of organized observation and theorizing, which we may call the early clinical phase. It had its center in the psychiatric generalizations of men like Kraeplin, the father of medical psychology in Germany; Janet, his counterpart in France; and Freud. But it also included philosophers or academic men specializing in personality, like William James in America, Ward, and Klages.

3. The quantitative and experimental phase, which did not begin (as far as personality, rather than other aspects of psychology, is concerned) until the turn of this century, is only beginning to show its fruits in the last decade.

It is this third stage of development to which we address our problem. Taking as our basic assumption that theories or hypotheses about personality (normal or abnormal) must be tested, it is the next step to set up research designs that enable us to explore old theories and discover new insights. The development of mathematical-statistical methods such as factor analysis has enabled us to take natural data, much as the clinician has long done, and find laws and associations related to the structure and functioning of personality. Leighton, Clausen, and Wilson [9] recognized that there was a need to develop rather than to dismiss nosology. In the first edition of *Explorations in Social Psychiatry* they presented a theoretical model for defining patterns of symptoms. The present project is an attempt to make these concepts operational.

Our research application of CASE involved two basic steps:

1. Determination of the factor structure of the categories in the dictionary. In essence this described the co-occurrence of tags in the sample of 120 respondents. The statistical model for this step was factor analysis.

2. Determination of the predictive validity of the factors derived in the previous step. The classification based upon the CASE tags and factors was compared to the classification of the psychiatrists who rated the respondents as A (high probability of being a psychiatric case) or D (high probability of being symptom-free). The statistical model for this step was multiple discriminant analysis. The rationale and a brief description of the procedures for each step will follow.

Factor analysis tests the degree of association between the tags within the sample population. The advantage of this kind of analysis is that it yields a measure of the co-occurrence of tags. The factors are patterns of symptoms that define the underlying dimensions in the sample. The type of factor analysis used was a principal components analysis and a Varimax rotation. Forty-seven tags from the possible ninety-seven were used in this analysis. Tags with greater than 20 percent occurrence were used. This is not to say that the other categories, with less than 20 percent occurrence, are unimportant, but that we wanted to obtain stable co-occurrence factors that would help in determining the predictive validity of CASE.

Some tags that were logically related to each other were combined to form a new category. For example, schizophrenic label, suicidal label, and undifferentiated psychotic indicators all had low frequencies of occurrence as separate tags. They were grouped under a new category called psychotic indicators. The new grouping permitted us to include this important set of behaviors in our analysis, since the frequency of the grouped category was substantially higher than for the separate tags. The net result of our grouping efforts was that twenty-six low-frequency tags were grouped under four new categories, each having a significantly greater amount of occurrence than before. In all, sixty-nine tags (categories) were used to form the forty-seven categories used for analysis.

The next statistical procedure was the application of multiple discriminant analysis to the data. This is a form of pattern recognition which utilizes the a priori classification of the respondents (by the psychiatrists) to obtain a validation "hit" rate for the sample. There are a number of steps to this procedure. The first step utilizes the factor scores from the factor analysis and determines the factors that are statistically related to the separation of the A and D groups.[5] If the factors are related to the classification, then one or more discriminant functions are derived that give each respondent a probability score of belonging to the independent groups. From these data a hit-miss table can be constructed to note the agreement between the computer classification and the psychiatric criterion. The following sections will describe the results of the factor analysis and the discriminant function analysis. Each of these steps are part of the sequential validation process of the computer model.

RESULTS OF THE FACTOR ANALYSIS

Six factors were derived from the factor analysis of the forty-seven tags. These six factors accounted for 37 percent of the total variance. This is a respectable amount of variance considering the fact that the tags were chosen so as to be as independent as possible. The results which represent the co-occurrence of behaviors of psychiatric interest are therefore higher-order dimensions.

As shown in Table 19.2, Factor I is a psychoneurotic factor that is clearly defined by the presence of both anxiety and depressive elements. The cardiovascular loadings include both symptoms (lower-order complaints) and actual disorders. Factor I represents a factor commonly found in many diverse samples.[1] The involvement of both psyche and soma are clearly illustrated in this dimension. In terms of the present factor analysis it is the dimension that accounts for the 28 percent of the common variance.

Factor II in Table 19.3 illustrates a set of symptoms related to allergic conditions. The psychological elements are less specified in this factor than in Factor I. This factor, like Factor I, has been isolated in other samples. It accounts for 18 percent of the common variance.

367

TABLE 19.2

Factor I: Anxiety-Depression with
Physiological Components

TAG	LOADING
Anxiety Physiological	.71
Cardiovascular Symptom	.69
Mood Disturbance	.61
Depressive Label	.58
Subjective Body Sensations	.53
GI Disorder	.52
GI Symptom	.52
Cardiovascular Disorder	.48
Respiratory Symptom	.41
Anxiety Generalized	.40
Worry	.40
Headache Ordinary	.40
Musculoskeletal Symptom	.39

Factor III, Table 19.4, is a close representation of the conversion hysterical syndrome reported in early clinical literature. In order of importance, Factor III accounts for 16 percent of the common variance. It is interesting to note that this cluster of symptoms has not disappeared from the clinical scene but is not as prominent as the anxiety-depression dimension.

Factor IV, Table 19.5, is an interesting combination of behaviors and complaints representing a personality-state dimension that appears to be a sub-

TABLE 19.3

Factor II: Allergy–Skin–Nerves

TAG	LOADING
Allergy	.69
Skin Disorder	.58
Drug Use (Therapeutic)	.53
Respiratory Disorder	.45
Nervousness	.45
Trouble Sleeping	.40
GU Symptoms	.40

clinical cluster. Factor IV accounts for 13 percent of the common variance. This dimension is a complex of outer-directed (aggressiveness) urges and inner tensions. The basic complaints are based on anemia and low blood counts. The relationship of this is unclear at the present.

Factor V, Table 19.6, defines a dimension that comes closest to a psychotic syndrome. This dimension combines social difficulties (either drinking, antisocial acts, or dyssocial acts) with psychotic indicators. The minus sign attached

TABLE 19.4

Factor III: Psychosomatic–Conversion–Hysterical

TAG	LOADING
Conversion Symptoms	.63
Headache Sick	.58
GU Symptoms	.52
Anxiety Physiological	.49
General Motor Disturbance	.48
Overweight	.44
Respiratory Symptom	.41

to hypochondriasis on this dimension means that this tag is negatively associated with the others. Individuals who score high on this dimension are likely not to have hypochondrical complaints, but rather to act out their tensions and conflicts. Factor V accounts for 12 percent of the common variance.

TABLE 19.5

Factor IV: Outer-Directed–Tension State

TAG	LOADING
Agressiveness	.76
Tense	.44
Hemic Disorder (Anemic)	.44
Anger	.38
Undifferentiated Complaints	.34

Factor VI, Table 19.7, represents a bipolar dimension in which there are both positive and negative relationships among the tags. One end of the dimension defines a group of behaviors related to high general activity (high involvement in work or other time-consuming activities over and above the norms for

TABLE 19.6

Factor V: Social Deviancy–Psychotic Indicator

TAG	LOADING
Restlessness	.62
Social Difficulties	.59
Psychotic Indicators	.36
Respiratory Disorder	.36
Hypochondriasis	−.39

this group of people) and social isolation (insulation of the self from the social network). The other pole of the dimension defines behaviors related to low intellectual functioning, passivity, anxiety, and physiological involvement. Factor VI accounts for 12 percent of the common variance.

TABLE 19.7

Factor VI: Reserved Compulsivity–High Intellect
Versus Passive–Intellectual Deficiency

TAG	LOADING
High General Activity	.49
Social Isolation	.33
Intellectual Deficiency	−.45
Anxiety General	−.40
Trouble Sleeping	−.40
Cardiovascular Disorder	−.39
Nervousness	−.35
Passive Attitude	

Factors V and VI account for 24 percent of the common variance and appear to be clinically relevant factors in defining more severe forms of behavior disturbance. Descriptions of the factors were kept to a minimum because of space limitations. A complete interpretation and clarification of the meanings of the factors goes beyond the scope of this chapter. The factors that emerged, however, have both practical and theoretical significance. It is our purpose to demonstrate that computer-derived evaluations in combination with statistical analyses have both discriminative and structural properties.* The structural aspects (the theoretical relationships of the factors) have been described in the previous paragraphs.

The next section will attempt to describe the results of the steps taken to demonstrate the predictive (discriminative) validity of the computer-derived factor dimensions. In this step each respondent was given a factor score for each of the six factors as described above. The a priori classification of the respondents into either the A group (psychiatrically defined as a case) or the D group (symptom-free) was used as the criterion for prediction based upon the six factors.

RESULTS OF THE DISCRIMINANT FUNCTION ANALYSIS

The discriminant function analysis indicated that the six factors, when combined into a statistical function, were meaningfully related to the separation of the groups. The results of the discriminant analysis were significant at less than the .0001 probability level. Table 19.8 contains the means for each of the two groups based upon the six factor scores, and the scaled vector weights for each factor contributing to the discrimination between the groups.

When each respondent was scaled according to the weights derived from the discriminant function analysis and assigned probabilities of belonging to either the A or the D group, the agreement between the computer assignment (CASE)

* Meehl has proposed that there are two basic uses of statistics: (1) the structural (or analytic) use which describes constructs to "explain" the behavior; and (2) the discriminative-validating use which confirms the relationship of certain constructs to other criteria.[11]

TABLE 19.8
Means for the A and D Groups

FACTORS	A GROUP	D GROUP	SCALED WEIGHT
I	53.4	46.0	.66
II	52.9	46.6	.55
III	52.1	47.5	.41
IV	52.3	47.3	.44
V	50.9	48.8	.19
VI	51.8	47.9	.34

Scores are based upon a mean of 50 and standard deviation of 10. The scaled weights are a measure of the combination of the factor toward discrimination of the two groups.

and psychiatrist assignment was 80 percent. These results are presented in Table 19.9.

In the present instance we found a 20 percent disagreement between the computer classification and the psychiatric grouping. In cell b of Table 19.9, CASE classified the respondents as D and the psychiatrists as A. In cell c the re-

TABLE 19.9
Case Factors as Predictors for Psychiatric Classification

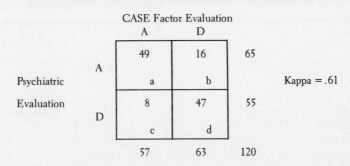

CASE Factor Evaluation

		A	D		
Psychiatric	A	49	16	65	
		a	b		Kappa = .61
Evaluation	D	8	47	55	
		c	d		
		57	63	120	

verse was true. It is possible to run retrievals on these cases and to identify the types of discrepancies. In our original study we identified four forms of potential errors:

1. Judgment differences—in which the tenets of the operational definition were not adhered to by the clinical raters. This type of discrepancy (JD) is found in cells b and c.
2. Dictionary error—in which the CASE dictionary did not have the appropriate words, idioms, or combinatory routines to assess a given category. These errors (DE) are found in cell b. When such omissions are found, they are added to the dictionary.
3. Editing error—discrepancies which occur in the editing of the document. It is really random error, and is found in both b and c cells.
4. Residual error—unidentified differences (RE).

Once the discrepancies are identified, then corrective steps can be taken to improve upon the prediction ratio. For example, if a judgment error has been found, rethinking of the concept may take place or the judgment of the computer accepted as more reliable. Adjustment of dictionary error is a reiterative process that continues as long as new language samples are accumulated in our research. As one can see, use of the computer is synergistic rather than mechanistic and is based upon feedback loops.

The successful prediction of an external or concurrent criterion adds greater validity to the CASE dictionary and the resulting factor patterns from the tags. More elaborate analyses of the factors could reveal the types or patterns of illness and wellness that exist in the sample. Although the results are not presented in this chapter, we have found that the A group has at least seven types of combinations of the various factors. These represent clinical syndromes in the usual sense that they are recurring individual types rather than dimensions across people.

In summary, we found that the CASE dictionary had validity at the tag level and at the factor level. The conceptual model of behaviors of psychiatric interest proved to be useful in classifying individuals at the most fundamental level of ill versus well.

Implications and Further Development

A content analysis dictionary is a collection of content analysis categories. However, the focus of the categories is on a specific line of theory that links the dictionary together. In the present research, the implicit assumption behind the dictionary is that there are phenomenal behavior patterns of psychiatric interest that can be measured independently of each other. The classification or assessment procedure precludes etiological considerations and matters of impairment, although impairment can be determined for any given category, based on the information pertinent to it. Differential diagnoses are not the aim of the assessment procedure; instead, an array of independently measured symptoms or behaviors is assessed. It is in this sense that the CASE dictionary is a specific research tool for survey epidemiological studies in the area of psychiatric or psychological disorder.

Collection of these independent categories permits the user to correlate the behaviors of psychiatric interest with demographic, social, and other associated variables of concern. Each category has explicit operational criteria for measurement of the concept. Factor analysis of the tags or lower-order concepts permits us to clarify the relationship of the behaviors of psychiatric interest. This study has only scratched the surface of the problem and opens up for future concern the nosology of psychological and psychiatric disorders. One of the positive results has been the realization that a computer model can reliably codify psychiatric interviews at a high level of agreement with external criteria.

Other possibilities include the expansion of the number of categories into areas such as coping mechanisms and social attributes of the respondent. This is a matter of defining the categories and then recycling the same procedures used in the current study.

Analysis of the data does not stop at category tagging. Once you have obtained valid measures of your concepts, multivariate analyses of the data are possible, and the multivariate techniques may be as complex as analysis of variance, factor analysis, or discriminant function analysis. In addition to analyzing the group data by the abovementioned techniques, the data from CASE for any one individual can be used with data from other sources. In the Stirling County study, for example, physicians are interviewed regarding their knowledge of the health of a respondent. If the respondent had reported nonspecific symptoms, the doctor may offer a precise diagnosis of the disorder. Conversely, the physician's report may negate the physical disorder reported by the individual. This would change the assessment of symptoms in the final analysis.

In addition to CASE we have constructed a computer program, called PROBE, that analyzes self-report or questionnaire data obtained from the respondent.[2] In this instance the questions are preceded into response categories (sometimes, often, or never). PROBE generates detailed symptom patterns, impairment, and CASEness. It is possible to utilize the different sources of data, self-report and interview, to obtain a combined assessment of a given respondent.

The model for this type of synergistic interplay between CASE and a questionnaire (as assessed by PROBE) is to: (1) administer a health survey questionnaire; and (2) have local physicians report on the psycho-social-medical status of our respondents. Each source of data represents a view of the person. In the case of the questionnaire, it is essentially the self-report of the individual plus some interviewer comments about the person. On the other hand, the physician comments are expert observer opinions about the individual. These data can stand alone as perspectives of the individual or they can be integrated to achieve a fuller picture of the psycho-social status of the respondent.

In some ways the physician's comments complement the survey information by corroborating physical or mental disorders mentioned by the respondent. On another level, they can amplify the report by the respondent. This is a clarifying function of MD comments. Again the inputs from the physician reports can nullify an erroneous impression from the questionnaire (especially in the sphere of physical disorder). We shall call this the correcting operation.

In Figure 19.1, the two computer programs, CASE and PROBE, operate

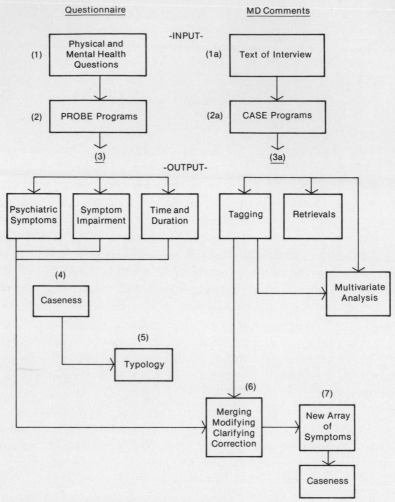

FIGURE 19.1. System flow for psychiatric evaluation.

independently until step 6 is reached. At that point a number of decisions have to be made. Basically three models of contingencies have been delineated: corroboration, contradiction, and complementation.

In the corroborating situation, the questionnaire evaluation parallels the MD comments evaluation and no adjustment is necessary. In a contradictory situation the symptom may be judged present by PROBE and absent by CASE, or vice versa. In this instance modification is based on the best estimate of information. If it involves the psychological state of the respondent, the PROBE evaluation stands. For example, if the respondent complains of anxiety and the doctor does not mention the symptom, the anxiety symptom is retained. If the respondent denies anxiety and the doctor describes the respondent as anxious, the anxiety symptom given by the doctor is neglected because the symptom by definition involves phenomenological behavior of the respondent. On the other hand, a respondent is not likely to report personality disorder symptoms, while the doctor or other key informants may report them. In that case the symptom is recorded. Each symptom has a different set of possibilities if there is contradictory information. A set of logical decision trees can be written for each contingency.

In the complementary contingency the symptom is reported by both CASE and PROBE, but different information is provided by the two sources. For example, if CVS is present in both CASE and PROBE, the contributing subsymptom in PROBE may be high blood pressure, while in CASE the doctor reports high blood pressure along with an actual reading and whether it is essential hypertension or due to renal involvement.

There is another possible merging of the two programs, and that is at the input level. It may well be that the signs presented by a respondent are subthreshold for the presence of a symptom. The doctor may also present marginal evidence. The elements in the questionnaire and the physician's comments could combine to reach suprathreshold proportions for the symptom.

This interaction between two programs is another example of the proposed uses for the computer to foster reliable and valid assessments of field survey data.

REFERENCES

1. Benfari, R. C., and Leighton, A. H. "Comparison of Factor Structures in Urban New York and Rural Nova Scotia Population Samples: A Study in Psychiatric Epidemiology." In *The Community as an Epidemiologic Laboratory*, edited by I. J. Kessler and M. L. Levin. Baltimore: Johns Hopkins Press, 1970.

2. ———. "PROBE: Computer Instrument for Field Surveys in Psychiatric Disorder." *Archives of General Psychiatry* 23(1970):352,358.

3. ———; Beiser, M.; and Coen, K. "CASE: Computer Assigned Symptom Evaluation." *Journal of Nervous and Mental Disease* 154 (1972):115–124.

4. Cattel, R. B. *The Scientific Analysis of Personality*. Chicago: Aldine, 1965.

5. Cooley, W. W., and Lohnes, P. R. *Multivariate Procedures for the Behavioral Sciences*. New York: Wiley, 1962.

6. Cronbach, L. J., and Meehl, P. E. "Construct Validity in Psychological Tests." *Psychol. Bull.* 52(1955):281–302.

7. Leighton, A. H. *My Name is Legion*. New York: Basic Books, 1959.

8. ———, and Leighton, D. C. *Handbook for the Psychiatric Evaluation of Personal Data*. Harvard School of Public Health. Mimeographed. 1965.

9. Leighton, A. H.: Clausen, J. A.; and Wilson, R. N. *Explorations in Social Psychiatry*. New York: Basic Books, 1957.

10. Leighton, A. H.; Leighton, D. C.; and Danley, R. "Validity in Mental Health Surveys." *Canadian Psychiatric Association Journal* 11, no. 3, May–June 1966, pp. 166–177.

11. Meehl, P. E. *Clinical versus Statistical Prediction*. Minneapolis: University Minnesota Press, 1954.

12. Stone, P. J., and Kirsch, J. *User's Manual for the General Inquirer*. Cambridge, Mass.: M.I.T. Press, 1968.

13. Stone, P. J.; Dunphy, D. C.; Smith, M. S.; and Ogilvie, D. M. *The General Inquirer*. Cambridge, Mass.: M.I.T. Press, 1966.

Part V

Future Issues

WHAT ARE the future issues for social psychiatry? Can a healthier social environment be created? Can we improve our ways of conceptualizing and measuring the key social and psychological processes that reveal important aspects of social system effectiveness? These are persistent questions that require the application of our best imaginative minds. They form the foci of the two chapters in this concluding section.

The following is a set of future questions to consider:

1. In the evolution of the study of the relationships between sociocultural environment and psychiatric disorder, we are still confronted with the problem of a more adequate conceptualization of the duality posed by the founding fathers, Durkheim and Freud. Durkheim focused on social etiology; Freud on inner dynamics. What new theories are emerging? Can we better reduce theory to reality-testable propositions?

2. Can we provide a more adequate conceptualization of the social process risk factors for psychiatric disorder? What are the social equivalents in the area of psychiatric disorder to the high predictive value of blood pressure, cholesterol, heavy cigarette smoking, and body weight for the risk of having a myocardial infarction? Intuitively, social support, coping skills, and public and private self-esteem appear to be the social analogues to the predictive power of blood pressure and cholesterol in coronary heart disease.

3. What are the symptomless patterns of health?

4. How do people begin to show signs of illness and how can we better prevent psychiatric disorder by recognizing early signs?

5. What are the effects of healthy leaders or healthy individuals on other

people around them? Conversely, what is the effect of mentally ill people on others in their environment?

6. What are the best areas for preventive opportunities, e.g., at work, in school, and so on?

7. What are the best theoretical frameworks for looking at the relationship between the social environment and psychiatric disorder? For example, what are the global variables such as urbanization and industrialization? What are the institutional variables such as primary socialization groups, voluntary association, and social class? What are the social psychological constructs such as personal values, norms, expectations, status dimensions, role definition needs, and sentiments, all of which conceptualize the relationships of individuals and institutions? What are the basic psychological constructs such as anxiety, hostility, and happiness?

8. Is there such a thing as mental health? What are the possibilities and limits of actually altering the social environment to be more promotive of psychological health?

9. Do we have an adequate theory of socialization throughout the life cycle?

10. Culture is important, but how important? Are there patterns of mental disorders in all populations regardless of culture?

11. Are there social psychological developmental universals that contribute to social psychological health? In thinking of coping, what are the layers of defense, e.g., individual, interpersonal, and social systems protective of other social systems?

12. The longest social psychiatric investigation has been the Stirling County study, directed by Alexander H. Leighton. What contributions are needed in order to do more effective life histories, to better study socialization, to better conceptualize and test a tree of hypotheses about sociocultural determinants, and to better conceptualize community models of sentiments? What do we need to know about supportive-expressive behavior? Finally, what do we need to learn with respect to the developmental changes of noxious social areas?

13. What do we need to do better to conceptualize and measure the variety of dependent variables which are reflective of psychological stress?

14. Finally, what are the specific types of indicators of social disintegration related to psychiatric disorder?

There is a great need for more extensive and intensive study devoted to the search for shared psychosocial health.

Editorial Note

The concern of this chapter is with that ancient and elusive question: "How do you measure mental health?" Of course, rooted in this question is the equally difficult problem of defining the dimensions of both mental health and mental illness. Leighton and Rolland review the evolution of the difficult scientific process of increasing our approximations to the measure of mental health or illness in such a way as to make the things we say about the prevalence and incidence of mental illness far more valid and reliable than they have been in the past. We are now moving toward multiphasic, multiple criteria.

In approaching the measurement of mental health, we are confronted with the probability that if you scratch almost anyone deep enough, varying degrees of the despair, fear, and anxiety which are the human condition will be seen. Perhaps a certain amount of suffering, depending on our natures, our temperaments, and our experiences, is the human lot. Maybe we are really just discovering scientifically what the prophets of old already knew.

B. H. K.

CHAPTER 20

New Indicators of
the Dependent Variable

ALEXANDER H. LEIGHTON
JOHN S. ROLLAND

VIRTUALLY all presently existing methods of assessing the dependent variable (mental illness) are based on what people say about themselves and on third-party observation of their behavior. There exists, however, the possibility of another approach that utilizes physiological and biochemical indicators. If this could be shown to have validity and feasibility, it would have enormous advantages and would open new areas in psychiatric epidemiology.

The clue to the possibility is in the HOS (Health Opinion Survey) and other similar methods of identifying psychiatric disorder. Relying heavily on questions that ask if the respondent has been bothered by psychophysiological sensations, the questionnaire is able to distinguish populations of treated mental patients (mainly psychoneurotic) from representative samples of community populations. In surveys of community populations, it has been able to separate groups of people as psychologically "ill" and "well" so as to achieve agreement with a psychiatrist working independently.[3]

The derivation of the questions employed in the test has been empirical. That is, the questions do not come from any theoretical expectation, but emerged from a series of investigations in which many kinds of questions were tested for their ability to distinguish populations of people known on clinical grounds to be mentally ill.

Four hypotheses may be put forward as explanatory. First, pyschoneurotics may misperceive themselves as having physiological symptoms that they do not actually have. Second, psychoneurotics may be more keenly aware of physiological sensations which they actually share with normals. Third, psychoneurotics may in fact manifest more psychophysiological symptoms than normals and perceive this difference correctly. Fourth, the subjectively perceived differences may be incomplete, and it could be that physiological-biochemical measurements would reveal still further differences.

The third and fourth hypotheses raise the possibility of using physiological measurements as markers which could support, refine, supplement, or possibly substitute for the HOS type of questionnaire. The possibility calls strongly for investigation.

The notion of trying to see if this or that physiological variable correlates with one or more types of psychiatric disturbance is far from new. Most endeavors along this line have not, however, proved very fruitful. Work with such variables as blood pressure and skin resistance illustrate the point.

The HOS, however, offers a further clue and suggests a line of action. The HOS questions constitute a battery which covers a number of bodily systems such as cardiovascular, gastrointestinal, skin, and so on. The method of scoring is based on the net effect, not on any one particular system. This rouses the expectation that if physiological and biochemical tests have promise as indicators of psychiatric disorders, it will most likely be as a battery.

The approach, therefore, might be to start with making physiological comparisons of normal controls and psychiatric patients. A hospital allows for sophisticated tests to be performed. This would facilitate the comparing of: (1) gross and fine measurements individually to psychophysiological complaints; and (2) gross to fine measurements in terms of correspondence and complementarity.

Another possibility would be to utilize the multiphasic screening laboratory panel conducted on hospital admissions and many outpatients. Retrospectively and prospectively, this would supply individual and group baseline data that could be repeated serially and correlated with reporting of changes in quality of severity of psychophysiological symptoms in psychiatric and nonpsychiatric patients. Something analogous to this is being investigated at the University of Florida College of Medicine.[1] Gordon and his associates have constructed what is called "Automated Multiphasic Health Testing" to help screen psychiatric patients at a local VA hospital. They used a battery of tests to see if they could accurately predict on two dimensions: (1) whether a patient was admitted or not; and (2) to which service he was assigned: psychiatric, medical, surgical, and so on. Included in the test battery were: (1) general history (including psychiatric);

(2) psychiatric screening questions drawn from the HOS and Rahe; and (3) various physical, physiological, and biochemical measurements. Their preliminary results are encouraging and we are impressed by the overall method of combining psychophysiological questions with various physiological measurements. It would be expedient from our viewpoint to begin by picking specific physiological tests that correspond to the HOS psychophysiological questions.

There are numerous difficulties lying in the way of exploring the frontier we have sketched. The most formidable are probably concerned with developing the physiological and biochemical tests. Assuming that a battery is found which does have a high correlation with psychiatric disorders, there still remains the enormous task of reducing these tests to forms which are suitable for administration in epidemiological surveys without invoking high refusal rates, and which can be done without prohibitive laboratory costs.

Other problems have to do with what one can expect from the instrument once it is developed. Llewelyn Thomas,[4] in an article that reviews this approach to the dependent variable, states: "All living things respond to changes in the world around them by changes in themselves, and all emotional changes are correlated with some physiological change."

The core of the issue raised in this is the problem of separating organic from psycho-social-cultural stimuli as originators in the course of events leading to the final common pathway of physiological change. Although we accept Thomas's idea of social-cultural stimuli as conceptually separate from organic, we would refine his notion so as to include both internally created stimuli (i.e., memory, imagination, foresight) and physical stimuli that undergo a psychological transformation prior to response. The link between an organic illness (response) and a physical cause (i.e., microbial stimulus) can be strengthened or diminished, we would assume, by psychological intermediaries. Hinkle and Wolfe[2] found a clustering of many kinds of individual illnesses around periods of stressful life experience, especially in those who had the greatest difficulty in adapting to the situation. They hypothesized that the number of illnesses is correlated with the individual's psychological state, which in turn is correlated with the person's *perceived* current life situation. This was found to be independent of age, sex, race, and cultural or social background.

Another issue involves more specifically the relationship of physiological response to mental health and illness. Certain degrees of fear ("anxiety") and physiological concomitants may represent a state of alertness and receptivity for certain roles in society. Similarly, a lack of physiological response, when connected with certain affectless conditions (e.g., in some forms of sociopathy), could be as pathological as overreaction.

We raise these issues not to discourage but to keep us aware of the importance of context and the need for ancillary data. On the asset side is the first-order importance of developing a test battery for a significant portion of the mental disorder field, a battery that is independent of language and the vast possibilities for misperception that are inevitably tied to it.

In addition to epidemiological usefulness, there is the possibility that this area of research might have significant implications for primary prevention. Manifestations of stress, that is, strain, may surface physiologically in certain instances prior to their subjective awareness. This would permit intervention at an earlier, less complex level of an unfolding psychological problem. It might also, eventually have use in following the course of psychological disturbances. Generally, it seems that initiation of empirical studies of individuals will lead to population norms (some age- and sex-based, some sociological) and ultimately cross-cultural comparisons. From this a revised theory and, in turn, a refined comprehensive mental health index can emerge.

REFERENCES

1. Gordon, R. E.; Bielen, L.; and Watts, A. "Psychiatric Screening with Automated Multiphasic Health Testing in the VA Admission Procedure." *American Journal of Psychiatry* 130(1973):46–48.

2. Hinkle, L. E., Jr., and Wolfe, H. "Ecological Investigations of the Relationship Between Illness, Life Experiences, and the Social Environment." *Annals of Internal Medicine* 49 (1958):1373–1388.

3. Macmillan, A. M. "The Health Opinion Survey: Technique for Estimating Prevalence of Psychoneurotic and Related Types of Disorder in Communities." *Psychological Reports* 3 (1957):325–339.

4. Thomas, E. L., "The Possibility of Using Physiological Indicators for Detecting Psychiatric Disorder." In *Approaches to Cross-Cultural Psychiatry*, edited by A. H. Leighton and J. M. Murphy, pp. 161–187. Ithaca, N.Y.: Cornell University Press, 1965.

Editorial Note

Jane M. Murphy begins this chapter with one of the fundamental questions in social psychiatry: What are the social causes of mental illness? Under what social conditions does the individual or group of individuals become "unglued"? What are the specific social processes that contribute to either instabilities in social relationships or intrapsychic distress?

Durkheim is still one of the seminal contributors to this area of inquiry. His major social etiologic factors can be described as follows. First is the anomic situation, in which the individual is at loose ends in identifying values and appropriate norms to give direction to life. The second factor is egoistic, in which socially the person is thrown excessively on his own resources. The third major social etiologic factor is the altruistic, in which the individual's ego effectively belongs to the group and he is excessively dependent on group approval. These "social causes" are still interesting concepts. A major focus, however, in all of Durkheim's etiologic causes is the problem of social bonds, or interferences in social bonds, or defects in social bonds, or inadequate need-meeting facilities in social bonds. These problems are ancient and are still with us.

The main social stresses may be located in such variables as culture, acculturation, economic position, rural or urban living patterns, the family, and alienation. Murphy pays particular attention to the question of whether culture is causative. The evidence is unclear. Is mental illness ubiquitous? This chapter also pays attention to acculturation as a source of stress. Economic position has long been thought to be a factor in mental illness; it is certainly clear that the stress of poverty is very real. The rural-urban stress hypothesis, under the rubric of "alienation," raises questions about those old stereotypes of rural life being charming and urban life being deleterious to psychological well-being. In any case, atomistic social settings are probably pathogenic, whether they are rural or urban.

Alienation has been another frame of reference for looking at the quality of human relationships and at certain types of stress, particularly those stresses associated with affiliative needs. Another consideration is that of "labeling" and the stigma of being labeled. If we could unlabel the mentally ill, would the problem fade away? The evidence is clear, however, that the concept of mental illness is practically universal. In Murphy's view, we should bury the ideas of cultural differences and rural-urban differences, but labeling, economic stress, alienation stress, and acculturation stress remain possible causative factors.

In looking to the future, she urges us to pay careful attention to the uses of *social indicators which monitor change in society, the importance of social networks, and the specifics of behavior settings.*

Finally, we are challenged to take into consideration what the author calls social genetics, that is, that human behavior is influenced by both environmental and hereditary considerations. The importance of genetic factors as necessary but not sufficient causes is crucial to the future development of this field.

B. H. K.

CHAPTER 21

Social Causes:
The Independent Variables

JANE M. MURPHY

A MAIN PURPOSE of research in social psychiatry is to answer the question: "What are the social causes of mental illness?" Most effort in this direction has been guided by the methods of epidemiology. The other choices for research strategy are clinical and experimental. The nature of the question and the limited number of humane experiments which can be performed to answer it have made epidemiological techniques imperative. In addition to developing case-finding methods (for the dependent variables), this means locating the naturally occurring events in human societies (for the independent variables) which offer the opportunity for what Claude Bernard called "experimental reasoning." [15] To be useful, the "experiments of nature" need first of all to be relevant to sound theories of social etiology; they need to be open to creating research designs which can compare outcomes from natural experimental groups with outcomes from natural control groups; and they need to apply to large enough populations so that probability statistics can be used.

In the context of this field, mental health epidemiology, I will discuss past and future perspectives regarding independent variables, that is, the social experiences which can be hypothesized to play a major role in the causes of mental illness. In reviewing work already accomplished, I will mention the variables of culture, acculturation, economic position, rural-urban residence, family, alienation, and labeling. In looking to the future I will mention three additional promising approaches: social indicators, social networks, and behavioral settings. I will conclude with comments on the need for social genetic investigations.

The beginning of social experiences for human beings takes place in utero. For purposes of independent variables, however, we usually mean those events which happen to an individual from birth onward and which stem from the fact that he is a member of society. Further, we mean those experiences which are not determined by his psychiatric status but rather are genuinely antecedent to and therefore potentially causative of mental illness.

In regard to theory, most studies have employed *social stress* as a frame of reference and have been influenced by formulations from anthropology, psychology, and sociology. Stress consists of those events which are external to the persons in question and which threaten psychological well-being.* The popularity of stress theory is not a measure of its having been used in a consistent and standardized manner. To the contrary, it has often been abused, and it remains controversial even if largely unreplaced by other approaches.

A chief problem is the lack of a comprehensive view of the multitudinous and multifaceted experiences which are necessary to psychological well-being. Nevertheless, recognition is now widely given to the fact that there are potentially many social causes of mental illness and that they may have effect all along the course of life. Search for the critical events of early childhood which would inevitably lead to a damaged adult personality is now mainly a matter of history and probably represents the decline of Freudian theory as the primary source of hypotheses in the mental health field.

The stress theories currently used in epidemiology tend to reflect the view that mental health is promoted by social situations in which there are adequate resources for creature needs as well as needs for affiliation with others, for coherence in values, for social role training, for self-expression, and for recognition as a unique and valued human being. Stress involves the external social forces which threaten a person in regard to these needs, either in terms of depriving him of necessary supports or taxing him beyond the limits of his psychological vitality.

Culture

It is not surprising that *culture* itself was one of the early and still provocative independent variables to be considered in social psychiatric research. The vast diversity of cultures in human populations lends itself to comparative research,

* See references 27, 53, 56, 77, and 91.

and the concept of culture is eminently well-suited to population studies. Moreover, culture, as the social heritage of a group of people, is antecedent to any given individual who is its carrier, and culture can be studied in terms of the stress framework.

For a time there was a proliferation of culture comparisons which represented the effort to place different cultures in a stress taxonomy: tough and easy cultures, continuous and discontinuous cultures, competitive and cooperative cultures.[3,14,58,68] Much of the research using these seminal ideas was, however, loose and speculative regarding enumeration of the dependent variables of mental illness.*

Looking back over the three-quarters of a century during which ideas about cultural difference have influenced human research, it is remarkable that they have produced so few positive results regarding differences in mental illness. On the other hand, they have engendered the investigations which now allow us to put forth with considerable confidence that no group of people large enough to be self-perpetuating as a culture is protected from mental illness.† There is also some evidence that similarity in the types and frequency of mental illnesses is more noteworthy than the difference.[74] This suggests that if social stress has anything to do with mental illness, it must be of a type which is ubiquitous in human populations.

Acculturation

The view that mental illness is a disease of civilized and industrialized society has not died easily.[34,36] The fantasy of the noble savage is deeply embedded in Western heritage. If mental illness exists everywhere it may be due to the fact that even remote societies have come under the corrupting influence of modernization. Indeed, perhaps it is the process of cultural change that accounts for the fact that primitive groups appear to have an equal share of mental illness. Thus the *acculturative stress* hypothesis has come into existence.[26,47,101] Conflict in values, ambiguities about roles, and change too rapid for adjustment are some components of the acculturation process thought to be stressful. The hypothesis had some support in the early mental hospital studies carried out in developing countries.[18,71] However, the concentration of Westernized people among these patient populations was probably the outcome of their greater awareness of and

* See references 13, 38, 46, 52, 65, and 66.
† See references 19, 25, 48, 55, 72, 73, and 76.

access to such institutional facilities, rather than their illness being caused by Westernization.

A few epidemiological studies have sought evidence on the acculturative stress theme using normal community populations and employing a variety of measures of mental illness. There is as yet no clear-cut answer. On balance it appears that indicators such as Western education, urban residence, industrial work, and religious conversion are not, in and of themselves, associated with mental illness.[42, 75] These studies have suggested, however, that under certain circumstances acculturation may indeed be a state of risk concerning psychological well-being, as, for example, living in a city but not having the security of an industrial job, or being educated but not having work which utilizes it. These findings are sufficiently intriguing to crystallize a need for more sophisticated and complex change theories.

Economic Position

The difference in way of life implied by the global level of cultural contrast is by no means the sole focus of research concerning social etiologies. As a matter of fact, the evidence available on the relationships between social conditions and mental illness has mainly derived from investigations among populations who share the common features of being Western societies. One of the main interests in this research has been the attempt to see if *economic position* is related to mental illness.

There is currently a nearly unequivocal literature pointing to an association between high prevalence of mental illness and low socioeconomic status.* This has been found in a sufficiently large number of studies carried out by independent researchers in different countries to make it safe to generalize that in an economically underprivileged group it is very likely that there will be a higher proportion of the mentally ill than among the more advantaged. This is undoubtedly one of the most important findings produced in the field of social psychiatry.

The picture is not equally clear as to whether the stress of poverty causes mental illness, or whether being mentally ill leads a person to move downward in the socioeconomic structure. If the latter is true, the association would lend support to social selection theories rather than stress. Selection theory is applied to

---

* See references 28, 41, 60, 94, and 97.

open and competitive societies. It holds that individuals who are mentally ill for reasons as yet unknown but probably biogenetic in origin are sifted into the disadvantaged and undesirable positions of society. Some evidence favoring selection theory is that schizophrenic males tend to be in occupations of the same or lower skill levels than their fathers.[98] This finding occurs at a time when the mainstream of change is overwhelmingly in the opposite direction. Educational opportunity is increasing, and the skill levels of the service occupations, which now are the most common form of work, are higher than was true of the extractive and industrial occupations. That men suffering from schizophrenia do not keep up with this general trend suggests that it is not the external events (stress) but rather the problem of personality itself which accounts for the relationship.

On the other hand, there is some research indicating that the "social class-mental illness" correlation is not universal.[61] In a Swedish study using occupational level as the index of social class, people in the low levels of a skill and prestige hierarchy were not found to have higher prevalence, prevalence here referring to all kinds of mental illnesses. Due to welfare benefits, the annual income of individuals at this level was not proportionately small but rather was similar to that of the middle occupations. This is one of those natural experiments which open a window through which a new perspective on the issue is revealed. If economic deprivation is not imposed by the skill level of a subject's work, it appears that the influence on mental illness is not deleterious. Of course, this is not proof of the economic stress hypothesis. A further step toward its demonstration awaits an accumulation of data from studies in which natural "before-after" experiments are enacted.

An optimally useful experiment would be to study people who were, to begin with, mentally healthy and economically secure. If some became economically deprived through war, disaster, job obsolescence, or other process beyond their control, and then developed symptoms of mental illness, this would be an important addition to knowledge on the effects of economic stress. It is obviously a difficult design to execute due to the problem of knowing where to mount baseline studies, and because most industrial societies provide relief in such circumstances. Chronic economic depression is less likely to receive or respond to government programs but is also less useful for this kind of research.

However, since the goal of much national planning is toward improving economic conditions, there are opportunities for alternate though less precise designs. If a group of economically insecure people exhibiting a high prevalence of mental illness at the beginning of a longitudinal study is relieved of economic stress during the years of the investigation and then found to have a lower frequency of illness at the end of the study, this finding would be better support for the economic stress hypothesis than anything we have to date. It would strongly suggest that when the stress of poverty is removed, damage to mental health is lessened.

Rural-Urban Residence

Another key concern of social psychiatry in Western cultures has been to locate individuals in the geographic structure of society to see if differences in settlement pattern and spatial distribution are important regarding mental illness. This interest was greatly stimulated by the Chicago sociologists who characterized the *rural-urban continuum* in terms of differential qualities of interpersonal relationships. Rural communities were presented as the type of social milieu in which intimate, cooperative, face-to-face relations prevail; cities were the places in which impersonality, anonymity, and competition are the norm.* This led to the view that urbanism is injurious to personality functioning through a type of stress which can be called social alienation.

In the crowded, hurried environment of cities, the affiliative supports necessary for psychological well-being were thought to be absent.[29] The rural-urban hypothesis has received some support in epidemiological studies. On the other hand, there are several instances when it has not been born out.[12,54,60,77,94] I suspect that this failure is not a matter of the *alienation stress* hypothesis being wrong, but rather that the rural-urban dichotomy does not represent it. Like a culture, a large urban or rural area is too diverse within itself to have the same impact on all its carriers or dwellers. In line with this is the fact that a few studies have shown a prevalence difference between types of areas within a city, and types of communities within a rural locale. High prevalence in the "rooming house" areas of the central city and in disintegrated rural neighborhoods is a case in point.[32,43,60] It seems likely that smaller units such as these are homogeneous and specific regarding the fabric of human interactions, and the psychiatric findings indicate that indifferent and atomistic social settings are potentially pathogenic.

Alienation

A great deal of interest in social psychiatry has focused on the quality of human relationships. I used the phrase "social alienation stress" in a general way to represent this interest. The choice of term emphasizes the importance of affiliative

* See references 81, 83, 84, and 103.

needs—"people need people"—and points to the fact that to be socially alienated and excluded from the resources of human groups marks a serious risk for mental and emotional viability. To be alienated is to lack moral support, as contrasted with economic support. To be alienated is to be demoralized in the large sense of not being a part of a group process in which there are supportive and reliable interpersonal relations, inhibition of self- and group-defeating behaviors, and stimulation for alertness and involvement. In an intense form, alienation means to experience cruelty and neglect from the significant others who make up the social environment.

Family

In regard to alienation, there is no idea more commonly held than that the quality of relationships within a family has something to do with mental health.* A broken home has often been thought the most damaging of environmental conditions. The family of orientation has received much attention, for the obvious reason that it is more likely to be independent of the psychiatric status of a subject than the family of procreation. Even among adults, however, the quality of marital relationships and the fracturing of family life through widowhood or divorce have been put forth as threatening to the maintenance of mental health.

From the epidemiological point of view there is evidence that marital instability of parents is associated with juvenile delinquency,[35] that the absence of a father from the home during the formative years is related to subsequent suicide,[80] and that divorce or separation of parents is among the stresses which, when taken together in an additive sense, are associated with the more common and milder forms of mental illness found in normal adult populations.[53] Both community and hospital epidemiology indicate that there is strong probability for the rates of mental illness to be higher among the single, divorced, and separated than among those who are married.[30,60,85,94]

One of the weaknesses of family research in psychiatric epidemiology is reliance on structural rather than functional attributes of family. This is indicated in the use of variables such as marital status, physical absence of a father, rank in family of orientation, and, in cross-cultural studies, the differences in marriage patterns involved in monogamy and polygyny.[20,59] These are the kinds of variables about which it is possible to gain reliable data on sizable numbers of subjects and are therefore immediately relevant to epidemiology. They do not, how-

* See references 21, 22, 24, 62, and 69.

ever, reveal how a collection of biologically and affinally related people function as a family in terms of the quality of interpersonal interactions. Studies of family interaction abound in clinical research, but it has been exceedingly difficult to translate these models into investigations of a large number and wide range of natural family settings.

There appears to be a limit to the number of families which can be studied as whole units by traditional and highly intensive participant observation techniques. Efforts have thus far ranged from about twenty to sixty families.[17,49] The need for larger samples has usually been accompanied by a shift to questionnaire surveys of individuals. When this takes place, the results need to be tested for correspondence between the self-report of attitudes and experiences from one person and the actual functioning of a family as a whole. The latter task has often failed in accomplishment. Nevertheless, some innovative questionnaire scales have been developed for the purpose of measuring, for example, consensus in values and division of responsibility between marriage partners, patterns of sociability, and the practice of joint obligation and mutual respect.* If applied in mental health epidemiology such information might contribute further understanding of the role of social alienation in family relations.

Another problem is the possible contamination of family variables by the psychiatric characteristics of a subject. The question of whether stress or selection offers the best explanation is as pertinent to marital status as to economic position. Due to prior mental illness, a person may not be chosen as a marriage partner, or if he enters such a relationship his illness may interfere with its maintenance to the extent that divorce or separation result. Two types of longitudinal studies are needed to deal with the question of contamination, one as it pertains to disrupted relations in the family of orientation and the other to disruptions in the family of procreation.

A few long-term studies of the growth and development of children are underway, with attention being given to mental and emotional as well as physical factors.† If studies such as these were to include reliable observation of valid indicators of the quality of family interaction in which the children are born and grow up, they would represent an important leap forward on two accounts: They would reveal the quality of interpersonal relations before being influenced by the health or illness of a child subject, and they would not depend on retrospective and possibly distorted accounting of childhood by an adult subject. A main obstacle to this design is the need for large numbers and adequate representation of the family styles which actually occur in populations. Since the methods are expensive and time consuming, this is clearly a large order. The other kind of longitudinal study is to follow adults whose mental health had been investigated

* See references 16, 23, 33, 82, and 95.
† See references 31, 44, 45, 67, 93, and 100.

as part of a baseline study in order to trace psychiatric changes as the subjects undergo various kinds of family processes. High incidence following widowhood or divorce would be evidence for alienation stress.

Labeling

A final idea which has come into prominence recently concerns the stress of stigma and prejudice through psychiatric labeling.[86,89,90,96] The theory is that symptoms of mental illness are stereotypes perpetuated by the psychiatric establishment, and that if these behaviors were unlabeled the mental illness problem would disappear.

Although this iatrogenic-sociogenic idea has captured a great deal of interest, it has not yet generated the kind of epidemiologic research which has clarified other themes in social psychiatry. Furthermore, it is an exceedingly difficult theory to test. One way of investigating it would be to find societies in which there is absolutely no idea of mental illness, and therefore no negative view of it, and then carry out an epidemiologic search for behaviors which are called psychiatric in the Western system of thought. If the signs and symptoms of mental illness were absent in groups which also lacked the concept, it would suggest that mental illness is indeed a myth and that believing in it creates the negative sanctions which actually cause mental illnesses.

Unfortunately for the theory, such societies have not been found. As ethnographic knowledge expands it has become increasingly apparent that, at a minimum, the idea of "insanity" is universal. Where adequate investigation has been made, almost all kinds of major mental illnesses are known and occur at about the same frequency as in Western groups. A society without a mental illness ideology appears to be as mythical as mental illness itself is believed to be in labeling theory.

There is no doubt that in the history of man, false beliefs have promoted the exercise of inhuman atrocities, beliefs such as the inferiority or superiority of certain groups or "races" of people. There is also no doubt that some people have unjustly been called "insane." But as a concept, mental illness is probably not a hazardous assumption. It has evolved everywhere, as far as we can tell, in recognition of certain forms of aberrant behavior and certain kinds of symptoms; to propose discarding the whole idea for humanitarian goals is comparable to refusing to be aware of the differences between men and women in an effort to increase sexual equality.

The labeling theory is inimical to research for other reasons as well, such as the fact that any design would require the application of criteria regarding those behaviors and symptoms which would be counted as pathological. This is, of course, an act of labeling. Furthermore, stigma is so recalcitrant as an antecedent and independent variable that it seems wiser to accept it for what it probably is, a reciprocal and associated variable. In other words, there is strong likelihood that a greater number of mentally ill persons will have been the victims of stigmata than is characteristic of a random population, and also that mental illness and stigma probably have a circular relationship. Symptoms of mental illness elicit social disapproval and then negative sanction reinforces the symptoms, which in turn leads to more disfavor, and so on and on.

It would be valuable to explore stigma as a social attitude process which, if realigned through public education to tolerance and positive orientation, might foster recovery and allow opportunity for adjustment to self, others, work, and community life on the part of those who are or have been mentally ill. In this regard there is a natural experiment in process which may throw light on the topic. For several years the populations of state mental hospitals have been progressively reduced through discharges of long-term patients. Since being or having been a mental hospital patient is a main form of the labeling process, it should be possible to follow and evaluate large numbers of people in order to determine the patterns of outcome resulting from hospital release. If the environments into which they are released were identified on a range from relatively stigma-free to relatively stigma-saturated, it would be possible to compare rates of symptom remission and improved functioning in such a way as to gauge the influence of negative sanction more accurately than hitherto.

To summarize past endeavors regarding independent variables, it appears that there are one or two ideas which can safely be buried, at least one which is in limbo, and two or three which are good leads. I put cultural difference and rural-urban settlement in the first category, labeling in the second, and economic stress, alienation stress, and acculturation stress in the third.

Looking to the future, there are three concentrations of interest in the behavioral sciences which may profitably be attended in building on the past and launching further exploration. These are social indicators, social networks, and behavior settings. As far as I have been able to discover, none of these has been a central focus in any psychiatric epidemiology published so far, and yet each is in the wind.

Social Indicators

In recognition of the fact that modern society is a changing society, a field of scientific inquiry has developed called *social indicators*.[11,92,102] This began with the census, was formalized in economics, and is currently in the attention of the human sciences. The indicator field is concerned with measures which can be used to monitor change and thereby show us something about where our society has been and where it is going.

Already it has been documented through the routine reporting services of various private and governmental agencies that life expectancy is increasing, the size of families is decreasing, educational achievement is higher, the standard of living is rising, geographic mobility is commoner, leisure time is mounting, population is concentrating in the cities and suburbs, and so on. Regarding mental health it is known that the use of mental hospitals in the United States increased steadily from the mid-1800s until 1955, when a dramatic decline came into effect, and further that much of this utilization was and is by people over sixty-five suffering from the mental illnesses which appear to be characteristic of senescence.[50,51]

Employment of hospital statistics does not, of course, reveal trends in the true prevalence and incidence of mental illness. A few community epidemiology investigations got started twenty and thirty years ago and can be used as baseline data for small-scale trend analysis regarding whether or not mental illness is increasing, decreasing, or staying at the same level of frequency.* Hopefully, other studies will be instigated and maintained so that in the future it may be possible to have a larger, more generalizable base for mapping psychiatric trends and seeing how they relate to trends in other social and health indicators.

The indicator movement is an effort to systematize descriptive information on key variables regarding the quality of contemporary life. The expansion and improvement of indicators means that we will have an enormously useful picture of how trends in different areas of life are related. As a hypothetical example, an increase in urbanization occurring in the same historical period as an increase in mental hospitalizations does not mean that one is cause and the other effect. But as a backdrop against which to develop questions and formulate research, the value of indicator trends cannot be discounted.

Social Network

Another frontier is *social network* research.† A social network consists of the people with whom a given subject associates and who are significant to him in a variety of ways. It is at the heart of the matter concerning interpersonal relationships,

* See references 30, 39, 57, 63, and 64.
† See references 1, 2, 10, 17, 78, and 99.

and its relevance to social psychiatry rests in the fact that it may provide a next step in understanding the role of affiliative needs and alienation stress.

There is a steadily accumulating body of information about social networks as they apply to human relations in families, in industrial institutions, in political processes, and in psychotherapeutic group procedures. The development and promotion of the concept has, until recently, been the work of British anthropologists in the years since World War II. Their numerous applications in both European and African societies give confidence that networks can be extremely useful in cross-cultural studies.[70]

Investigation thus far shows that a network almost always includes some family members. This is not a requirement of the concept but an empirical finding. In view of this I would include in this topic the needed expansion of family life investigation. The emphasis, however, is on network, because network is a more general concept and can be applied to people at different stages in the life cycle, irrespective of type of family constellation or lack of family which may pertain. Since we know that there is a preponderance of single, divorced, and separated persons among the mentally ill, it seems advisable to choose, as a means of studying interpersonal relations, a concept which is not limited to consanguineous and affinal ties.

Network analyses also indicate that there is high probability for some neighbors to be included, although the concept is not tied to a particular residence pattern any more than it is to family. Like a suitcase, a network is carried by a person from place to place as well as from phase to phase over the life arc. This is especially important in societies in which geographic mobility is common. If networks were found useful to mental health studies, it would mean that people in rural, urban, and suburban environments could be compared in the same social frame of reference.

In addition to family and neighbors, a network can and often does include friends, work associates, and co-workers in various interest activities, as well as people of a variety of other kinds of relationships, both formal and informal. A physician, a welfare officer, or a teacher could be as critical a network member as a friend or relative. Network means the effective social milieu in that it refers to those others to whom a given individual, as an index subject, is linked in terms of influencing or being influenced by, supporting or being supported by, depending on or being depended upon, and so on. It is not, however, a corporate entity with a formal membership and a boundary. A network has neither, and therein is both an asset and a liability. The advantage is that a network crosscuts the many boundaries and memberships which make up a person's social existence and selects those individuals who are important to him. The disadvantage is that, lacking a clear-cut line of inclusion and exclusion, no one has yet come up with a generally accepted criterion for deciding who should be "in" and who "out".

Regarding alienation stress in terms of network, it can be pointed out that two attributes for which reliable measurement can probably be developed include the size of a network and the frequency with which the links between constituents are activated. In this regard, zero network means total alienation. This is probably a rare phenomenon, but we do not actually know its distribution in populations or its relationship to psychiatric epidemiology. It is possible that dearth of network is as characteristic of persons who suffer mental illness, or some forms of mental illness, as are the civil statuses of being single or divorced. It would seem useful, therefore, to have descriptive data on size and frequency for very large samples in order to begin defining the range of differences for these basic dimensions of network. If a positive relationship were found between lack of network and high prevalence, such information would be useful to clinicians and policy makers irrespective of its value as an independent variable. Community- and family-oriented therapeutic approaches often assume that a network exists and the need is for mobilization. But existence of network may indeed be questionable for some segments of the population.

Most of the work on networks has focused on dimensions which pertain when existence is not in question and which become evident when dealing with networks of a certain minimum size and density of interaction. These dimensions concern the collective functioning of a network and are therefore worthy of consideration as independent variables. Much of this interest has concerned variability in the capacity of a network to meet a crisis being experienced by one network member, and to maintain the norms of the social environments in which the network is embedded. These collective qualities act to inhibit demoralization and alienation. The underlying characteristics which appear to support these functions include features such as "connectedness" and the "plex" of network strands, as well as several others which will not be described here. Connectedness is a measure of the degree to which the associates of one person, the index case, are also associates of each other. At one extreme is the person with a highly compartmentalized network, and at the other the person with a closed circle of friends. The plex of a network refers to the role relationships involved in the linkages. A uniplex strand has a single role definition, while a multiplex strand includes such overlapping as a formal associate also being an informal friend. These dimensions appear to be useful indicators of the success with which a network carries out group functions of support and influence.

A significant and still-unanswered question is whether certain kinds of networks are characteristic of different socioeconomic levels. This is important in mental health epidemiology in view of the strength of the economic position findings. Considerable is already known about differences in life style correlated with economic position, and it is not unlikely that network variation also applies. Further research on the three variables (class, network, and mental health), if conducted in coordination, may throw light on the question of what it is that is stressful about economic position over and above material deprivation.

Behavior Setting

With regard to *behavior setting* we encounter another post–World War II concept, this one developed mainly by a group of American social psychologists.* Like social network, its cross-cultural applicability has been shown. A behavior setting is composed of three highly interlinked parts: places, people, and actions. The behavior settings of communities are identified by such familiar labels as town meetings, church worship services, committee meetings, local baseball games, doctor's office visits, the annual picnic, and the school's senior prom. In reporting news, whether through local newspapers or institutional newsletters, human behaviors are almost always described in terms of settings. This is a thumbnail indicator of the fact that behaviors stemming from social relationships are highly patterned to fit a particular setting. By entering a setting, a person comes under the command of that setting for certain behaviors in relation to the other occupants and to the physical environment.

The accumulated work on behavior settings indicates that environments vary greatly in terms of the quantity and quality of their settings. Many aspects of these differences have been found to be measurable. The environments most carefully studied thus far are small natural communities and schools, but the concept can clearly be applied to other institutions such as households, hospitals, factories, or prisons. The problems of application increase, though possibly not by insurmountable degree, when focus is directed to an urban agglomeration as a whole.

Various features of behavior settings appear to have influence on certain aspects of human behavior which may be relevant to mental illness. The feature I consider most important in this regard is the pressure emanating from settings for amount and kind of participation. In keeping with the terminology of behavior setting analysts, I will use the phrase "redundancy stress" to refer to settings which exert minimal force in stimulating and utilizing human resources.

The specific meaning of redundancy in this regard can be amplified by an illustration. In a valuable study on high schools of different-sized student bodies, it was found that the ratio of settings to students was higher in a small school than in a big school.[7] In range of activities and behaviors engendered, however, the

* See references 4, 5, 6, 8, and 9.

two different-sized schools were very much the same. Each had classroom lectures, science laboratories, lunchroom sessions, sports meets and practices, debating contests, and band or orchestra performances. Although each school functioned in terms of this basically similar composition, the small school settings were undermanned, the big school settings were overmanned. The impact of the small school appeared to be an environment requiring students to enter a large number of different kinds of settings and to play central roles in them. The settings in the large school functioned by the participation of a smaller proportion of students; participation for any one student tended to involve a specialized rather than varied repertoire of behaviors; a larger proportion played the role of onlooker in more settings; and some settings survived with many of the students not even being needed as onlookers. In other words, the large school was an environment in which many students were superfluous to the maintenance of the institution and may have experienced redundancy stress.

The psychological needs likely to be frustrated in such situations are primarily those for stimulation. There is considerable evidence, of course, that stimulus deprivation at the sensory level is a threat to psychological stability. At the social level, the lack of pressure to be alert and involved, to develop and practice interpersonal behavior, appears to be equally important. A deterioration of personality sometimes identified as "the social breakdown syndrome" is known to occur in the back wards of mental hospitals, and is believed to relate in part to lack of stimulation and lack of settings which demand participation.[37] Also, it is not simply random and erratic action that needs to be stimulated; rather, the actions and behaviors stimulated need to be useful and significant to the immediate group. In regard to network and alienation I used the expression "people need people." Here it may be appropriate to introduce the expression "people need to be needed."

Behavior settings and social networks can be compared in various ways. An attractive aspect of each is that it has quantifiable dimensions. Each has more direct and proximal impact on individuals than concepts such as culture, urbanization, and community. At the same time, neither requires assessment of the intimate nuances of private relationships which, however important they may be, are not the kinds of researchable independent variables appropriate to epidemiology at this stage.

The emphasis in network is on people and the nature of the links between them. The starting point is a subject and the interpersonal strands outward from him into the social universe. These will take him to multiple places and involve different actions. The emphasis in setting is on the tight alliance between site and behavior. The starting point is a place or places in the sociophysical environment, and this leads immediately to the people who occupy this space and the joint actions they carry out. The reason I have suggested that both be considered in future social psychiatric studies is that, if used together, a researcher would be confident that he was attending both to the nature of the available environment (settings) and to how this environment is utilized by individuals in relation to other individuals (networks).

The future needs for research on the possible social factors in mental illness involve first of all baseline and follow-up investigations. The ideal longitudinal study would have several features. It would be guided by more complex formulations of stress theory than has been true of much early work. It would be built on the existing findings regarding poverty and mental illness. This means that new work needs to select populations for sufficient representation of different levels of socioeconomic status, so that statistical testing can be carried out regarding the interaction of economic position with other social variables such as those described here. The research currently ongoing in the fields of indicators, networks, and settings shows that techniques are being matured which will be appropriate for studying large groups of people. Modifications will be needed, but guidelines exist for application to epidemiology.

Social Genetics

There is one other highly important endeavor which needs to be mentioned, even though it is not exclusively concerned with social causes. It is remarkable for the amount of lip service it receives and at the same time for the meagerness of effort to deal with it. I call it *social genetics*. This phase is in line with the wide recognition that human behavior is influenced by *both* environmental and hereditary considerations. Yet when it comes right down to it, most investigations concern "either" or "or," and the hyphen between nature-nurture is increasingly a barren land.

A considerable amount is known about the social correlates of the full range of mental illnesses, neurotic to psychotic, mental retardation to senility. This is also true of the genetic correlates of illnesses such as schizophrenia and mental retardation.[79,87,88] There may also be a genetic component in the milder forms of mental illness as well—the psychoneuroses and psychosomatic disorders. But the relationships of genetic predisposition and social experiences in mental illness are very little understood.

Just as the research on social causes must hold to high standards of excellence for design, noncontaminated variables, experimental reasoning, long-term follow-up, and so on, research on genetic causes cannot afford to, and obviously will not, change its basic direction. There is continuing need for biochemical exploration at the laboratory level, for using such natural experiments as monozygotic twins and aborted fetuses, and for work in countries where birth registration is enforced. But perhaps the ground between the two traditions can be usefully plowed, at least initially, by less precise methods.

I have in mind that the techniques developed by anthropologists for extensive recording and computerization of kinship in total communities may be helpful in building up relevant data banks on populations in areas where official registers do not exist. Even though the accuracy may not be as good as in areas where registration is enforced, such information would greatly expand possibilities for inspecting genetic trends in different kinds of environments. Knowledge is also weak regarding the social forces at work in mate selection, and yet this is a point of critical linkage. We have no idea what natural experiments might become evident if we had better maps for this terrain.[40]

In the few long-term psychiatric epidemiological studies of relatively stable community populations, it ought to be possible to begin answering the question of balance between environment and heredity as it applies to different kinds of mental illnesses, and to suggest some of the mechanisms whereby the two are joined. In two such studies, the Lundby study in Sweden and the Stirling County study in Canada, psychiatric evaluations exist for large numbers of people, representing in some instances three and four generations of the same consanguineous line and representing birth and residence in different kinds of social environments.[30,39,57] In view of this, an interesting question can be asked: Are the psychiatric characteristics of a subject's blood relatives *or* the interpersonal qualities of his friends, neighbors, and affinals the source of greatest difference in the probability of his becoming mentally ill?

As a concluding comment, I believe social cause questions should be asked in partnership with genetic cause questions. Does the balance tip toward genetics in all or only some forms of mental illness, and if only some, which? Does the balance tip toward social experiences in all or only some forms of mental illness, and if only some, which? And if social factors account for part of the phenomena, which kinds of stresses make the greatest difference—economic impoverishment, stigma, acculturation, understimulation, alienation, or human redundancy?

REFERENCES

1. Adams, B. "Interaction Theory and Social Network." *Sociometry* 30 (1967):64–78.
2. Aldous, J., and Strauss, M. "Social Networks and Conjugal Roles: A Test of Bott's Hypothesis." *Social Forces* 44 (1966):576–580.

3. Arsenian, J., and Arsenian, J. "Tough and Easy Cultures, A Conceptual Analysis." *Psychiatry* 2 (1948):377–385.

4. Barker, R. G. *Stream of Behavior.* New York: Appleton-Century-Crofts, 1963.

5. ———. "Explorations in Ecological Psychology." *American Psychologist* 20 (1965):1–14.

6. ———, and Barker, L. S. "The Psychological Ecology of Old People in Midwest Kansas and Yoredale, Yorkshire." *Journal of Gerontology* 16 (1961):144–149.

7. Barker, R. G., and Gump, P. *Big School, Small School.* Stanford, Calif.: Stanford University Press, 1964.

8. Barker, R. G., and Schoggen, P. *Qualities of Community Life.* San Francisco: Jossey-Bass, 1973.

9. Barker, R. G., and Wright, H. F. *Midwest and Its Children.* New York: Harper & Row, 1955.

10. Barnes, J. A. "Class and Committees in a Norwegian Island Parish." *Human Relations* 7 (1954):39–58.

11. Bauer, R. *Social Indicators.* Cambridge, Mass.: MIT Press, 1966.

12. Beiser, M.; Ravel, J. L.; Collomb, H.; and Egelhoff, C. "Assessing Psychiatric Disorder Among the Serer of Senegal." *The Journal of Nervous and Mental Disease,* Vol. 154, No. 2, 1972, pp. 141–151. This is the first of a series of articles which will present the results of an epidemiologic study among the Serer, half of whom were rural and half urban dwellers. In personal communication, 1974, Beiser indicates that scores on a psychoneurotic inventory were similar in the two groups.

13. Benedict, R. *Patterns of Culture.* New York: Houghton Mifflin, 1934.

14. ———. "Continuities and Discontinuities in Cultural Conditioning." *Psychiatry* 1 (1938):161–167.

15. Bernard, C. *An Introduction to the Study of Experimental Medicine.* Translated by H. C. Greene. New York: Macmillan, 1927.

16. Blood, E., and Wolfe, D. *Husbands and Wives.* New York: Free Press, 1960.

17. Bott, E. *Family and Social Networks.* London: Tavistock, 1957.

18. Carothers, J. C. *African Mind in Health and Disease. A Study in Ethnopsychiatry.* Monograph Series No. 17, Geneva World Health Organization, 1953.

19. Caudill, W., and Lin, T., eds. *Mental Health Research in Asia and the Pacific.* Honolulu: East-West Center Press, 1969.

20. Caudill, W., and Scholer, C. "Symptom Patterns and Background Characteristics of Japanese Psychiatric Patients." In *Mental Health Research in Asia and the Pacific,* edited by W. Caudill and T. Lin, pp. 114–147. Honolulu: East-West Center Press, 1969.

21. Cheek, F. E. "The 'Schizophrenogenic Mother' in Word and Deed." *Family Process* 3 (1964):155–177.

22. Cleveland, E., and Longaker, W. "Neurotic Patterns in the Family." In *Explorations in Social Psychiatry,* edited by A. H. Leighton, J. A. Clausen, and R. N. Wilson, pp. 167–200. New York: Basic Books, 1957.

23. Croog, S.; Lipson, A.; and Levine, S. "Help Patterns in Severe Illness: The Roles of Kin Network, Non-Family Resources and Institutions." *Journal of Marriage and the Family.* 34 (1972):32–41.

24. Cumming, J. "The Family and Mental Disorder." In *Causes of Mental Disorders: A Review of Epidemiological Knowledge, 1959,* pp. 153–180. New York: Milbank Memorial Fund, 1961.

25. de Reuch, A. V. S., and Porter, R., eds. *Transcultural Psychiatry, CIBA Foundation Symposium.* London: J. & A. Churchill, 1965.

26. DeVos, G., and Miner, H. "Oasis and Casbah—A Study in Acculturative Stress." In *Culture and Mental Health,* edited by M. Opler, pp. 333–350. New York: Macmillan, 1959.

27. Dohrenwend, B. P. "Social Status, Stress and Psychological Symptoms." *American Journal of Public Health* 57 (1967):625–632.

28. ———, and Dohrenwend, B. S. *Social Status and Psychological Disorder.* New York: Wiley, 1969.

Part V / *Future Issues*

29. ————, and Dohrenwend, B. S. "Psychiatric Disorders in Urban Settings." In *American Handbook of Psychiatry*, 2nd ed., edited by Silvano Arieti, pp. 424–447. New York: Basic Books, 1974.

30. Essen-Möller, E. "Individual Traits and Morbidity in a Swedish Rural Population." *Acta Scandinavica Psychiatrica et Neurologica*, Supplement 100 (1956):1–160.

31. Falkner, F., ed. *A Base-line of Investigations for Longitudinal Growth Studies of the Child*. Paris: International Children's Center, 1954.

32. Faris, R. E. L., and Dunham, H. W. *Mental Disorders in Urban Areas*. New York: Hafner, 1960.

33. Feldman, H., and Brightman, L. "The Family Setting." In *Psychiatric Disorder and the Urban Environment*, edited by B. Kaplan, pp. 189–212. New York: Behavioral Publications, 1971.

34. Freud, S. *Civilization and Its Discontents*. London: Hogarth, 1949.

35. Glueck, S., and Glueck, E. *One Thousand Juvenile Delinquents*. Cambridge, Mass.: Harvard University Press, 1934.

36. Goldhamer, H., and Marshall, A. W. *Psychosis and Civilization—Two Studies in the Frequency of Mental Disease*. New York: Free Press, 1949.

37. Gruenberg, E.; Snow, H.; and Bennett, C. L. "Preventing the Social Breakdown Syndrome." *Social Psychiatry* 47 (1969):179–195.

38. Gussow, Z. "Pibloktok Hysteria Among the Polar Eskimos." In *Psychoanalytic Study of Society*, edited by W. Muensterberger. New York: International Universities Press, 1960; pp. 218–236.

39. Hagnell, O. *A Prospective Study of the Incidence of Mental Disorder*. Norstedts, Svenska: Bokforlagel, 1966.

40. Harrison, G. A.; Hiorns, R. W.; and Küchemann, C. F. "Social Class and Marriage Patterns in Some Oxfordshire Populations." *Journal of Biosocial Science* 3 (1971):1–12.

41. Hollingshead, A. B., and Redlick, F. C. *Social Class and Mental Illness*. New York: Wiley, 1958.

42. Inkeles, A., and Smith, D. "The Fate of Personal Adjustment in the Process of Modernization." *International Journal of Comparative Sociology* 2 (1970):81–113.

43. Jessor, R., et al. *Society, Personality and Deviant Behavior: A Study of a Tri-Ethnic Community*. New York: Holt, Rinehart, 1968.

44. Jones, H. F., and Bayley, N. "The Berkeley Growth Study." *Child Development* 12 (1941):16–173.

45. Kagen, J. "American Longitudinal Research on Psychological Development." *Child Development* 35 (1964):1–32.

46. Kardiner, A., ed. *The Individual and His Society*. New York: Columbia University Press, 1939.

47. Kellert, S., et al. "Culture Change and Stress in Rural Peru." *Milbank Memorial Quarterly* 45 (1967):391–415.

48. Kiev, A. *Transcultural Psychiatry*. New York: Free Press, 1972.

49. Koos, E. L. *Families in Trouble*. New York: King's Crown Press, 1946.

50. Kramer, M., et al. *Mental Disorders: Suicide*. Cambridge, Mass.: Harvard University Press, 1972.

51. ————. "Patterns of Use of Psychiatric Facilities by the Aged: Past, Present, Future." In *The Psychology of Adult Development and Aging*, edited by C. Eisdorfer and M. P. Lawton, pp. 428–528. Washington, D.C.: American Psychological Association, 1973.

52. Kroeber, A. "Psychosis or Social Sanction." In *The Nature of Culture*. Chicago: University of Chicago Press, 1952, pp. 310–319.

53. Langner, T. S., and Michael, S. P. *Life Stress and Mental Health*. New York: Free Press, 1963.

54. Leacock, E. "Three Social Variables and the Occurrence of Mental Disorder." In *Explorations in Social Psychiatry*, edited by A. H. Leighton, J. A. Clausen, and R. N. Wilson, pp. 308–340. New York: Basic Books, 1957.

1

55. Lebra, W. P., ed. *Transcultural Research in Mental Health*. Honolulu: University of Hawaii Press, 1972.

56. Leighton, A. H. *My Name is Legion*. New York: Basic Books, 1959.

57. ———. "Poverty and Social Change." *Scientific American* 212, no. 5 (1965):21–27.

58. ———, and Murphy, J. M. "Cultures as Causative of Mental Disorder." In *Causes of Mental Disorders, A Review of Epidemiological Knowledge, 1959*, pp. 341–365. New York: Milbank Memorial Fund, 1961.

59. Leighton, A. H., et al. *Psychiatric Disorder Among the Yoruba*. Ithaca, N.Y.: Cornell University Press, 1963.

60. Leighton, D. C., et al. *The Character of Danger, Psychiatric Symptoms in Selected Communities*. New York: Basic Books, 1963. In this rural study, 20% were found to be or to have been impaired by psychiatric disorder, p. 142.

61. Leighton, D. C., et al. "Psychiatric Disorder in a Swedish and a Canadian Community: An Exploratory Study." *Social Science and Medicine* 5 (1971):189–201.

62. Lidz, T.; Fleck, S.; and Cornelius, A. *Schizophrenia and the Family*. New York: International Press, 1965.

63. Lin, T. "A Study of the Incidence of Mental Disorder in Chinese and Other Cultures." *Psychiatry* 16 (1953):313–336.

64. ———, et al. "Mental Disorders in Taiwan Fifteen Years Later: A Preliminary Report." In *Mental Health Research in Asia and the Pacific*, edited by W. Caudill and T. Lin, pp. 66–91. Honolulu: East-West Center Press, 1969.

65. Linton, R. *Culture and Mental Disorders*. Springfield, Ill.: Charles C. Thomas, 1956.

66. Malinowski, B. *Sex and Repression in Savage Society*. New York: Harcourt, Brace, 1927.

67. McCammon, R. W. *Human Growth and Development*. Springfield, Ill.: Charles C. Thomas, 1970.

68. Mead, M., ed. *Cooperation and Competition Among Primitive Peoples*. New York: McGraw-Hill, 1937.

69. Mischler, E., and Waxler, N. *Interaction in Families: An Experimental Study of Family Processes and Schizophrenia*. New York: Wiley, 1968.

70. Mitchell, J. C., ed. *Social Networks in Urban Situations*. Manchester, England: Manchester University Press, 1969.

71. Murphy, H. B. M. "Social Change and Mental Health." In *Causes of Mental Disorders: A Review of Epidemiological Knowledge, 1959*, pp. 280–329. New York: Milbank Memorial Fund, 1961.

72. ———; Wittkower, E.; and Chance, N. "A Cross-Cultural Survey of Schizophrenic Symptomatology." *International Journal of Social Psychiatry* 9 (1963):237–249.

73. ———. "The Symptoms of Depression—A Cross-Cultural Survey." In *Cross-Cultural Studies of Behavior*, edited by I. Al-Issa and W. Dennis, pp. 476–493. New York: Holt, Rinehart, 1970.

74. Murphy, J. M. "A Cross-Cultural Comparison of Psychiatric Disorder: Eskimos of Alaska, Yorubas of Nigeria, and Nova Scotians of Canada." In *Transcultural Research in Mental Health*, edited by W. Lebra. Honolulu: University of Hawaii Press, 1972, pp. 213–226.

75. ———. "Sociocultural Change and Psychiatric Disorder Among Rural Yorubas in Nigeria." *Ethos* 1 (1973):239–262.

76. ———, and Leighton, A. H. *Approaches to Cross-Cultural Psychiatry*. Ithaca, N.Y.: Cornell University Press, 1965.

77. Murphy, J. M., et al. "Psychological Responses to Stress." In *Beliefs, Attitudes and Behavior of Lowland Vietnamese—A Study of the Effects of Herbicides in South Vietnam*, pp. VIII-1 to VIII-50. Washington, D.C.: National Academy of Sciences, 1974. For a comparison of a rural site in Canada and an urban site in the U.S., see pp. VIII-23.

78. Nelson, J. "Clique Contacts and Family Orientation." *American Sociological Review* 31 (1966):663–672.

79. Nora, J. J., and Fraser, F. C. *Medical Genetics, Principles and Practice*. Philadelphia: Lea and Febiger, 1974.

80. Paffenbarger, R. S., and Asnes, D. P. "Precursors of Suicide in Early and Middle Life." *American Journal of Public Health* 56 (1966):1026–1036.

81. Park, R. E.; Burgess, E. W.; and McKenzie, R. D. *The City*. 4th ed. Chicago: University of Chicago Press, 1967.

82. Rapoport, R., and Rapoport, R. *Dual Career Families*. New York: Penguin, 1972.

83. Redfield, R. *The Primitive World and Its Transformations*. Ithaca, N.Y.: Cornell University Press, 1953.

84. ———. *Peasant Society and Culture: An Anthropological Approach to Civilization*. Chicago: University of Chicago Press, 1956.

85. Redick, R., and Johnson, C. "Marital Status, Living Arrangements, and Family Characteristics of Admissions to State and County Mental Hospitals and Outpatient Psychiatric Clinics, United States 1970." NIMH Surveys and Reports Section, *Statistical Note #100*, February 1974.

86. Rosenhan, D. "On Being Sane in Insane Places." *Science* 179, no. 4070, 1973:250–258.

87. Rosenthal, D. *Genetics of Psychopathology*. New York: McGraw-Hill, 1971.

88. ———, and Kety, S. *The Transmission of Schizophrenia*. New York: Pergamon, 1968.

89. Sarbin, T. R. "The Scientific Status of the Mental Illness Metaphor." In *Changing Perspectives in Mental Illness*, edited by S. C. Plog and R. B. Edgerton, pp. 9–31. New York: Holt, Rinehart, 1969.

90. Scheff, T. J. *Being Mentally Ill: A Sociological Theory*. Chicago: Aldine, 1966.

91. Scotch, N., and Levine, S., eds. *Social Stress*. Chicago: Aldine, 1970.

92. Sheldon, E. B., and Moore, W. E. *Indicators of Social Change: Concepts and Measurements*. New York: Russell Sage Foundation, 1968.

93. Sontag, L. W. "The History of Longitudinal Research: Implications for the Future." *Child Development* 42 (1971):987–1002.

94. Snole, L., et al. *Mental Health in the Metropolis*. New York: McGraw Hill, 1962.

95. Sussman, M., and Burchinal, L. "Kin Family Network: Unheralded Structure in Current Conceptualizations of Family Functioning." *Marriage and Family Living* 24 (1962):231–240.

96. Szasz, T. *The Myth of Mental Illness: Foundations of a Theory of Personal Conduct*. New York: Hoeber-Harper, 1961.

97. Taylor, L., and Chave, S. *Mental Health and Environment*. London: Longmans, Green, 1964.

98. Turner, R. J., and Wagonfeld, M. O. "Occupational Mobility and Schizophrenia: An Assessment of the Social Causation and Social Selection Hypotheses." *American Sociological Review* 32, no. 6 (1967):104–113.

99. Udry, J. R., and Hall, M. "Marital Role Segregation and Social Networks in Middle-Class, Middle-Aged Couples." *Journal of Marriage and the Family* 27 (1965):392–395.

100. Valadian, I., and Reed, R. "Influence of Nutritional Factors During Early Adolescence on Reproductive Efficiency." In *Congenital Defects—New Directions in Research*, edited by D. T. Janerich, R. G. Skalko, and I. H. Porter, pp. 57–71. New York: Academic Press, 1974.

101. Vallee, F. "Stresses of Change and Mental Health Among the Canadian Eskimos." *Archives of Environmental Health* 17 (1968):565–570.

102. Wilcox, L. D., et al. *Social Indicators and Societal Monitoring, An Annotated Bibliography*. San Francisco: Jossey-Bass, 1972.

103. Wirth, L. "Urbanism as a Way of Life." *American Journal of Sociology* 44 (1938):1–24.

Index

INDEX

Aaron Complex, xix

Accommodation: in competent community, 202-03

Accountability, 328-29

Acculturation: acculturative stress hypothesis, 388-89, 395; in developing countries, 142; as social cause of mental illness, 384, 388-89; violence, self-destructive behavior and, 143

Ackerly, William C., 210-28, 242

Action for Mental Health (report; Joint Commission on Mental Illness and Health), 57, 58

Acutely disordered: services for, in hospital-centered community mental health programs, 52-53

Adams, John E., 157-75, 228, 242

Adaptive behavior, *see* Coping

Adaptive process: health as, 179-80

Addiction: dependence and, distinguished, 274; *see also* Drug dependence

Administrators: as essential skill of, 40; total health care and, 40-41

Admissions, *see* Hospital admissions

Adolescence: coping strategies in, 161-64; drug dependence and development of, 279-81; drug use and concept of essential striving sentiments in, 11

Advisory boards: citizen, 65

Affective states: correlates of (table), 188

Age: in health measurement model, 295; well-being and, 185-89

Albee, George W., 232

Alcohol: use of, 142, 278-79; *see also* Drug dependence

Alcoholics Anonymous, 115

Alienation: as social cause of mental illness, 384, 391-92; social network and, 398

Allergy-skin-nerves (table), 368

Ambulatory services: in hospital-centered community mental health programs, 53-54

Anderson, Richard, 55

Annual Report (Commonwealth Fund), 47

Anticipatory detachment: as coping strategy, 161-62

Anticipatory grief: as coping behavior, 171

Anticipatory guidance: described, 157, 172-73; organizational model of, 242

Antidepressant medications: introduction of, 33-34

Anxiety-depression with physiological components (table), 368

Articulateness: in competent community, 201

Aspiration: modifying level of, as coping strategy, 162

Astrology, 112

Automated Multiphasic Health Testing, 381-82

Awareness: clarity of situational definitions and self-other, 200-01

Bandler, Bernard, 66, 67

Baylis, L. E., 181

Behavior covariation diagram, 292-96

Behavior settings, 399-401; social networks and, 400-01

Behavioral conditioning therapies: rise of, 235

Beiser, Morton, 176-92, 200-306

Beisser, A., 230

Bell, G. M., 51

Benfari, Robert C., 290-306, 354-76

Bennis, W. G., 242

Berger, Gaston, 268

Bernard, Claude, 386

Bethel school, 266

Bindman, A. J., 230

Bion, W. R., 247, 264

Bloom, Bernard, 228

Blue Ridge (Kaplan), xviii

Boardman, Virginia, 197n

Boards of trustees (boards of directors): citizens on, of state facilities, 39-40

Borne, xviii

Borstal system, 54

Bowen, W. A. L., 64

Bower, Eli M., 239

Boyer, L. Bryce, 142

Bradburn, Norman, 180, 184, 189

Brenner, B., 190

Bridesmaid principle, 211, 224-25

Brodie, H. Keith H., 157-75, 228, 242

Brown, Bertram, 63

409

Index

Cambridge-Somerville Youth Study, 50-51

Camus, Albert, 157

Capital: for developing countries, 134-36

Caplan, Gerald, 51, 59-61, 230

Cardoza, Victor G., 210-28, 242

Carrel, Alexis, 252

CASE (Computer Assigned Symptom Evaluations), 356-57; *see also* Computer use

Case factors: as predictors for psychiatric classification (table), 371

Case report: community action, 218-25

Case studies: for evaluating mental health center programs, 533-35

Case-study method, 314-15

Caseload: in child guidance clinics, 48

Catalytic: term, defined, 217

Catalytic model: of community action, 215-17

Catalytic role: sociotherapist as, 242-43

Catchment areas: and community mental health service model, 62-64; and mental health center programs, 323-25; and state mental health model, 38-40

Cattel, R. B., 293, 365

Center for the Study of Responsive Law, 324

Chemical restraints, *see* Drugs

Child guidance clinics, 47-51; effects of and problems with the model, 50-51; fiscal support for, 50; model of, 47-50; purpose of, 47

Children's Guidance, Bureau of (Commonwealth Fund), 48-49

Ciarlo, James A., 345

Clan Brotherhood (Rhodesia), 142

Clausen, J. A., xix, 76, 85; work of, xiv, 3, 4, 13, 14, 366

Clinical approach: to consultation programming, 230-33

Clinical classifications: empirical types and, for health measurement (table), 304

Clinical ratings: over five-year period (table), 303

Clinical survey: of normal population (table), xiii

Cohen, Raquel, 66, 68, 69

Collaborative coprofessionals: roles of, 68-69

Collomb, H., 142

Colorado study, 330-31

Colonialism: effects of, 133

Commitment: in competent community, 198-99

Commonwealth Fund, 47, 50

Communication: in competent community, 201-02

Community: child guidance clinics and cooperation of, 49 (*see also* Child guidance clinics); conceptual propositions aiding analysis of competence of, 12 (*see also* Competent com-

munity); corollary issues of social psychiatry and mental health of, 5-6; defined, 95-96; defining nature of, 7; effects of stress in, 213-14; individual and, 19-21; inertia in, 70; mental health and contribution of, 183-91; mental hospital as mental health center and, 35-36; population growth and size of, 20; psychiatric register and coordination of care in, 96, 98-100; psychiatric register and objectives of care in, 96-97; structure and sentiments in, 213; types of mental health care in, in northern Europe, 52

Community action, 210-28, 242; case report on, 218-25; catalytic model of, 215-17; felt needs, defined, 216; further questions raised by study, 225-26; high-risk groups in, 215, 216; leadership in, 216-17; model for Somerville elderly program, 224; problem involved with, 213-15; Somerville Mental Health Center and, 217-18; term catalytic, defined, 217

Community home, 36

Community Mental Health Center (Denver General Hospital), 345

Community mental health center model, 56-64; background of, 56-58; comprehensive, 37-40; comprehensive, federal government in, 37-38; described, 35-37, 58-62; problems and viewpoints over, 62-64; as professionally controlled, 63-64

Community mental health center programs: client-therapist contingency contract treatment goal setting in, 343-45; concrete goal-setting in, 342-43; criticism of, 324-25; development of methods for evaluating, 331-33; early evaluation strategy on, 328-29; evaluation of effort in, 329-31; failure to implement, 71-72; funding for, 328; goal attainment follow-up guide (table), 339; goal attainment scaling of, 337-38; goal-oriented automated progress note, 340-41; impact on community structure of, 333-35; measurement of effects of, 322-53; methods of measuring treatment outcomes, 335-45; outcome value per unit cost in, 348-49; positive effects of, 323-24; problem of evaluation of, 325-28; prospective on, 349-51; systems approach to evaluation of, 345-48; *see also* Child guidance clinics; Community mental health center model; Community mental health and human services model; Hospital-centered community mental health programs; Psychiatric registers

Community mental health centers: creation of (1963), 114; decline of, 42; placed in

410

Index

Demoralization: alienation as, 391-92; demoralization hypothesis, 122-24; as target of all psychotherapies, 110, 112; see also Disintegration

Denial of deviance, 87

Dependence, see Drug dependence

Dependent variable: assessing, 379-83; see also Mental illness

Detribalization: effects of, 142

Developing countries, 130-53; economics of, 133-36; education in, 146, 148; groups vulnerable to mental illness in, 142; health problems in, 145-48; mental health orientation in, 136-40; need for adaptation to industrial civilization in, 251; needs of children in, 148-49; psychiatry, folk medicine and development process in, 150-52; psychiatry's role in, 132-33; rural development in, 149-50; social change and mental illness in, 140-43; strategy for, 143-50

Deviant behavior, 77-88; in corrective role failure, 82-83; defining, 77, 84-86; dangerous behavior as limit of tolerance in, 83-84; elements of theory of, 77-78; in expressive role failure, 79-81; in instrumental role failure, 78-79; recognition of illness legitimates, 86; in representational role failure, 81; social deviancy-psychotic indicator (table), 369; treatment issues in, see Treatment; types of coping responses to, 87-88; in unpredictable role performance, 82

Deviant role: as variant of corrective role, 83

Diagnostic and Statistical Manual (American Psychiatric Association), 25

Dictionary, psychiatric, 356-57; see also Computer use

Different: sick differentiated from, 169

Directory of Psychiatric Clinics for Children, 50

Disintegration: defined, 214; in developing countries, 141; flocculation and, 22-23; intervention in processes of, 228; mental health movement adversely affected by, 43; outcome of, 22; teaching point of, 18-19, 20-21; see also Demoralization

Disorganization: unpredictability and, 82

Displaced roles, 79

Division of labor: instrumental roles and, 78-79

Divorce, 392

Dostoyevsky, Feodor, xviii

Drug abuse: defined, 275

Drug dependence, 272-85; addiction and dependence, distinguished, 274-75; adolescent development, youth culture and, 279-81; drug use in U.S., 275-76; drugs of abuse, 276-79; education, development of competence and, 281-85; evaluative methods and, 332-33; mean percentage of students who have ever used drugs as of 1972 (table), 277

Drugs (chemical restraints; medications): affecting moods and emotions, 15; in custodial mental hospitals, 32; introduction of antidepressant medications, 33-34; see also Drug dependence

Dunn, Halbert, 176

DuPuy, H., 230

Durkheim, Emile, 289, 377, 384

Dynamic equilibrium concept, 17-19

Eastern Middlesex Opportunities Council, 223

Economic Opportunity, Office of, 200

Economic position: as social cause of mental illness, 384, 389-91, 395; see also Socioeconomic status

Economics: of developing countries, 133-36

Edgerton, J. Wilbert, 307, 321-53

Education: conceptual propositions aiding understanding of problems in, 11-12; concerns with, of child guidance clinics, 47-48; drug dependence and, 281-85; education programming, 229, 233-36; mental hospitals as mental health centers and, 37; positive mental health and, 186-87; as requirement in developing countries, 146, 148; well-being and, 185-89

Elderly Planning Committee (Somerville), 225

Empirical groups: and social interaction variables in health measurement (table), 304

Empirical types: and clinical classifications for health measurement (table), 304

Encounter groups (personal growth centers): community mental health compared with, 118-19; counterculture values and, 120-21; described, 116-17; education programming and, 235; leaders of, 115; therapist-patient distinction blurred in, 121-22

Environmental influences: and concept of essential striving sentiments, 11

Epidemiology: approach to, 105; computer use in, see Computer use; in developing countries, 141-42; emergence of, 56; as evaluative research, 314; psychiatric register and, 107-08; see also Social causes

Erikson, Erik, 272

Essen-Möller, E., xiii

Index

Harvard School of Public Health, 218

Hawthorne Effect, 307

Health: disease and, as sociological concepts, 181; *See also* Health measurement; Mental health; Mental illness

Health, Education and Welfare, Department of (HEW), 323, 328

Health Amendment Act (1956), 56

Health measurement, 289-306; clinical ratings over five-year period (table), 303; characteristics of O-types in sample (table), 301; composition of rural panel (table), 297; description of samples for, 296-97; empirical groups and social interaction variables in (table), 304; empirical types and clinical classifications (table), 304; model for analysis in, 291-96; O-types in urban sample for (table), 300; urban sample age and sex distribution for (table), 297; trying out the model for, 296-306

Health Opinion Survey (HOS), 380-83

Hennepin County Mental Health Center, 337, 338

Heroin, *see* Drug dependence

HEW (Health, Education and Welfare, Department of), 323, 328

High-risk groups: in community action study, 215, 216; drug dependence and, 274; elderly as, 220-23; preventing mental illness and, 218

Hilgard, E. R., 258

Hinkle, L. E., Jr., 382

Hoffmann, Albert, 276

Hollingshead, A., 56

Hollister, William G., 157, 210-11, 228-41, 243

Home treatment service, 36

Hope: in coping strategy, 169, 171

HOS (Health Opinion Survey), 380-83

Hospital admissions: catchment areas and, 324; mental hospitals as mental health centers and, 37; psychiatric register and, 100-01; and recognition of illness, 85

Hospital-centered community mental health programs, 51-56; ambulatory and rehabilitation services in, 53-54; preventive and consultative services in, 54-55; problems of, 55-56; services for acutely disordered in, 52-53

Hostility: among patients with serious physical impairments, 166

Human interaction: as key component of community, 7

Human services model, 45, 66; *see also* Community mental health and human services model

Hunt, Robert C., 52

Huntsville-Madison County Mental Health Center, 343

Hypnotism, 113

Identification: as foundation of change, 256-57

Ideology: change and, 20, 43; consultation programming and, 232-33; education programming and, 233-34; prevention programming and, 236-38

Impairment Index, 333

Inadequacy: feelings of, in coping behavior, 165

Inceptive groups, 246

Independent variables, *see* Social causes

Indigenous nonprofessionals, 118

Individual freedom: human services model and, 69; limits of, 21-22

Individualized goal attainment methods, 336-45; Concrete Goal-Setting in, 342-43; Contingency Contract Treatment Goal-Setting in, 343-45; Goal Attainment Scaling and, 337-39, 350; Goal Attainment Scaling follow-up guide in, 339; Goal-Oriented Progress Note in, 340-41

Industrialization: effects of, 250-51; *see also* Developing countries

Innovation: psychiatric register and community care, 96

Insight: change and, 259

Institute for Child Guidance (Commonwealth Fund), 49

Institutional changes: in developing countries, 138-39

Instrumental roles: failure of, 78-79

Integration: in health measurement model, 295-96; as key issue, xv-xvi; *see also* Conceptual perspectives

Interagency Network measure, 334-35

Interpersonal patterns: propositions on sociocultural environment and, 10

Intervention, *see* Sociotherapy

Introspection: change and, 259

Jackson, J. K., 84

Jacoby, A., 236

Jahoda, M., 179

James, William, 366

Janet, 366

Jarett, M., 347

Joint Commission on Mental Illness and Health, 37, 56, 57

Index

Mental illness (*continued*)
ing sociocultural patterns to, 11; psychiatric register function of studying determinants and outcome of, 102 (*see also* Psychiatric registers); social change and, in developing countries, 140-43; social class and different conceptions of, 56, 84-85; table of disorders, 25, 27; *see also* Social causes

Mental Retardation Facilities and Community Mental Health Centers Act (1963; PL 88-164), 58

Mertens, Charles J., 130, 242-71

Mescalero Apache (tribe): crime rate among, 142

Mesmer, Franz Anton, 113

Mesmerism, 113

Message-centered intervention: defined, 259, 262

Meyer, Adolf, 43, 53, 71

Miasma theory, 228

Middle class: in developing countries, 133, 139, 148

Midtown study, xiii, 25

Migration: in developing countries, 139-40, 142, 144, 147, 149-50; as problem of communities, 20

Milbank Memorial Fund conference (1955), 54-55

Mind-altering use of drugs, 275-78

Mingo-County experience, 206

Minnesota Multiphasic Personality Inventory (MMPI), 356

Monitoring function: of psychiatric registers, 97-100

Morale: of individual and group, 123

Morbidity measurement: level of health in populations and, 289, 291; *see also* Health measurement

More for the Mind (Canadian committee report), 57, 58

Moses, xviii-xix

Moses Complex, xviii-xix

Multidisciplinary teams, 66-69

Multivariate analysis, 373, 374

Murphy, H. S., 84

Murphy, Jane M., 290, 306, 384-406

Murray, Henry A., xviii, 157

Nader, Ralph, 324

National Bureau of Health Statistics, 230

National Commission on Marihuana and Drug Abuse, 274-75, 277, 278

National Committee for Mental Hygiene, 47, 49, 50

National health insurance, 41-42, 351

National Health service (England), 55

National Institute of Alcohol Abuse and Alcoholism, 332

National Institute of Mental Health (NIMH), 56, 161, 324, 328-30, 333, 335

National Mental Health Act (1946), 56, 114

Nationalism: in developing countries, 139

Navajo (tribe), 151

Network analysis, 347-48

New careerists, 118, 120

Nietzsche, Friedrich, xviii

Night hospitals, 36

NIMH (National Institute of Mental Health), 56, 161, 324, 328-30, 333, 335

Nixon, Richard M., 42, 322

Nonprofessionals, 115-22

Normal people: in natural settings, empirical studies of, 182-83

Nuttin, J., 258

O-analysis, 293, 294, 299-305

O-types: characteristics of, in sample (table), 301; in urban sample (table), 300

Organizational change, 242; *see also* Sociotherapy

Outer-directed-tension state (table), 369

Outpatient services, 36, 53-54

Output Value Index, 348-49

Pages, M., 250

Parents: of leukemic children, coping behavior of, 169-71

Parsons, Talcott, 82, 86, 181-82

Participation: in competent community, 203; evaluating, 333-35; level of health in populations and social, 289, 291 (*see also* Health measurement); machinery for facilitating participant interaction in competent community, 205

Patients: conceptual propositions aiding understanding of patienthood, 11

Peace Corps: preparation of volunteers for, 172-74

Peer counseling: described, 157, 173-74

Peer groups: drug dependence and, 279-81

Perceived danger: and need for social control, 84

Index

Redlich, F., 56
Redundancy stress, 399-401
Rees, T. P., 51, 53
Registers, *see* Psychiatric registers
Rehabilitation services: in hospital-centered community mental health programs, 53-54
Religio-magical healing, 112
Religion: in coping behavior, 170
Remedially oriented responses, 87
Rennie, T. A. C., xiii
Report On The World Social Situation (United Nations), 148
Representational role failure, 81
Reserved compulsivity-high intellect versus passive-intellectual deficiency (table), 370
Responsibility: in coping behavior, 165, 170
Rieker, Patricia Perri, 307-21
Right: view of mental health movement by the extreme, 121
Role complementarity: learning through, as coping strategy, 163
Roles: as basic unit, 16-17; community mental health programs and, 64-65; modification of, social change and, 252-53; positive mental health and effective performance in major social, 183; rehearsal of, as coping strategy, 162; social disintegration and, 21; sociotherapist in catalytic, 242-43; *see also* Deviant behavior
Rolland, John S., 379-83
Rollman Psychiatric Institute, 342
Rosenberg, M., 190
Rule-breaking behavior: deviance as, 77
Rural development: in developing countries, 149-50
Rural panel: composition of (table), 297
Rural-urban residence: as social cause of mental illness, 391, 395

S-analysis, 294, 295
Sample and data base: for computer use, 358-59
Samples: description of, in health measurement, 296-97
Sanctioning mechanisms, 87
Satanism, 112
Schiller, Friedrich von, xviii
Schwartz, C. G., 84
Seclusion: in custodial mental hospitals, 32
Secondary prevention: defined, 47
Seeking activity: as coping strategy, 161

Selective service rejections (by 1945), 51
Self-image: continuity with present, as coping strategy, 161-62
Self-interest: and competent community, 199
Self-other awareness: and clarity of situational definitions in competent community, 200-01
Separation: and coping behavior, 165
Sex: distribution by age and, in urban sample (table), 297; in health measurement model, 295; sexual problems of patients with serious physical impairments, 165-66; well-being and, 185-89
Shona (tribe), 142
Sick: "different" differentiated from, 169
Sick role: defined, 82
Situational definitions: self-other awareness and clarity of, 200-01
Sivadon, P., 245
Slater, P. E., 242
Smith, M. Brewster, 197n
Social breakdown syndrome: demoralization and, 123; *see also* Demoralization; Disintegration
Social change: in developing countries, 137-43; experience of the effect of, 258-59; general resistance to, 252-53; and means of reducing stress, 214 (*see also* Community action); as planned change, 307; unawareness of processes underlying, 251 (*see also* Sociotherapy)
Social class: correlation of mental illness and, 390; in developing countries, 133-35, 139, 148; different conceptions of mental illness in different, 56, 84-85; ills of lower, in developing countries, 139; large lower, in developing countries, 138; middle, in developing countries, 133, 139, 148; type of psychotherapy and, 116-17
Social causes of mental illness, 384-406; acculturation as, 384, 388-89, 395; alienation as, 391-92, 395; behavior setting as, 399-401; culture as, 384, 387-88, 395; family as, 392-94; labeling as, 394-95; rural-urban residence as, 391, 395; social genetics and, 401-02; social indicators and, 395-96; social network research and, 396-99
Social deviancy-psychotic indicator (table), 369
Social disintegration, *see* Disintegration
Social genetics, 385, 401-02
Social indicators, 395-96
Social institution: psychotherapy as, 119-22
Social interaction variables: empirical groups and, in health measurement (table), 304
Social milieu: as therapeutic force, 34

418

Index

Temporary society, 242

Theory of Social and Economic Organization, The (Weber), 321

Therapeutic community, 52

Therapeutic egalitarian model of state mental hospitals, 33-35

Therapeutic staff: in custodial authoritarian model, 31-32; and mental hospital as mental health center, 35-37; therapeutic egalitarian model and, 34-35; *see also* Professionals

Thomas, Llewelyn, 382

Thomas, W. I., 82

Thorndike, 258

Threshold phenomena: defined, 18

Titnuss, Richard, 55

Toffler, A., 242

Total health care model, 40-42

Total health insurance plan, 41-42, 351

Training programs: mental health center, 118-19; for psychotherapists (since World War II), 113-15

Tranquilizers: introduction of, 33-34

Transcendental meditation, 112

Treatment: concept of, in community mental health centers, 118; definitional function in issues of, 89-90; efforts at, as coping response, 87; social diagnosis in issues of, 88-89; social therapy in issues of, 89; *see also specific treatment forms, for example*: Psychotherapy; Sociotherapy

Tribal associations: in urban areas, 149-50

Tribal customs: in developing countries, 147-48

United Community Services of Greater Boston, 225

United Nations, 136

United Nations conferences (1964; 1968), 251

Unpredictable role performance, 82

Urban-rural residence: as social cause of mental illness, 391, 395

Urban sample: age and sex distribution in (table), 297; O-types in (table), 302

Urbanization: in developing countries, 138-40, 142, 144, 147, 149-50

V-analysis, 293-94, 298-99

Values: change and, 20, 43; encounter groups and counterculture, 120-21; health and, 181-82; measurement as laden with, 321;

objectives set by, 317; *see also* Conceptual perspectives

Van Bockstaele, J., 246

Veroff, J., 179-80

Visiting Nurses' Association, 223

Volunteering: in mental hospitals, 35

Walk-in clinics, 36

Wallace, A. F. C., 181

Ward, Barbara, 133, 134, 136, 366

Weber, Max, 321

Well-being: level of health in populations and feelings of, 289, 291; measure of, 184-85 (*see also* Health measurement); studies related to sense of, 183-91

Wet-sheet packs: in custodial mental hospitals, 33

"Where Should We Attack the Problem of the Prevention of Mental Defect and Mental Disease?" (Meyer), 71

White, Robert W., 176, 193, 196n-97n

White Mountain Apache (tribe), 142, 143

Whitmer, C. A., 83, 84

Wilson, M. L., 215

Wilson, Robert N., xviii; on conceptual perspectives, 4-13; work of, xiv, 3, 4, 13, 14, 366

Wing, John K., 54

Winton, F. R., 181

Witchcraft, 112

Witmer, H. L., 48-50

Wolfe, H., 382

Wolfe, S., 256

Wolford, J. A., 323

Work programs: burgeoning of, 36; explorations of use of, 33; law on, in England, 54; positive mental health and, 187

Working class: in developing countries, 139-40

Worry: usefulness of, as coping strategy, 162

Yarrow, M. R., 84

Yolles, Stanley F., 63

Youth culture: drug dependence, adolescent development and, 279-81; encounter groups and values of, 120-21

Zeigarnik, B., 258